FOOD ALLERGY
AND
GLUTEN-FREE
WEIGHT LOSS

Control Your Body Chemistry
Reduce Inflammation
and Improve Your Health

NICOLETTE M. DUMKE

FOOD ALLERGY AND GLUTEN-FREE WEIGHT LOSS
CONTROL YOUR BODY CHEMISTY, REDUCE INFLAMMATION AND IMPROVE YOUR HEALTH

Published by
Adapt Books
Allergy Adapt, Inc.
1877 Polk Avenue
Louisville, Colorado 80027
303-666-8253

©2011 by Nicolette M. Dumke
Printed in the United States of America

Publisher's Cataloging-in-Publication
(Provided by Quality Books, Inc.)

Dumke, Nicolette M.
    Food allergy and gluten-free weight loss : control
your body chemistry, reduce inflammation and improve
your health / Nicolette M. Dumke.
    302 p. 24.6 cm.
    Includes bibliographical references and index.
    LCCN 2011920154
    ISBN-13: 978-1-887624-19-0
    ISBN-10: 1-887624-19-8

    1. Reducing diets. 2. Food allergy--Diet therapy.
3. Gluten-free diet.   I. Title.

RM222.2.D86 2011   613.2'5
          QBI11-600013

DEDICATION

To Mark, Joel, and John
who fill my life with love

and to the memory of those
who loved me first

my father, Eugene Jiannetti,
my mother, Mary Jiannetti,
and my grandmother
Maria Savioli Jiannetti.

DISCLAIMER

The information contained in this book is merely intended to communicate food preparation material and information about possible treatment options which are helpful and educational to the reader. It is not intended to replace medical diagnosis or treatment, but rather to provide information and recipes which may be helpful in implementing a diet prescribed by your doctor. Please consult your physician for medical advice before embarking on any treatment or changing your diet.

The author and publisher declare that to the best of their knowledge all material in this book is accurate; however, although unknown to the author and publisher, some recipes may contain ingredients which may be harmful to some people.

There are no warranties which extend beyond the educational nature of this book, either expressed or implied, including, but not limited to, the implied warranties of merchantability, fitness for a particular purpose, or non-infringement. Therefore, the author and publisher shall have neither liability nor responsibility to any person with respect to any loss or damage alleged to be caused, directly or indirectly, by the information contained in this book.

If you do not wish to be bound by the above, you may return this book to the publisher for a full refund.

TABLE OF CONTENTS

Menu for a Quick Start

Perhaps you want to slim down or decrease your inflammation *now* and don't have a lot of time to read this book. Here's a reading menu and a how-to menu so you can easily start in your own way.

READING

If you would like to be able to implement the healthy eating plan presented in this book now and understand it later, read "Putting Principles into Practice: Your Customized Healthy Eating Plan," page 71. If you have time for one more how-to chapter, read "Practical Tips for Success," page 84.

If you have been disappointed with the results of previous weight loss diets and want to know why they failed and why this one will succeed, read "The Problem with Diets," page 15. For more answers to the "why?" question read "What Determines Our Weight?" page 22.

If you want a brief explanation of the physiology of how this healthy eating plan can help you, read "The Principles of Glycemic Control Weight Loss," page 26, and "Inflammation is Part of the Problem," page 33. For a more in-depth understanding, read "Control Your Hormones to Control Your Hunger, Weight, and Inflammation," page 36, and possibly eventually read the whole book.

WHAT TO DO

Make a decision. Think about why you want to try this eating plan. List your reasons and personal pros and cons. Make a deliberate decision and keep your list where you can easily see it.

Wrap your mind around planning, shopping, and doing a little cooking. Even using this quick-start menu, it will take a little work to get started on your eating plan. However, this eating plan will not involve hunger or deprivation and, with the increased energy it should give you, the work will not be burdensome. Make a mental commitment to planning what you will eat on a weekly basis (for meal and snack ideas see pages 102 to 158), shopping for the foods you need, preparing snacks and probably a lunch to take along with you when you leave home, and doing a little cooking.

Just do it! To start your healthy eating plan, here is a "most important" list of things to do. These will stabilize your hormone levels and allow you to burn fat.

1. **Every morning eat a linked-and-balanced protein-containing breakfast** as early as you can, hopefully within the first hour after arising.

2. **Eat protein-containing snacks three times a day**, mid-morning, mid-afternoon, and at bedtime. They don't have to be large, and after your blood sugar and insulin lev-

els stabilize, you can simplify snack-packing by having an apple instead of a multi-food snack.

3. **Eat linked-and-balanced meals.** Try to have carbohydrates which are low on the glycemic index as much as possible. Keep your carbohydrate intake at or below two units (30 grams at 15 grams per carbohydrate unit) per meal and balance it with the same or a greater number of units of protein (7 grams per protein unit). Add a little fat (if the protein food doesn't provide some) and enough additional protein and vegetables to satisfy your hunger.

4. **Think nutrients.** Eat plenty of the anti-inflammatory foods listed on pages 262 to 264 and consider taking a supplement which provides general nutritional support as well as the nutrients most important for control of insulin levels and inflammation. See page 90 for more about this.

5. **If you have an apple shaped body, you are over-producing cortisol.** This is the root of your problem. Controlling your blood sugar and insulin levels will help your cortisol level, but you might also consider taking a supplement[1] such as Relora™ to ease your way by addressing the cortisol problem directly, at least during the early weeks of your healthy eating plan. See page 90 for more about this.

6. **Do some moderate exercise** or brisk activity. Intense or prolonged exercise, especially without food, can cause your body to hold onto fat and burn muscle, which will decrease your metabolism and make weight loss more difficult. See pages 265 to 268 for more about exercise.

7. **Listen to your body** and use your good common sense to decide what is best for you.

To your health! That's what this is all about.

---

[1] Although Relora™ comes recommended by a holistic M.D. whose medical expertise I trust, you are an individual. Consult your health care practitioner for personal advice about changing your diet and taking supplements. This book is meant to be used for education, not to be taken as medical advice.

GRANDMA

My grandmother could have used this book. Grandma Jiannetti, who died when I was six months old, was described to me as five-by-five – five feet tall and five feet wide. (Judging from the pictures, such as the one below of her with my dad, maybe her width was exaggerated). When my parents traveled to Italy for the first time when I was 14, they met her brother, Pietro Savioli, who was six-by-three, literally. Grandma, her brother, and several members of my paternal extended family had and have what family members call "the Savioli body type."

My mother used to say, "Grandma was big, but my, how she could move." Then she would describe the sound of her rapid footsteps and how quickly she covered ground when she walked. My father told stories about how she could hoe a row of vegetables with lightning speed. He described her bending straight from the waist to wrap and tie bunches of the Paschal celery which was the family's cash crop. She could wrap several bunches in the time it took him to do one as he worked with her when he was in his teens.

Not only did Grandma work hard on the family farm, she did everything else vigorously because of her personality and perhaps also because she had so much to do. My father was born later in her life. His sister, Louise, was fifteen, and because Grandma needed to get back to the fields to work, my aunt left school after the eighth grade to take care of my father. Although my aunt was a very intelligent woman and wanted to attend high school, she never seemed to regret having given up her personal opportunities to help raise my father.

I remember hearing a conversation between my mother and Aunt Louise when I was young. My mother said that Grandma was stubborn. My aunt said, "No, she just had determination." Determination, along with a dedication to hard work, is very much a part of the Savioli personality. Grandma, in her "determination," didn't let anyone push her around. When a salesman came to the house, she would open the door, say, "No speak-a the English," and slam the door in his face. She was an independent thinker, and some things just had to be done her way.

However, the most significant characteristic of the Savioli personality was and is a passionate love for family. When my father's family moved from the coal mining country of southern Colorado to the Denver area to farm, Grandma insisted that they live near a school so her children could receive a good education. They bought a parcel of land with a hundred-year-old farm house just three blocks from a good primary school.

When I was born, Grandma was dying of cancer. In those days, it was thought that if a person were told that she had a terminal illness, she would give up and die quickly. Thus, nobody told her what she had. My mother said that Grandma's greatest joy would have been to hold me, her newborn granddaughter, in her arms. Unfortunately, she never held me because she was afraid that she would give me her illness. Instead she sat by my cradle and rocked me while singing to me in Italian.

When my father was dying of cancer many years later, he became anemic and the doctors suggested that blood transfusions would give him more energy. I told him that I wanted to donate blood as a way of giving back just a little to him for his lifetime of love and hard work for me. He told me that he had said the same thing to his mother years before, and she told him to pass the love on to his children instead. My dad said that he wouldn't take blood from me because I needed my strength to keep up with my two young boys. (My younger son, John, was a very frisky two-year-old at the time). He told me that the best way I could thank him would be to pass on the legacy of love to his two beloved grandsons.

This book is dedicated to the memory of my grandmother and father, two of the originators of the legacy of love, to my husband and sons who love me now as I love them, and to all readers of this book who have the Savioli body type. To you I say – you are important. You were put here for a reason and a purpose. There are people who need you, and/or there will be those who need you in the future. When you find it difficult to take charge of your health for your own sake, let your love for those who need you be your motivation. If you are an independent thinker with the Savioli "determination" as well as the body type, rest assured that this book will not dictate to you. It is designed to be flexible and therefore practical for those on special diets, and this flexibility allows you to personalize it to insure enjoyment of your food as well. You can use it to do things *your way* as you lose weight and improve your health.

THE STORY OF THIS BOOK

This book, the title notwithstanding, is not as much about weight loss as it is about health. When she had cancer, my grandma used to say, "If you have your health, you have everything." In order to enjoy life fully and fulfill the purpose for which we are here, good health is essential. Truly optimal health manifests in a healthy weight (not necessarily the weight of a model), a good energy level, restful sleep, and the absence of chronic illness or inflammation. Thus, overweight is a symptom of a problem, the lack of optimal health, rather than the root problem itself.

I have been told that I lack the qualifications for writing a book about weight loss because I am not overweight. However, I do understand the frustration of not being able to maintain your desired weight from having Crohn's disease and food allergies severe enough to make me underweight off and on over the last 25 years, and I did struggle with overweight in my early 20s. However, in spite of my appearance, I am an excellent candidate for the eating plan in this book because of health problems associated with chronic inflammation such as allergies, Crohn's disease, and osteoarthritis.

Because I have written food allergy and gluten-free cookbooks, I frequently talk to or exchange emails with individuals with food intolerances. They very rarely mention being overweight in the list of their health problems, and for many years I assumed that this was because overweight wasn't a problem for those on restricted diets. In recent years, however, with the rising incidence of diagnosed celiac disease, I have been receiving phone calls from people who have eaten rice, rice, rice until they become allergic to rice. (Hence my book *Gluten-Free Without Rice*). They sometimes mention in passing that they gained weight when they switched from eating wheat to eating rice at every meal and snack. Eventually I concluded that someone who has a new, hopefully temporary weight problem might mention it, but those who are chronically overweight, especially if it has been a problem from childhood, do not because they feel shame about their weight. (See page 22 for more about why they shouldn't feel shame about their weight). As I began researching this book, I discovered why people tend to gain weight when they change from eating wheat to eating rice for every meal. Rice is the only grain which in whole grain form has a high (fat deposit inducing) glycemic index value. (You will hear all about the glycemic index later in this book).

In addition, within the last few years I have developed a close email friendship with a woman in England who takes low dose immunotherapy shots for severe multiple food allergies. If she goes too many months between shots, she can "lose" so many foods that she really struggles. Last fall she had a series of lung infections which kept her from taking her shot as scheduled. Then she had a mild heart attack.

Her doctor told her that she absolutely had to get her weight, cholesterol, and blood pressure down, so she joined Weight Watchers.™ By the time she was finally able to take a shot in the spring, seeds had become her only protein foods. Over the last several months I have been listening to stories about counting points in the context of her food allergies. Weight Watchers™ is do-able for her because it does not dictate food choices absolutely, meaning if seeds are the only protein you can eat, that's O.K. She also benefits greatly from the social support the group offers.

Listening to her made me remember the time in my early 20s when I struggled to lose weight. I grew up on a Mediterranean type of diet. We ate almost no fried food, and sweets were reserved for special occasions. My husband, however, grew up in a family that truly loves sugar and fat. When my mother-in-law dieted, she gave up most nutritious foods but made sure that candy was generously represented in the low number of calories she ate. On our honeymoon, my husband introduced me to the pleasure of picking something from the restaurant's dessert cart every night. The trend continued after we settled in the city where he was attending graduate school about 1000 miles away from my home. When my parents came to visit us for Christmas after we had been married about six months, my mother looked at my behind and said, "You better watch out. You're going to end up looking like…" and she mentioned the names of my relatives who inherited the Savioli body type.

I took my mother's warning seriously and tried to lose weight with a standard low-calorie, low-fat diet. I carried a small spiral notebook with me, recorded everything I ate with the calorie count, and kept my food intake at 500 calories less than the books said I needed per day. According to the experts, I should have lost weight, but I didn't, so I boosted my supposed calorie deficit to 1000 per day. I began doing a lot of swimming and still didn't lose very much weight. I was starved all of the time, but surprisingly, if I went swimming when hungry I was less hungry when I got out of the pool. (The explanation for this, which is not good for health or weight loss, is on pages 267 and 42). Yet I just could not lose weight without a tremendous struggle.

An office assistant at work who was about 40 (which seemed old to me at the time) but was very slim and stylish followed a high-protein, ultra-low-carbohydrate diet routinely. I decided to try that. The first day I didn't feel that great by mid-afternoon, but I stuck with it. I lost weight but never really felt right. Then my uncle died and I flew home for the funeral and the weekend. For four days I ate normally, including bread, fruit, and foods I hadn't eaten at all for a few months. When I flew back, my husband picked me up at the airport. He put his arm around my waist and said, "Gained a little weight, didn't you?" It was that obvious! I had gained back every pound that I had lost.

Then I found a book called *Low Blood Sugar and You* by Carlton Fredericks, PhD. I began to follow his diet which was more balanced and contained a moderate amount of carbohydrate, but not more than the equivalent of one-half to one thin slice of bread at any meal or snack. It directed that the dieter have a snack that contained protein three times a day, mid-morning, mid-afternoon, and at bedtime. I lost weigh slowly and was never hungry. When I had slimmed down, I stopped paying attention to portion sizes, but retained some of the basic habits from Dr. Fredericks' diet such as eating a snack when I was hungry between meals and listening to my body about what, when, and how much to eat. When my food allergies were diagnosed, I had to change what I ate drastically but I still ate nutritious between-meal and bedtime snacks.

I have heard about my email pen-pal's Weight Watchers™ experiences and received pictures of her getting progressively slimmer over the past months. She is doing a good job at improving her health outcome prospects, but I mentally compare the amount of struggle she has with the ease and lack of hunger I experienced losing weight on a plan which stabilized my blood sugar and insulin levels. I have thought, "There has to be a better way." People with food allergies or gluten-intolerance need to be able to lose weight with a system that allows the flexibility they need in order to stay on their special diets but doesn't require counting calories (points for my friend) or being hungry.

I began to do some research and discovered that in the last 30 years there has been a tremendous amount of progress made on the science behind the type of diet that worked for me. Back then, blood sugar and insulin were factors know to be involved in weight control. I've recently read about other hormones and chemical messengers now known to be equally important – cortisol, leptin, eicosanoids, and more. A major breakthrough in the application of this science to real-world weight loss has been the development of the glycemic index. All of these factors are pieces of the puzzle of weight control. Only when we make use of them all can we succeed at achieving and maintaining a healthy weight without constant struggle.

I was determined to find all the missing puzzle pieces so I read everything I could find about the glycemic index (GI), weight loss diets that employ principles which control blood sugar and insulin levels, and the physiology which explains how and why these diets work, and incidentally, also explains why it is so hard to keep weight off permanently when you lose it with low-calorie dieting. One book I came across was *The Fat Resistance Diet* by Leo Galland, MD. His diet is an extremely nutrient-dense unprocessed food diet that involves eating in a way that controls blood sugar levels. Although he mentions the glycemic index, he does not dwell on it or on insulin. Rather, he emphasizes different aspects of the physiology of weight loss such as the hormone leptin, the role of inflammation in contributing to overweight, and how excess body fat in turn causes inflammation. Since the control of chronic inflammation is at the heart of his diet, his book includes a list of 40 superfoods that dampen inflammation. He advises people to include these foods in their diets in generous amounts.

My diet for the last 30 years has been in fair compliance with the principles of glycemic control diets. I owe this to the habits I retained from Dr. Fredericks' book and my allergies to all grains and grain alternatives. However, my diet was not ideal. I would often eat, for example, a half pound of grapes for an afternoon snack without any accompanying protein to balance the carbohydrate. Because my arthritis has been worse than usual lately due to a very humid spring and summer, I decided to try an experiment. I gave up eating fruit alone for snacks and had a moderate amount of fruit with nuts instead. Although I am allergic to about two-thirds of the foods on Dr. Galland's superfoods list, I began eating generous quantities of those I can eat. I revised my rotation diet to include at least two of the superfoods on each rotation day.

Within a few days of changing my eating habits, I noticed that even though the humidity was still high on the weather reports and that there was visible moisture in the air or rain much of the time, my joints were no longer screaming, "Too much humidity!" at me. Most of them felt pretty good most of the time. Two weeks after I changed my diet, only my left knee was still a major problem.[1] This convinced me to make a thorough study of the physiology of glycemic control and inflammation and begin writing this book.

---

[1] My experience with diet change helping my arthritis does not guarantee that this eating plan will cure your arthritis or any other health condition. Other factors may also be contributing to the problem. If you have undiagnosed food allergies, you will need to diagnose them and eliminate those foods from your diet. Then too, even though Dr. Galland's superfoods are highly recommended, if you are allergic to some of them, you must avoid the problem foods or they will increase your inflammation. The story above is simply my experience. I am not totally immune to the effects of weather on my joints although the effect is less pronounced. This chapter and book are not meant to replace individualized medical advice from your health care professional.

My left knee has improved after physical therapy and a continued home knee exercise program, but the inflammation in that knee had progressed to damage of the cartilage on the back of the kneecap. However, with proper exercise and muscle strengthening, I hope to avoid further damage. I hope that you will take my experience with my left knee as a lesson that helps you decide to be pro-active and not put off addressing inflammatory issues and weight problems before they cause irreversible damage to your joints or health.

THE PROBLEM WITH DIETS

There is more to food than just nutrients. We derive pleasure and emotional satisfaction as well as physical sustenance from eating. The problem with most diets is that they involve a great deal of deprivation. In addition to sometimes making us overwhelmingly hungry, many weight loss diets leave us feeling psychologically and emotionally deprived, as if all pleasure vanished from our lives. That's a lot to give up.

A restrictive diet can be like a bossy, seemingly arbitrary teacher or parent wagging a finger and saying, "No!" to everything we want. The diet tells us what to do constantly and, at least as far as food goes, makes most of our decisions for us. Because eating is basic to satisfaction, even people without a Savioli-type mindset (i.e. those who are not super-independent thinkers) find this degree of control over their lives hard to endure for very long.

Hunger is the most significant problem with weight loss diets. If we muster up enough willpower, we can tolerate hunger for a few days, but soon it will seemingly overtake our lives. Because we are physically hungry, food will become an all-consuming passion. We will have difficulty concentrating on almost anything else because we will be thinking continually about how long it will be until the next meal and what we are or are not allowed to eat. A diet that regularly results in hunger is not a diet that anyone can live with for very long.

On some of the more reasonable diets, we may not actually be hungry all the time, but we may still feel deprived psychologically and emotionally. Some diets are nutritionally adequate but do not meet our needs for the pleasure which is normally derived from eating. The foods allowed on the diet may be boring, bland, or things that we hate to eat. We miss our favorite foods.

The most discouraging problem with weight loss diets is that many of them do not work long-term. We may lose weight and reach our goal, but as soon as we liberalize our eating habits, the pounds return. If the caloric restriction of a diet is extreme enough or if the diet promotes muscle loss, people may end up heavier than before they dieted because their metabolism has been reprogrammed to burn food more slowly and thus need less food. Unfortunately, most of the time weight loss diets fail to produce long-term weight loss.[1]

Many weight loss diets are time-consuming and complex. They require constant recording of the foods eaten. Then the calories, points, grams of carbohydrates, or fat grams consumed must be tallied up throughout the day to prevent exceeding one's daily allotment. I don't know about you, but my life is already too busy without adding "food math" to my to-do list!

---

[1] For more about why low-calorie diets fail, see this page: http://www.montignac.com/en/la_methode_scientifique_echec_regimes_hypo.php

Most weight loss diets have relatively narrow prescribed lists of allowed or preferred foods. If people with multiple food allergies cross off all the foods they are allergic to from the diet's list, the remaining food may be nutritionally inadequate.

So what must we do to lose weight? A non-diet – an eating plan that is not overly restrictive, supplies all of our nutritional requirements and permits choices that respect our need for the pleasure and emotional satisfaction that should come from food. This plan must accommodate our food allergies or gluten-intolerance and be such that we can comfortably follow it as a routine part of our daily lives. Hunger and pleasure deprivation cannot be part of any eating plan we expect to be able to stay on for more than a few days. In addition, the eating plan must "work" and result in a healthy weight that is easily maintained permanently.

We must have a healthy eating plan that lets us do things our way, both psychologically and physically, and that controls our body chemistry to eliminate hunger and promote the burning of fat. It must put us in touch with our bodies so that we work with our physiology rather than against it. It also must still enable us to receive pleasure from eating.

Keep reading to discover a healthy eating plan that is tailored to YOUR needs. Find out how you can do it your way.

Do It Your Way

A strong will and determination are good. They make us independent thinkers who have ability to know truth from falsehoods. They enable us to choose right over wrong, even when our choice may not be popular. They impart the drive we require to do difficult things. Although I'm generalizing from a limited sample (my relatives, my pen-pal in England, and other heavy friends I have known personally and well), it seems to me that many with the Savioli body type also have the Savioli personality. The benefits of the personality greatly outweigh the disadvantages of the body type. The disadvantages of the body type are superficial and cosmetic (although if you get too heavy, it may adversely affect your health). The advantages of this personality have long-lasting positive effects that extend to those around you, even to future generations. When determination, even in its negative extreme of stubbornness, is balanced with love – love for others and yourself – you can accomplish great things. This chapter addresses how to harness your determination to improve your health so you have more energy to do what you want to do on a daily basis and even to help insure a normal-length life span in which to accomplish your deeper goals.

Everyone prefers to do things his or her own way. For a weight loss program to work long-term, almost all of us have a better chance of success if we are able to do things our way, both physically and mentally. Your body should be the *only* "boss" that tells you if you absolutely must or must not eat a certain food, when to eat, and how much to eat. If you are hungry, that is a signal from your body that your blood sugar is dropping, and you need to eat a small, properly balanced snack to prevent the consequences of low blood sugar (which can lead to fat deposition) no matter what the clock says about mealtime. With a healthy eating plan that lets you do it your way, you will not feel deprived of food enjoyment either. Feeling deprived and hungry are two factors that make it difficult to slim down, so enjoy your favorite foods! Learn how to do it, how to make or eat them in a more healthy way, and have them within the limits of your food allergies or intolerances.

YOU must be the one to determine WHEN and WHY to embark on a healthy eating plan. The motivation must come from you, and the timing must be right. As explained on page 41, an especially stressful time in your life may not be the time to start this program, especially if you will be discouraged if your weight loss is slow due to high levels of stress hormones. (Of course, there is no period of life that is completely stress-free). Make the decision to embark on this plan thoughtfully and write down your reasons for wanting to change your eating habits. List both pros and cons. Keep this list handy. Perhaps put a copy on your refrigerator, in your desk, and/or on your computer so you can refer to the list easily and often.

In the course of preparing to write this book, I reviewed over a dozen diets that promote the control of blood sugar and insulin levels and/or inflammation. One discovery I made was that there are no absolute prohibitions common to all of the diets. For example, while they all discourage the over-consumption of caffeine (no trying to live on coffee to lose weight!), most allow coffee with breakfast for those who feel they really want or need it. In *The Fat Resistance Diet*, Dr. Leo Galland, MD recommends drinking green tea for its anti-inflammatory and antioxidant effects.[1] His daily menus of meals and snacks list "Slim Chai Green Tea" as a beverage several times a day. [2]

Several of the diets prohibit the use of artificial sweeteners. However, in *The Glycemic Index Diet*, Rick Gallop uses them freely and even includes them in recipes.[3] In *The Insulin Resistance Diet*, Dr. Cheryle Hart, MD, a specialist in bariatrics (weight loss) reports that although the sweet taste of artificial sweeteners causes a slight release of insulin by the pancreas, this is not a problem unless the sweeteners are consumed without any food, such as in drinking a diet soda without food. She says that if diet sodas are taken with food so the insulin has something to work on, they will not send one's blood sugar and hormones on a roller coaster ride.[4] However a more recent publication offered on Dr. Hart's website says that patients are allowed to drink diet sodas without food.[5] I suspect that with time she has come to the conclusion that tolerance for diet sodas in regard to weight control is an individual matter.

Sugar is another controversial food which is absolutely forbidden in some of the books I read. All of the authors agree that is should not make up the high percentage of our carbohydrate intake that it does in the standard American diet, but some of them recognize that the need for emotional satisfaction can be as important as the need for physical satisfaction and allow sugar as part of a "controlled splurge." On the glycemic index, a measure of the actual effect a food has on our blood sugar, table sugar scores lower than refined white bread and most types of rice. Therefore, if a sugar-containing treat is eaten in moderation and balanced with protein, it can be a part of a healthy eating plan. However, if you are actually allergic to sugar or have problems with candidiasis, you may have to avoid it. Don't despair though. There are other delicious ways to sweeten foods. See pages 197 to 225 for recipes for sugar-free treats.

The only absolute on foods that you must avoid are dictated by your own body – by your food allergies and intolerances. All of the sources I read that mentioned allergies

---

[1] Galland, Leo, MD, *The Fat Resistance Diet,* (New York: Broadway Books, 2005), 98.

[2] Although green tea is low in caffeine, it is not caffeine-free, and the total amount of caffeine in several cups of green tea can be more than in a single cup of coffee for breakfast. Dr. Galland moderates the caffeine by always having food consumed with the recommended green tea. See the recipe for "Caffeine-Controlled Green Tea" on page 229.

[3] Gallop, Rick, *The GI [Glycemic Index] Diet,* (New York: Workman Publishing, 2002), 27.

[4] Hart, Cheryle R., MD and Mary Kay Grossman, RD, *The Insulin Resistance Diet,* (New York: McGraw-Hill, 2001, 2007), 96.

[5] Grossman, Mary Kay, RD, *Foods by Chance or by Choice,* (Free download from irdiet.com, 2008), 12.

(*The Fat Resistance Diet, The Insulin Resistance Diet, The Complete Idiot's Guide to Glycemic Index Weight Loss, Your Hidden Food Allergies Are Making You Fat,* etc.) said that eating an allergic food causes inflammation and the release of adrenal hormones which start a hormonal cascade leading to the promotion of depositing food as fat.[6] Therefore, the only absolute "no" you will hear will be from your own body if you are intolerant of certain foods. If you are reading this book, you have probably already learned to listen to that "no" so that you can avoid allergic or celiac reactions and feel well.

Rather than presenting only do-not instructions, a few of the books told readers to DO things that you would not expect to see in a diet book. They advised that feelings of deprivation have to be managed, and that a good way to do this was to have planned, controlled splurges.[7] One example given was to eat an ounce of good (not cheap) dark chocolate containing 60 to 70% cacao. (Do not do this if you are allergic to chocolate! Have a non-allergenic fun food splurge instead. See recipes for treats on pages 200 to 225). The carbohydrates from the chocolate were to be balanced with protein to prevent a blood sugar spike and the portion size controlled, but since chocolate is an excellent feel-good food because it raises levels of neurotransmitters, Dr. Cheryle Hart reports that controlled chocolate splurges help people continue and succeed on a healthy eating plan rather than give up due to feelings of deprivation.

Your body – your physical need for nutrition and food allergies or intolerances – and your pleasure needs, combined with the science in the next few chapters, will help you to determine what is right for YOU. After you have followed your healthy eating plan and listened to your psyche's and body's response to it for a while, you will be able to refine the plan to fit you even better. You will find that increased energy, improved sleep, and possibly how you feel if you abandon the plan for a meal or a day, will convince you that you are doing the right thing for your health. With the improved health that results from working with rather than against your body will come a healthy weight.

WHO IS IN CHARGE?

Who is in charge of your diet now? If you are an adult and your diet is influenced by your spouse or other family members, you may need to start cooking for yourself or enlist their help with your eating plan. Chances are, they want to keep you alive and healthy and will do what they can to help.

If you are living alone, it may seem as if you are the only one who could possibly be in charge of your diet. Thus, you may blame yourself for your weight problem, and

[6] Rivera, Rudy, MD and Roger Deutsch, *Your Hidden Food Allergies Are Making You Fat,* (Rocklin, CA: Prima Publishing, 1998), 148-149.

[7] Beale, Lucy and Joan Clark, RD, CDE, *The Complete Idiot's Guide to Glycemic Index Weight Loss,* (New York: Alpha, 2005), 299, and Hart, Cheryle R, MD and Mary Kay Grossman, RD, *The Insulin Resistance Diet,* (New York: McGraw-Hill, 2001, 2007), 107.

think that you overeat because you have a character flaw or no willpower. THIS IS NOT TRUE! Your body chemistry and the food industry may be causing you to overeat, or you may be eating a reasonable or low amount of food but your hormones are causing it to be deposited as fat while leaving you short on energy.

For those with food allergies, eating an allergic food, known or unknown, will cause a hormonal cascade that can lead to weight gain. It also can cause allergic cravings which drive you to overeat. When you eat a problem food, you have an immune response which often involves making antibodies (usually of the IgG4 or IgE classes) that mediate the immune response to the food. Eating that food again ties up some of the antibodies and decreases allergic symptoms. Thus, some people unknowingly manage their allergy symptoms by getting regular "fixes" from eating their problem foods. If you suspect that you are having allergic cravings or notice that some foods make you feel better, you may be allergic to more foods than you currently know, and you should pursue the diagnosis of potential new food allergies. See www.food-allergy.org/diagnosis.html for more about this. You must eliminate all of your allergenic foods from your diet to control inflammation and lose weight.

If you have problems with keeping your blood sugar levels stable, which is likely if you're overweight, your blood sugar-controlling hormones may be making you very hungry between meals, which makes it hard to not overeat. This is especially likely to happen if a meal contains a large amount of high glycemic index carbohydrate. (This is why many people are famished two hours after eating at a Chinese restaurant). This book will show you how to be the boss and take charge of your blood sugar-controlling hormones.

In addition to the allergic and hormonal influences of your own body, there is another player that may be controlling what and how much you eat. This player is doing it for profit, and you rightly may be angry when you learn about how its control is being exercised over you. If you or your non-allergic family members or friends eat commercially-made processed foods or eat in restaurants, the food industry may be making you overeat. Former FDA Commissioner Dr. David Kessler, MD exposes the manipulative tricks used by the food industry in his book *The End of Overeating*.[8] His message, in a few words and possibly oversimplified, is that commercially made foods are laden with sugar, fat and salt, making them hyper-palatable, and thus provoking an almost addictive response in some people involving opiate-like brain chemicals.

Furthermore, he reports that food can be so highly processed that it is almost pre-digested. If the food is mostly carbohydrates, your body's hormonal response will result in the energy from the food being stored as fat and will make you hungry for more very soon. While we may be aware that white flour and sugar are highly processed, processing to the point of near pre-digestion can also be done to protein foods. Kessler describes

---

[8] Kessler, David, MD, *The End of Overeating*, (New York: Rodale, 2009).

interviewing food industry representatives about the chicken served at Chili's Restaurants. The former president of Standard Meat, the company Chili's buys its meat from, told Kessler that the marination-by-injection process they used for the chicken "essentially pre-chews" the meat although it still looks normal. This reduces the need to chew, making it easier for diners to eat much more food than is needed before they realize how much they have eaten. [9]

YOU MUST TAKE CHARGE!

If you want to lose weight successfully and permanently or to control chronic inflammation, you must take charge! Do it your way! You don't have to be hungry or deprived of pleasure. As my grandma did with the door-to-door salesmen, say, "No." Don't let the food industry control you and trick you into eating highly processed foods. Eliminate all of your allergenic foods so reactions do not lead to allergic cravings or to wild fluctuations in your blood sugar control hormones that make you so hungry that you overeat. Using the information in the next several chapters, design your own healthy eating plan and thus take control of dietary factors that cause blood sugar and hormone imbalances that lead to weight gain. Use your healthy eating plan to elicit the desired responses from the hormones that control fat deposition and thus tell your body to burn fat rather than store it. YOU can be in control!

---

[9] Kessler, David, MD, *The End of Overeating,* (New York: Rodale, 2009), 69.

WHAT DETERMINES OUR WEIGHT?

What causes overweight? Conventional medicine says it is all a matter of how much you eat and exercise. If you take in more calories than you use, the surplus is stored as fat. Indeed, some doctors point a finger at the overweight patient and say, "It's all your fault." Although calories do count, they are not the only or the major determiner of weight. This reasoning of conventional doctors and the diets they prescribe rarely produce sustained weight loss, but they do a great job of producing guilt and feelings of inadequacy when we either cannot lose weight or keep it off.

If conventional doctors were correct in their reasoning, the much-attempted standard American weight loss regimens of calorie counting accompanied by exercise and the abundance of low-calorie, low-fat diet foods in the stores would have slimmed us all down. Instead, the prevalence of obesity in the United States has been growing rapidly for the last 40 years.

I believe that the true cause of overweight can be summed up in the following statement by Leo Galland, MD, a well-known and respected nutritionally oriented doctor who takes a holistic approach to the practice of medicine. He says, "Your weight problem is not a matter of will or discipline, but a chemical imbalance that, once corrected, holds the key to permanent weight loss."[1] This imbalance can be corrected by changing what foods you eat (probably not drastically if you are already on an allergy diet and therefore not eating processed foods), how you combine them, and when you eat.

Dr. Galland's statements carry the weight of authority; he has practiced medicine for over 30 years. In *The Fat Resistance Diet,* he supports his assertions with numerous references to articles in respected medical journals. His holistic and nutrition-oriented approach has put him ahead of his peers on discerning the real causes again and again.

So how did we arrive at this state of chemical and hormonal imbalance and overweight? As with many of our characteristics, both genetics and our environment and experience play a role.

NATURE: GENETICS

This book began with a story about my Grandma Jiannetti and her heavy-around-the-waist Savioli body type (i.e., an apple-shaped body). Since her brother and several descendents had or have the same shape, it seems that genetics plays a role. Weight gain and shape patterns are obvious in my own family. On my father's side, my heavy relatives are all big around the waist, taking after Grandma Jiannetti. On my mother's side,

[1] Galland, Leo, MD, *The Fat Resistance Diet,* (New York: Broadway Books, 2005), 7.

most of my relatives are slim, and when the older women gain weight, it is in the hips. They have pear-shaped bodies.

Of the two body shapes in my extended family, the pear shape is statistically associated with little medical risk. Apple-shaped weight gain is associated with increased risk of cardiovascular disease, high blood pressure, and diabetes.

On a chemical level, apple-shaped people have higher levels of the adrenal hormone cortisol which negatively influences their ability to maintain stable blood sugar levels. (For more about this see pages 41 to 43). The healthy eating plan in this book addresses balancing blood sugar and insulin levels. However because of their inherited higher cortisol production, some apple-shaped people, under their doctor's supervision, my also benefit from using supplements to moderate their production of cortisol. (See page 90 for more information about these supplements).

A family history of type II diabetes is another genetic factor that can lead to overweight. People who eventually develop type II diabetes may have blood sugar regulation difficulties for years before they develop overt disease. However, if when they begin gaining weight (a symptom of blood sugar control problems) they take charge, follow an eating plan which controls blood sugar levels, and thus reduce the strain on their pancreas, full-blown diabetes might be averted.

Other genetic factors which influence our body size can be positive. Some people have thick heavy bones, large rib cages, and wide pelvises. At an ideal level of body fat, these people may be called "stocky," but their body type carries advantages. Those heavy bones are less likely to break in a fall, especially as bone density decreases with age. If you are musical, a large rib cage may allow you to sing opera or play a large wind instrument well and powerfully. A woman with a wide pelvis will appreciate her body type during childbirth, especially if the baby is large. So if this eating plan brings your body mass index (BMI) to a normal level and you still do not have the shape of a model, actor, or actress, be glad to be healthy again and accept your genetically determined shape for the advantages it offers.

NURTURE: ENVIRONMENT AND EXPERIENCES

Our environment and previous experiences also influence our weight. Some environmental factors are social. For example, each year in November and December, many of us attend family Thanksgiving dinners and holiday parties. During these months we are repeatedly put in social situations where we are surrounded by an overabundance of delicious foods. We don't want to offend our favorite aunt or employer's wife by turning down the food she has worked hard to prepare, so we almost feel forced to indulge a little. And who can sit at a baseball game without wanting a hotdog? We don't want to miss out on the fun, and in our past experience, a hotdog has been part of the fun!

If your allergies allow, these social situations are the time to plan ahead for a controlled splurge. Do not unnecessarily deprive yourself of experiences that add fun to life! However, you can plan ahead to limit portion sizes to what will satisfy but not stuff you. Also determine to balance whatever carbohydrate you eat with protein. If you are allergic to too many foods to indulge in the party goodies or a hotdog, planning ahead is even more important. Bring your own food, and try to make it something that you will really enjoy. Watching those around you eat delicious treats while you go hungry can make you so ravenous that it will be impossible to maintain control when you get home.

Television viewing can be another environmental trigger that leads to overeating. We tend to munch mindlessly while we watch TV. It is best to not come to your favorite program hungry. If you just ate, it's easier to ignore the food commercials, but if you are physically hungry, you will want to eat every food advertised. If you find yourself craving the foods displayed on TV and getting hungry, try a healthy snack which will stabilize your blood sugar level such as an apple or a handful of nuts. Do not take the whole bag of nuts back to the TV with you however, or you may eat more than you need to satisfy your physical hunger.

If your problem with watching TV is not actual hunger but rather than you have been in the habit of eating while you watch, consider starting a new TV habit. I enjoy doing needlework while I watch TV. Perhaps the best TV habit for weight loss is to do some exercise while you watch. Pedal a stationery bicycle (but not necessarily at breakneck speed) or do stretching exercises. See pages 265 to 268 for information about aerobics versus moderate exercise, which is actually the best way to burn fat, and is why you should not bicycle too hard for too long.

Past experiences can profoundly influence our weight; old eating habits can be hard to break. When you are tempted to slip back into old habits, look at the list you made of motivating reasons for embarking on a healthy eating plan.

Past eating habits may also have changed us in ways that promote overweight. Over-consumption of sugars and processed carbohydrates may have over-taxed your pancreas. Thus, you may have trouble maintaining a stable blood sugar level. If you have lost muscle mass due to past low-calorie dieting, your metabolism may be lower than it otherwise would have been. This can be overcome by building muscle, however. Eat plenty of protein and begin an appropriate exercise program to build muscles. (See pages 265 to 268 for more about exercise).

The final and most important factor that impacts our weight is chronic inflammation. Overweight and inflammation form a vicious cycle, but this cycle can be broken. Excess body fat contributes to inflammation and inflammation causes hormonal problems that promote further weight gain.[2] However, by addressing the problems of over-

---

[2] Galland, Leo, MD, *The Fat Resistance Diet,* (New York: Broadway Books, 2005), 12.

weight and inflammation simultaneously, the cycle can be broken and both problems can be resolved. See pages 33 to 35 for more about this.

If you are reading this book, there is a good chance that you have been on a weight loss diet in the past. You have exerted more willpower and endured more hunger than any genetically thin person will ever understand. Now that you have read about the genetic and environmental factors that contribute to overweight in this chapter and about the food industry's manipulative practices in the last chapter, it is time to abandon self-recrimination over past dieting failures (most of which are due to the type of diet). Banish guilt, take charge, and move on. Have determination! Re-read Dr. Galland's statement at the beginning of this chapter. Copy it and put it on your refrigerator or add it to your list of motivations for changing your eating habits that you have saved on your computer or in your desk. You are not a failure; you are a valuable person. Your health is important. Move on and begin taking steps to correct the chemical imbalance which has caused to you to gain weight and/or led to inflammatory health conditions. You can do it!

The Principles of Glycemic Control Weight Loss

When we hear the word "hormones," our first thought is about sex hormones. However, the hormones discussed in this book are not sex hormones. An endocrine hormone is actually any chemical messenger that travels from where it is produced through the bloodstream to another part or parts of the body where it exerts its effect. Our hormones interact with each other to create a fast-acting chemical control system for our entire bodies. For weight control, hormones rule!

What happens when you eat a piece of bread? As you chew, an enzyme in your saliva begins breaking down the starch in the bread into single sugar units (monosaccharides). The digestive process continues in the stomach and small intestine and the monosaccharides that are released from the digesting starch are absorbed from the small intestine into the bloodstream. If the monosaccharide is glucose, it is ready to be used by body cells immediately. Monosaccharides other than glucose and also any protein we consume that is in excess of our protein needs for body building and repair are absorbed from the bloodstream into the liver. There they are converted into glucose to supply our cells with fuel. This glucose is released from the liver into the bloodstream, but the conversion process takes time so proteins and monosaccharides other than glucose (such as fructose) are not available to be used by our cells as quickly as glucose is.

The hormone **INSULIN** is needed for glucose to enter our cells and be used for energy. When the pancreas detects a rise in the glucose level in the bloodstream, it secretes insulin which allows glucose to enter the cells, and the level of glucose in the bloodstream returns to a pre-meal level. Glucose may be used by our cells for immediate needs or stored as glycogen (chains of glucose molecules) in the cells of the liver and muscles for future energy needs. The amount of glycogen we can store is limited, so within about two hours after a meal we will begin storing as fat any excess glucose over what we have used or saved for future use as glycogen. Glucose can be converted to triglycerides (the basic unit of fats) for storage by the liver. Insulin also allows glucose to enter into fat cells where it is converted to triglycerides and stored as fat.[1]

In an optimally healthy person, insulin secretion is correctly balanced with the amount of glucose entering the bloodstream from the small intestine and liver. In some people, however, the secretion of insulin is excessive. This results in an abnormally rapid drop in the blood glucose (also called blood sugar) level after a meal if the pancreas overshoots on insulin production. The result is too little glucose in the blood; this condition is called reactive hypoglycemia. It is hypoglycemia (low blood sugar) in response to a

[1] Hart, Cheryle R., MD and Mary Kay Grossman, RD, *The Insulin Resistance Diet,* (New York: McGraw-Hill, 2001, 2007), 5; also www.montignac.com/en/la_methode_scientifique.php .

meal rather than as a result of a pancreatic tumor. Conventional medicine traditionally has not believed that reactive hypoglycemia is a significant problem. However, the person experiencing it may become weak, irritable, dizzy, or develop a headache. They will probably also become very hungry with an hour or two after a meal and crave sugar or starchy foods. Another dose of carbohydrates will start this cycle over again. Thus, appetite is out of balance with the body's actual need for food, and the glucose that is being driven out of the bloodstream and into the cells by the excess insulin will be stored as fat.

A high level of insulin also activates an enzyme called lipoprotein lipase. This enzyme catalyzes the production of triglycerides from any fatty acids (digested fat units in the form that is absorbed by the intestine) eaten in a meal. Thus, excess insulin promotes storage of any fat we eat by our fat cells rather than using it for fuel after our meal. In a person with normal insulin levels, any recently eaten fats could have been used for energy during the two hours after a meal. If insulin levels are high, dietary fat is more likely to be stored in the fat cells.[2]

In addition, high insulin levels in the blood inhibit the activity of the enzyme triglyceride lipase which breaks down stored fat for use as energy. Thus, if you have chronically high insulin, you cannot burn your own body fat![3]

If a person continually over-produces insulin, a state of insulin resistance may result in which insulin becomes less effective in getting glucose into the cells to be used for energy or stored. Since blood sugar levels do not drop as readily after a meal in a person with insulin resistance, the pancreas keeps secreting more insulin which becomes less and less effective in doing its job. Insulin resistance is a pre-diabetic state. It can result in weight gain and other symptoms which characterize metabolic syndrome such as high blood pressure and abnormal blood fat levels. Paradoxically, fasting or skipping meals can also cause insulin resistance, possibly by increasing cortisol levels.[4] (See page 41 for more about this).

Other hormones also affect the insulin-glucose balancing system. One such hormone is **CORTISOL**, which is produced by the adrenal glands. Some cortisol is present in our blood at all times; the levels follow a daily cycle, peaking between 6 and 8 a.m. and being lowest in the evening. The adrenal glands produce a spurt of cortisol when we encounter stress and must respond quickly to a crisis. This is known as the "fight or flight" response, and cortisol levels return to normal when the crisis has passed. However, chronic stress can result in chronically high cortisol levels. Chronically high cortisol can cause chronically high insulin levels (hyperinsulinism), which leads to weight gain. Cortisol can also deplete the level of the brain neurotransmitter serotonin which can

[2] www.montignac.com/en/la_methode_scientifique.php .

[3] Hart, Cheryle R., MD and Mary Kay Grossman, RD, *The Insulin Resistance Diet,* (New York: McGraw-Hill, 2001, 2007), 5; and www.montignac.com/en/la_methode_scientifique.php .

[4] Hart, Cheryle R., MD and Mary Kay Grossman, RD, *The Insulin Resistance Diet,* (New York: McGraw-Hill, 2001, 2007), 19.

result in difficulty in sleeping, depression, and anxiety.[5] This is how stress disrupts our sleep and makes us miserable and fat! I hope understanding it makes you feel better about it. It should because there are things you can do to minimize the effects of stress. (See below and pages 42 to 43 for more about this).

Cortisol causes a type of weight gain that is visibly different from over-all weight gain, namely the apple-shaped gain around the mid-section of the body. Here's the Savioli body type again! Some people are genetically pre-disposed to high cortisol levels which may explain why apple-shaped bodies tend to run in families.

Because insulin production increases cortisol production and cortisol production increases insulin production, bringing insulin levels under control can moderate cortisol production. Stress reduction and relaxation techniques are discussed in some glycemic control diet books as a way to help with weight loss.[6] Supplements may also be helpful, especially for those who are genetically predisposed to excess cortisol production.[7] (See page 23 for more about this). Phytonutrients in foods such as fruits, vegetables, nuts and seeds can also help moderate cortisol production.[8] See the superfoods list on pages 262 to 264 for foods that will help.

Body fat is not inert. It plays a role in the hormonal regulation of weight.[9] (See pages 43 to 44 for more about the hormones **LEPTIN** and **ADIPONECTIN**). Those with more body fat tend to have higher cortisol levels and are more likely to be insulin resistant. A rough test for insulin resistance can be preformed with a tape measure. A waist measurement of more than 35 inches for women or more than 40 inches for men indicates that it is likely that the person is insulin resistant.[10]

However, the good news about body fat and hormones is that as you lose weight, insulin resistance lessens, blood glucose levels are easier to keep stable, and weight loss becomes easier due to improved hormonal factors. In fact, Dr. Galland finds that many of his patients who achieve normal weight on the very healthy diets he prescribes maintain a permanent self-regulating normal weight due to the re-establishment of normal hormonal control of their weight.[11] Dr. Galland's focus is on the role of inflammation in weight problems and on hormones besides insulin such as leptin. These topics will be discussed in detail in the next chapter.

---

[5] Hart, Cheryle R., MD and Mary Kay Grossman, RD, *The Insulin Resistance Diet,* (New York: McGraw-Hill, 2001, 2007), 23.

[6] Ibid., 222-227.

[7] Ibid., 228-229.

[8] Galland, Leo, MD, *The Fat Resistance Diet,* (New York: Broadway Books, 2005), 8 and Hart, Cheryle R., MD and Mary Kay Grossman, RD, *The Insulin Resistance Diet,* (New York: McGraw-Hill, 2001, 2007), 229.

[9] Galland, Leo, MD, *The Fat Resistance Diet,* (New York: Broadway Books, 2005), 5, 26, 29.

[10] Hart, Cheryle R., MD and Mary Kay Grossman, RD, *The Insulin Resistance Diet,* (New York: McGraw-Hill, 2001, 2007), 15.

[11] Galland, Leo, MD, *The Fat Resistance Diet,* (New York: Broadway Books, 2005), 5.

Other hormone-like substances that affect weight include **EICOSANOIDS**. (These are not technically hormones because they act right where they are produced and last only a few seconds rather than traveling through the bloodstream). Barry Sears, PhD, was originally an eicosanoid researcher and became the author of the series of *The Zone* diet books. He espouses rigidly maintained ratios of protein, carbohydrate and fat at every meal to "enter the zone" of optimal eicosanoid production. His take on the how hormones influence weight is that insulin exerts its influence by determining whether good or bad eicosanoids are produced.[12]

A final chemical messenger that can affect your ability to lose weight is active in the brain rather than actually affecting fat storage directly and is the neurotransmitter **SEROTONIN**. The amino acid tryptophan and carbohydrates are both necessary for the production of serotonin. In *The Feel Good Diet,* Dr. Cheryle Hart tells about patients who have been on strict low-carbohydrate diets and come to her with depression and even symptoms of mental imbalance such as compulsive behavior. They also struggle to stay on a diet. This is because without sufficient carbohydrates in their diets their brains have been depleted of serotonin. While balancing their insulin and blood sugar levels with a link-and-balance eating plan, she allows more carbohydrate to fuel the production of serotonin and "controlled splurges" on their favorite high-carbohydrate foods. With higher serotonin levels and improved mental health, they do not feel deprived or depressed and are able to stay on the weight loss program she prescribes.[13]

This multitude of opinions about hormones and weight reminds me of John Godfrey Saxe's poem about the blind men and the elephant. One felt his tail and thought an elephant was like a rope, one felt his side and thought an elephant was like a wall, one felt his knee and thought an elephant was like a tree, etc. While all the authors of the books I reviewed agree that insulin plays a major role in weight problems, some focus on other body chemicals as well. Dr. Galland, with his 30-plus years of experience in a medical practice which includes many allergy patients, sees leptin and inflammation as the central players. Dr. Sears focuses on eicosanoids. Dr. Hart sees insulin and serotonin as crucial. All of these chemical messengers are involved, and they can all be controlled by the same healthy eating plan.

TAKE CONTROL OF YOUR HORMONES

Don't despair if the first several pages of this chapter sound like a series of vicious cycles reminding you of the old song, "There's a Hole in my Bucket." There *is* a way to escape problems with your weight-controlling hormones. The most basic way to break the hormonal cycles that lead to overweight and inflammation is to moderate insulin

[12] Sears, Barry, PhD, *Enter the Zone,* (New York, Regan Books, 1995), 38.

[13] Hart, Cheryle R., MD and Mary Kay Grossman, RD, *The Feel-Good Diet,* (New York: McGraw-Hill, 2007), 6-7.

levels. Insulin can be controlled by taking charge of what you eat, when you eat, and how you combine foods.

You do not have to be hungry, deprived, or give up your favorite foods. The solution to your problems is to balance the types of foods you combine and to eat most of your carbohydrates in the forms they were in a hundred years ago rather than the way they are now.[14] Years ago, grains were stone ground; therefore bread and other foods made from the resulting flour were digested slowly. As the glucose from this bread entered the bloodstream, it provided sustained energy, rather than jolting the pancreas at every meal the way today's over-processed, fluffy, chemically stabilized white bread does. The bread of a hundred years ago would not cause insulin resistance. Sugar was an infrequent luxury food, and thus was not harmful because it was not a large part of the daily diet as it is now. In addition to being better for us, bread and desserts prepared the "old way" with less-refined sweeteners and flour taste better and are more satisfying than modern processed foods. See pages 179 to 225 for recipes for low to moderate GI breads and desserts.

THE GLYCEMIC INDEX AND WEIGHT LOSS

How then can we control our insulin levels? By determining that we will eat wisely and in harmony with what our bodies actually need rather than by following conventional nutritional doctrine. A most important tool for making wise decisions about what to eat is the glycemic index (GI). The glycemic index will be discussed fully on pages 47 to 53, but for the purposes of this chapter, you should know that the glycemic index is a system of scoring foods based on how they affect the blood sugar levels of real people. The GI score of a food reflects what actually happens to our blood sugar level when we eat that food. Testing to determine the glycemic index of a food requires human volunteers; calorie determinations are made by a machine, a calorimeter.

The glycemic index has been clinically proven to be useful in its application to diabetes, weight loss, appetite control, and coronary health.[15] It is used in Australia, Canada, the UK, France, Italy, Sweden, and other countries. The United States remains officially opposed to the glycemic index.[16]

---

[14] The major contributors to the rising level of obesity and diabetes in the United States are industrialized food production and processing (Michael Pollan, *In Defense of Food: An Eater's Manifesto,* (New York: The Penguin Press, 2008), 85-87, 91-92) and the standard high-carbohydrate, low-calorie weight loss diet (http://www.montignac.com/en/la_methode_scientifique_echec_regimes_hypo.php).

[15] Brand-Miller, Jennie, PhD, Thomas Wolever, MD, Kay Foster-Powell. MND, and Stephen Colaguiri, MD., *The New Glucose Revolution,* (New York: Marlowe and Company, 2003), 31, also www.montignac. com/en/la_methode_scientifique.php and www.montignac.com/en/la_methode_regime. equilibre.php.

[16] Brand-Miller, Jennie, PhD, Thomas Wolever, MD, Kay Foster-Powell. MND, and Stephen Colaguiri, MD., *The New Glucose Revolution,* (New York: Marlowe and Company, 2003), 30.

To control spikes in blood sugar and weight-depositing spikes in insulin or chronically high insulin levels, it is best to choose most of your carbohydrates from those that are low on the glycemic index with a GI score of 55 or less. Foods with an intermediate score of 56 to 69 can be eaten in moderation.[17] For best blood sugar and insulin control, high GI foods with scores of 70 or above should be eaten only occasionally. However, there are ways to enjoy favorite high-GI foods more often by making them with a healthier recipe that results in a moderate or even low GI score.

All high carbohydrate foods should be eaten at the same time as a balancing serving of a protein food. The very sensible, balanced diet in *The Insulin Resistance Diet* by Dr. Cheryle Hart, MD and Mary Kay Grossman, RD links each carbohydrate unit containing 15 grams of carbohydrate with a protein unit containing 7 grams of protein.[18] The various *Zone* diets, which are more restrictive, allow 9 grams of carbohydrate for each 7 grams of protein.[19] The amount of protein required to balance carbohydrate can vary from person to person. (See more about how to determine this on page 91). However, carbohydrate IS important for weight loss. As mentioned previously, in *The Insulin Resistance Diet* Dr. Hart reports that diets insufficient in carbohydrate inhibit the brain's production of the neurotransmitter serotonin, and the effect of this on one's mental state makes it difficult to stay on a weight loss program.[20]

In most of the diets I researched, some foods, such as non-starchy vegetables, need not be balanced with protein because they are not concentrated forms of carbohydrates. (Yet *The Zone* diets even require vegetables to be counted in the carbohydrate you are balancing with protein). Furthermore, a few foods such as yogurt and cooked dried beans (legumes) need not be linked and balanced because they contain the right ratio of carbohydrate to protein and also because the carbohydrate in yogurt has been changed to lactic acid by the yogurt-producing bacteria and much of the carbohydrate in beans is indigestible fiber.

The amount of carbohydrate eaten at any one meal or snack should be limited to two carbohydrate units, or 30 grams of available carbohydrate. (Available or net carbohydrate is the total carbohydrate minus the amount of fiber in a food). Each unit of carbohydrate should be eaten with a unit of protein, so if you eat 30 grams of carbohydrate at a meal, such as two slices of stone ground whole grain bread for a sandwich, you need

---

[17] Interestingly, white sugar falls in the intermediate range with a GI of 68. This is because each sucrose molecule is made of two monosaccharides, one glucose and one fructose. The fructose must be processed into glucose by the liver, thus slowing the release of glucose from that half of the sucrose molecule into the bloodstream.

[18] Hart, Cheryle R., MD and Mary Kay Grossman, RD, *The Insulin Resistance Diet,* (New York: McGraw-Hill, 2001, 2007), 64.

[19] Sears, Barry, PhD, *Mastering the Zone,* (New York, Regan Books, 1997), 30-35, 331.

[20] Hart, Cheryle R., MD and Mary Kay Grossman, RD, *The Insulin Resistance Diet,* (New York: McGraw-Hill, 2001, 2007), 92.

to balance it with two protein units, or 14 grams of protein, which is found in about two ounces of meat or cheese. However, more protein can be eaten at the same meal to satisfy hunger plus as many vegetables as you want, excluding corn, potatoes and a few exotic vegetables which are dense sources of carbohydrates. (See the list of these starchy vegetables on page 79). This system eliminates spikes in blood sugar and insulin and results in consistently lower and more stable insulin levels. Low and stable insulin levels, through the action of the enzyme triglyceride lipase, tell you body, "Go ahead and burn fat."

Hunger and fasting (as in skipping breakfast) are taboo on a healthy eating plan designed to control your blood sugar and insulin levels. They raise insulin levels which says to your body, "Blood sugar is low and falling. We're living in a land of famine. Hold on to that fat!" The stress of hunger and low blood sugar causes the secretion of cortisol and adrenaline (epinephrine) by the adrenal glands, which causes the breakdown of glycogen into glucose. This causes the blood sugar to rise and stimulates the release of more insulin. High insulin inhibits the burning of fat. If you fail to eat before your glycogen stores are depleted, muscle will be used for fuel rather than fat. Less muscle mass lowers your metabolic rate, making it harder to lose weight. The moral of this is that hunger, along with being unpleasant, really does not help you become healthier or reduce body fat while retaining muscle. Any weight loss achieved with excessive or prolonged hunger is an unhealthy reduction in pounds only and often reflects loss in muscle mass. When you are hungry, a small snack of a few nuts or a little protein and carbohydrate combined will stop this hormonal cascade and allow you to burn fat more efficiently than if you did not have the snack. This is one of the reasons why calorie-counting diets which forbid snacks between meals work poorly.

The way of eating described above – balancing carbohydrate with protein and never allowing hunger to continue for long – is probably a much easier and more pleasant way to lose weight than what you have done in the past. Maybe, in the calorie math mentality, your current habit is no breakfast, no snacks, and lots of exercise leading to minimal weight loss. Why not give this healthy eating plan a try? More specifics about how to implement it are found on pages 71 to 83. A more complete explanation of the physiology involved is found on pages 36 to 46.

INFLAMMATION IS PART OF THE PROBLEM

You may be thinking, "I don't have any major problems with inflammation," and start to turn this page. Read a few paragraphs of this chapter and then decide whether it applies to you.

Sometimes inflammation is obvious – it causes redness, warmth, and/or pain. However, chronic inflammation can be silent. If you are overweight, you may not know it, but you are experiencing silent inflammation. As we gain weight, our bodies do not add more fat cells. The fat cells we already have become larger and are filled with more fat instead. They may leak as they are stretched more and more. Then immune cells called macrophages come in to clean up the mess. The macrophages release inflammatory chemicals in the fatty tissues as they are cleaning up.[1] This inflammatory response may be the mechanism behind many of the negative effects of overweight on health.

Your body counteracts this silent inflammation by producing anti-inflammatory chemicals. Some of these interfere with the function of the hormone leptin. In optimally healthy people, leptin is responsible for automatically maintaining weight at the right level.[2] Some people do not gain weight no matter what they eat. If they overeat, their well-functioning leptin control system boosts their metabolism and decreases their appetite to restore them to their best weight. When leptin is made ineffective by inflammation, the dysfunction is called leptin resistance, meaning that even though you have normal or high[3] levels of leptin your leptin does not work to suppress appetite and speed metabolism, thus maintaining a healthy weight.

This may sound like a depressing vicious cycle. Excess fat leads to inflammation and the chemicals that counteract inflammation (which are necessary to keep silent inflammation from causing symptoms) make it impossible for the body's weight-control hormone, leptin, to function properly. Don't despair though – there is a way to break this vicious cycle. There is also good news: As you slim down, leptin resistance abates and when you reach a healthy weight on the correct eating plan for you, you won't have to struggle to maintain a healthy weight. Your newly-functional leptin system will control your appetite and weight.

So how do we reduce inflammation? A very important way is to control the type of fat we consume. Prostaglandins and other eicosanoids are made from the fats we eat. Some of prostaglandins promote inflammation and some reduce it. (These anti-inflammatory prostaglandins are not the anti-inflammatory substances responsible for

---

[1] Galland, Leo, MD, *The Fat Resistance Diet,* (New York: Broadway Books, 2005), 33.

[2] Ibid., 32-33.

[3] Leptin levels are usually high among those who are overweight.

leptin resistance). The essential omega-3 fatty acids eicosapentaenoic acid (EPA) and docosahexaenoic acid (DHA) tip the balance toward the production of anti-inflammatory prostaglandins. Although optimally healthy people can make EPA and DHA from other omega-3 fatty acids, those with allergies often lack this ability so must get the EPA and DHA they need pre-formed. The best dietary source of these fatty acids is fatty fish. Most people need more omega-3 fatty acids than they can consume easily by eating fish so benefit from fish oil or krill[4] oil supplementation. How much fish oil you need is an individual matter; also various authorities disagree on the amount.[5] See page 57 for more about omega-3 supplementation.

Some foods also have anti-inflammatory properties because they contain powerful bioflavanoids and carotenoids.[6] These foods include ginger and related spices, cherries, blueberries, other dark berries, pomegranates, and some other fruits, vegetables, and seasonings. See pages 262 to 264 for a list of these foods. You can add them to your diet in generous amounts to control inflammation. The recipes in this book will help you add them in delicious ways.

Another and probably the most essential way to reduce inflammation is to reduce insulin levels. In *The Anti-Inflammatory Zone,* Barry Sears, PhD describes his work with members of the Stanford University swim team during one summer and how he improved their stamina and performance by giving them EPA and another fatty acid, gamma-linolenic acid (GLA) in individualized regimens. (GLA is another fatty acid important to the proper balance of eicosanoids). However, when the school year started, their performance deteriorated and they became easily fatigued. Dr. Sears began to suspect that the cause was their diets and that high-carbohydrate dormitory food was raising their insulin levels. Library research confirmed his suspicion when he found a study which demonstrated that high insulin activates an enzyme that increases the production of pro-inflammatory eicosanoids. He had the swimmers change their diets and their performance improved. His conclusion was that following an eating plan which controls blood sugar and insulin levels results in the balance of eicosanoids being more anti-inflammatory, resulting in less silent inflammation.[7] Although the goal of the swimmers was not weight loss, his findings apply to those who wish to lose because when silent inflammation decreases, leptin becomes more active, and we lose weight more easily.

---

[4] If you are allergic to shellfish, do not take krill oil. It comes from tiny marine crustaceans.

[5] Dr. Leo Galland recommends 2 grams per day with more to be taken only under a doctor's supervision. The most significant problem that can be associated with excessive omega-3 supplementation is bleeding. (Galland, Leo, MD, *The Fat Resistance Diet,* (New York: Broadway Books, 2005), 102). Barry Sears, PhD of the *Zone Diet* books recommends 5 grams per day for people who are overweight, 7.5 gram per day for those with arthritis, and 10 grams per day for people with neurological conditions. (Sears, Barry, PhD, *The Anti-Inflammation Zone,* (New York, Regan Books, 2005), 81).

[6] Galland, Leo, MD, *The Fat Resistance Diet,* (New York: Broadway Books, 2005), 92-94.

[7] Sears, Barry, PhD, *The Anti-Inflammation Zone,* (New York, Regan Books, 2005), 215-216

Many readers of this book have inflammation that is not silent. You have allergic reactions, asthma, arthritis, inflammatory bowel disease, etc. Following a healthy eating plan for glycemic control, taking fish oil in the correct dose for you, and adding anti-inflammatory foods to your diet will help your inflammation. Dr. Galland writes about putting patients on diets designed to reduce inflammation and "those who were overweight began losing weight without even trying" as they saw their asthma, arthritis, or other inflammatory conditions improve.[8]

Therefore, your healthy eating plan should include three tools to improve your health through controlling inflammation: eating in a way that eliminates blood sugar and insulin spikes and maintains insulin at a relatively constant low level; consuming enough omega-3 fatty acids; and the inclusion of a generous amount of anti-inflammatory foods in what you eat. If you eat this way to lose weight, your inflammatory health problems may improve, and if you do it to control inflammation, your weight should normalize. An additional benefit will be the reduction of your level of cortisol, the inflammation dampening adrenal hormone. This may reduce anxiety and depression and lead to better sleep because excess cortisol depletes brain chemicals such at the neurotransmitter serotonin.[9] The antidepressant drugs you see advertised on television are designed to have the same effect of raising serotonin levels, but they can have serious side effects. Rather than helping you make more serotonin, they just inhibit its uptake, and any fluctuation in medication dosage, etc. can cause imbalances in the brain's serotonin level which may lead to dangerously erratic behavior.

You have much to gain from an eating plan that controls blood sugar levels and inflammation: easier weight loss, improvement in inflammatory health conditions, better sleep, and relief from anxiety and depression caused by imbalances in brain neurotransmitters. (This healthy eating plan won't make you ignore a *real* problem or do something out-of-character though!) With all of this to gain, why not give it a try? Read on to discover how controlling your hormones can control hunger, which is a major reason most weight loss diets fail to produce permanent results. With an eating plan that avoids hunger, you can do it! You can slim down without the struggle and distress you may have experienced while trying to lose weight in the past.

---

[8] Galland, Leo, MD, *The Fat Resistance Diet,* (New York: Broadway Books, 2005), 32.

[9] Beale, Lucy and Joan Clark, RD, CDE, *The Complete Idiot's Guide to Glycemic Index Weight Loss,* (New York: Alpha, 2005), 23, 27.

CONTROL YOUR HORMONES TO CONTROL YOUR HUNGER, WEIGHT AND INFLAMMATION

Hormones rule when it comes to weight loss, and the various players on the "hormone team" are interdependent and influence each other. Although there are differences of opinion about which hormone(s) are most important for controlling weight, in reality, they all are important and they all influence each other and work together to determine the final outcome. To control our weight, we must bring all of our hormones into balance. The question is, how do we control our hormones?

INSULIN

Insulin can be managed by controlling the factors that stimulate its release, such as the rate and amount of glucose entering the bloodstream from the small intestine after a meal or snack. This is determined by how much carbohydrate is eaten, its GI score, and what it is eaten with. In *The Insulin Resistance Diet,* Dr. Cheryle Hart recommends that the amount of carbohydrate in a meal or snack be kept to 30 grams for most people. However, she says that a few people may need a lower carbohydrate limit per meal or snack.[1] (See pages 90 to 91 for more about this individual variation and indications that you should try decreasing the amount).

How rapidly the glucose from that carbohydrate appears in the bloodstream is just as crucial as how much is eaten. If you eat low GI carbohydrates with protein and/or fat, the rate of rise in your blood sugar will be slow and steady. In a Canadian study,[2] for six day periods (at different times separated by an "off" period) volunteers ate either (1) a glycemic control diet containing low GI carbohydrates balanced with protein and enough food to satisfy them, (2) a standard low-fat American Heart Association (AHA) recommended diet with the amount of food sufficient to be satisfied, or (3) an AHA diet with the caloric intake limited to the same as that eaten on the glycemic control diet. On the sixth day of each type of diet in the study the researchers measured blood sugar,

---

[1] Individuals who may need less carbohydrate will not notice improvement in energy level or hunger on a link-and-balance eating plan that contains the higher level of carbohydrate. Hart, Cheryle R., MD and Mary Kay Grossman, RD, *The Insulin Resistance Diet,* (New York: McGraw-Hill, 2001, 2007), 221-111.

[2] www.montignac.com/en/etude_scient_sur_meth_mont.php

insulin, triglycerides, and weight loss for all subjects. The results showed that subjects who ate the glycemic control diet had significantly lower blood sugar, insulin, triglyceride and cholesterol levels than the other subjects and lost an average of 2.4 pounds in six days. The subjects who ate an AHA diet with enough food to satisfy hunger ate about one-third more calories than the subjects on the glycemic control diet. During the 6-day test period they had the highest blood sugar and insulin levels, a 28% increase in triglycerides, a 10% decrease in HDL ("good") cholesterol, and they gained an average of 0.2 pounds. The subjects on the calorie restricted AHA diet had intermediate blood sugar and insulin levels, no significant change in their blood fats over the course of the 6-day test period, and they lost an average of 1.7 pounds.

The most impressive results of this study were in the blood sugar and insulin levels of the participants on the glycemic control diet during the course of the sixth and last day of the diet. Their blood sugar was measured every hour from 8 a.m. to 8 p.m. While there was a major rise in blood sugar and insulin after breakfast, their blood sugar and insulin levels were fairly stable for the rest of the day including after lunch and dinner.

On the eating plan recommended in this book each 15 grams of carbohydrate is balanced with 7 grams of protein. Blood sugar levels are kept on an even keel and insulin levels are kept steady and low by eating frequently, about every two to three hours. A breakfast containing both carbohydrate and protein should be eaten within an hour of getting up. Mid-morning, mid-afternoon, and evening snacks are recommended. A protein-containing evening snack prevents blood sugar from falling too low during sleep. This produces sounder sleep and prevents adrenal hormones from kicking in to raise low blood sugar levels in the middle of the night which can lead to a spike in insulin levels.

Hunger is a signal that your blood sugar level is falling low. If you get hungry and it has been two hours since a meal or snack, have a small protein and carbohydrate containing snack. This prevents your adrenal hormones from signaling your liver to produce glucose from stored glycogen and this surge of glucose released from your liver from causing a corresponding increase in your insulin level. As you become accustomed to listening to your body, you will be able to differentiate physical hunger from boredom, appetite (stimulated by a TV commercial perhaps) or thirst. Thirst can be perceived as hunger, so staying well hydrated is important. If it has been less than two hours since you ate, have a drink of water to see if you might be mistaking thirst for hunger. If you still feel hungry, your blood sugar and insulin levels may be fluctuating because of stress or having eaten carbohydrates too high on the glycemic index or in too large a quantity at your last meal. In that case, a protein-containing snack is what you need to help stabilize your blood sugar and insulin levels. If it has been less than two hours since your last snack or meal, do not eat more carbohydrate.

FLIP YOUR FAT SWITCH FROM STORE TO BURN

As you will recall from the "Principles of Glycemic Control Weight Loss" chapter, high levels of insulin activate the enzyme lipoprotein lipase which takes fatty acids from the blood and stores them as triglycerides in fat cells. Therefore, by preventing insulin spikes, you avoid storing recently eaten fat and leave it in your bloodstream to be used for energy.

Low blood insulin levels allow the enzyme triglyceride lipase to be active. This enzyme promotes the breakdown of the triglycerides stored in fat cells and liberates the fatty acids from them into the bloodstream to be used for fuel. Thus, by keeping your insulin levels stable and low, **you can flip your fat control switch from "store" to "burn."**[3] So the most effective way to tell your body to use your fat reserves for energy is to control your insulin levels by controlling the amount and glycemic index level of the carbohydrates that you eat and by balancing carbohydrates with protein.

OTHER FACTORS THAT INFLUENCE INSULIN LEVELS

Certain foods and supplements can affect your insulin levels in either beneficial or detrimental ways.[4] The mineral chromium is probably the most important nutrient that influences insulin. Chromium promotes stable insulin levels and helps your insulin function efficiently. A supplemental intake of 200 to 400 mcg of chromium is often recommended for diabetics and those who want to lose weight. In *The Insulin Resistance Diet*, Dr. Cheryle Hart reports that diabetics and those with insulin resistance are often deficient in chromium. She recommends 200 to 400 mcg per day of chromium taken in the chromium polynicotinate form (called Chromate™), especially for her patients who struggle with sugar cravings[5] Doses higher than 400 mcg per day should probably be used only under a doctor's care.

In recent years, vitamin D deficiency has become prevalent among Americans. Studies have shown that improving the vitamin D level of people who are deficient and also

---

[3] Stevenson, E.J., N. Astbury, E. Simpson, M. Taylor, I. Macdonald, "Fat Oxidation During Exercise and Satiety During Recovery Are Increased Following a Low-Glycemic Index Breakfast in Sedentary Women," *Journal of Nutrition*, May 2009, 139(5):890-7. In a 2009 study of sedentary women in the UK, the participants consumed either a low-GI breakfast or a high-GI breakfast. Three hours later they participated in one hour of walking exercise. Fat breakdown was higher both before and during exercise among the women who ate the low-GI breakfast. You can see the abstract of this article at www.ncbi.nlm. nih.gov/pubmed/19321590?itool=EntrezSystem2.PEntrez.Pubmed.Pubmed_ResultsPanel.Pubmed_ RVDocSum&ordinalpos=5 .

[4] Please consult your healthcare provider before taking supplements or making changes in your sun exposure as described in the next paragraph.

[5] Hart, Cheryle R., MD and Mary Kay Grossman, RD, *The Insulin Resistance Diet,* (New York: McGraw-Hill, 2001, 2007), 94.

have insulin resistance improves their insulin resistance. In one such study the optimal blood level of vitamin D for improved insulin resistance was 80 to 119 nmol/l, which is higher than the current recommended level, possibly indicating that the optimal blood level of vitamin D figures should be revised.[6] Because those of us with celiac disease or food allergies often have sub-optimal intestinal absorption, consider bypassing your intestine and getting some of your vitamin D the old fashioned way, from the sun.[4] Sunlight causes vitamin D precursors to be converted to active vitamin D3 in the skin. Recommendations that we wear sunscreen at all times when we are outdoors may be partly responsible for the current state of our vitamin D levels, as well as spending too much time in front of televisions and computers rather than outside in the sun. You know how readily your skin burns; only wear sunscreen if you are very fair-skinned and prone to burn, and then put it on after you have been outside for at least 20 minutes with legs and arms exposed. If you rarely burn and are not in intense sun situations (such as boating or other water exposure) and will not be outdoors for a long time, you might consider skipping the sunscreen entirely unless you have been advised otherwise by your doctor. In addition to improving insulin resistance, adequate vitamin D levels can help prevent heart attacks and some forms of cancer and even reduce blood pressure.

Studies have shown that cinnamon may improve insulin resistance by affecting the insulin receptors on cells to promote the uptake of glucose from the bloodstream.[7] In addition to its effect on insulin resistance, cinnamon also exerts an anti-inflammatory effect by inhibiting the release of arachidonic acid from platelets and thus reducing the formation of an inflammatory messaging molecule called thromboxane A2.[8] Cinnamon supplements are widely available. However, since this spice enhances the flavor of food, in the interest of pleasure and economy you may want to use it as a food instead of a supplement. The amount of cinnamon effective for the longest time in the studies was ¼ teaspoon; higher doses had a greater effect but the effect was more transient. The recommended amount of cinnamon to consume per day is ¼ to ½ teaspoon on or in your food. Cinnamon may come from a variety of sources. If it is labeled Saigon cinnamon, it is the very flavorful cassia variety. Most supermarket cinnamon is cassia cinnamon. Ceylon (true) cinnamon has a sweeter and more mellow flavor. Both varieties are reported to have a beneficial effect on insulin control. The Ceylon cinnamon is lower in natural anticoagulants, which may make it a better choice for those taking anticoagulant drugs. However, most of the studies were done using cassia cinnamon because it is more common. If you want to use cinnamon that comes from a known source (cassia versus

[6] Von Hurst P.R., W. Stonehouse, and J. Coad, "Vitamin D Supplementation Reduces Insulin Resistance – a Randomized Placebo-Controlled Trial," *British Journal of Nutrition,* 28(2009), 1-7.

[7] A list of these studies can be found at www.whfoods.com/genpage.php?tname=foodspice&dbid=68 and http://lowcarbdiets.about.com/od/nutrition/a/cinnamonbenefit.htm .

[8] Solomon T.P., and A. Blannin, "Changes in glucose tolerance and insulin sensitivity following 2 weeks of daily cinnamon ingestion in healthy humans," *European Journal of Applied Physiology,* (April 2009)105(6):969-76.

Ceylon) or just to have the most delicious cinnamon you've ever tasted, try Penzey's cinnamon. (See "Sources," page 282).

Other substances may influence your insulin level and its stability in a negative way. Most of the glucose control diets ban alcohol, saying that it acts like a rapidly absorbed (high glycemic index) carbohydrate in the body and may stimulate the appetite.[9] (A few, but not all alcoholic drinks contain carbohydrate). However, in *The Anti-Inflammatory Zone,* Barry Sears, Ph.D. recommends alcohol, especially a daily glass of red wine, as a means of promoting the synthesis of anti-inflammatory eicosanoids.[10] If you do indulge in alcohol, have it in moderation with protein-containing food rather than on an empty stomach (always a good idea), and listen to your body's reaction to it. If you are excessively hungry in a couple of hours or the next day, it may have destabilized your blood sugar and insulin levels. Beer has a GI of up to 110[11] (higher than pure glucose) so is best reserved for an occasional treat. If you indulge in alcohol regularly, it may be wise to stick to Dr. Sears' recommendation of wine which contains practically no carbohydrate.

Caffeine, nicotine, and possibly artificial sweeteners[12] can raise insulin levels. If taken without food, this rise in insulin will cause your blood sugar level to fall, which may lead to the release of adrenal hormones causing the breakdown of stored glycogen into glucose, and this rising glucose level can cause the secretion of more insulin. To avoid this roller coaster effect, use caffeine, nicotine, or artificial sweeteners with food and in moderation. Some of us cannot live without our morning coffee or a diet soda, and if not having them deters you from trying this type of healthy eating plan, or if you struggle to stay on your eating plan without them, by all means, go ahead and have them. However, always have them with food[13] to keep your blood sugar level from major fluctuations and listen to your body's reaction to them. For more about caffeine and artificial sweeteners, see pages 66 to 69.

---

[9] Beale, Lucy and Joan Clark, RD, CDE, *The Complete Idiot's Guide to Glycemic Index Weight Loss,* (New York: Alpha, 2005), 62.

[10] Sears, Barry, PhD, *The Anti-Inflammation Zone,* (New York, Regan Books, 2005), 90-91. Dr. Sears recommends that you have 1 ounce of cheese or four jumbo shrimp or chicken wings with each alcoholic drink.

[11] www.montignac.com/en/ig_tableau.php . The GI score of beer is lower in other tables.

[12] In their 2007 edition of *The Insulin Resistance Diet,* Dr. Cheryl Hart, MD and her co-author Mary Kay Grossman, RD say that diet sodas should always be consumed with food to prevent this hormonal roller coaster effect. However, in a 2010 download from their website (irdiet.com) Ms. Grossman says that patients may have diet sodas without linking them with a protein food. I feel that one's tolerance for diet sodas is an individual matter, and possibly that the download, *Foods by Chance or by Choice,* may not be an ideal dietary guide for those on food allergy and gluten-free diets. The intersection of the preferred foods in this document and what we can eat on restricted diets might leave us with little to eat. Also, they stress portion sizes and the restriction of fat and calories in the download without a major emphasis on the principles of hormonal control and listening to your body.

[13] Some people may "get away with" diet sodas without food. Monitor your progress if you try this, and if this eating plan is not working well, try going without the sodas.

ADRENAL HORMONES SUCH AS CORTISOL AND ADRENALINE

The adrenal glands secrete hormones such as adrenaline (epinephrine) and cortisol when you experience stress. This hormonal effect happens with both positive and negative types of stress and other stimuli such as:

A sudden fright such as a narrow escape from an automobile accident

Chronic low-grade stress such as feeling that you are in an impossible situation or have too many demands on your time

An exciting, happy surprise

Lack of sleep

An allergic reaction or

Exercise that is too intense or prolonged.

We also have a normal daily cycle of cortisol secretion. Some people are genetically predisposed towards secreting excess cortisol, and if overweight, they will usually have an apple-shaped body.

When adrenaline (epinephrine) is secreted in response to stress, the body breaks glycogen stored in the liver down into glucose which is released into the bloodstream. Insulin is secreted to drive this glucose into your cells to be used for energy. If you have to run away from a wild animal, you will use that glucose to give you the energy for running. However, if your stress does not involve physical activity, the glucose may be stored as fat. This is the chemical explanation of why it is nearly impossible for some people to lose or even maintain their weight during stressful times even if they do not overeat.

High levels of cortisol, which is secreted with adrenaline in response to stress, direct your cells to stop taking sugar up from the blood, in essence causing temporary insulin resistance. The resulting high blood sugar levels promote the release of more insulin which, by its action on various enzymes (see page 27 for more about this), can lead to the storage of fat.[14] This is another mechanism by which stress causes weight gain. Even if you don't succumb to comfort foods when you are stressed, this is why you may gain weight at stressful times in spite of healthy eating.

How can we control our cortisol and adrenaline levels? The most obvious way is to avoid stress, but this is often easier said than done with our hectic lifestyles. However, relaxation is important and can help you control your hormones. Try relaxation exercises, massage, warm baths or showers, soothing music, relaxing activities such as hobbies and crafts (I find the repetitive motion of knitting calming), prayer and meditation, and cultivating and maintaining a positive attitude to reduce the effects of stress.

---

[14] Hart, Cheryle R., MD and Mary Kay Grossman, RD, *The Insulin Resistance Diet,* (New York: McGraw-Hill, 2001, 2007), 5.

A very significant way to lower cortisol levels is to get adequate sleep. Studies have shown that people who regularly sleep less than 5 hours per night are more likely to be obese. This is probably due to lower levels of leptin and higher levels of the hormone ghrehlin which stimulates the appetite.[15]

Moderate exercise is a good way to relax and thus reduce cortisol production by removing your mind from troubling situations and relieving stress physically. It releases endorphins in the brain[16] and gives you a chance to do something nurturing for yourself. Moderate exercise also decreases inflammation, thus decreasing leptin resistance.[17] (See the next few pages for more about leptin resistance). It is also an excellent way burn fat, so if you garden, you can lose fat while decreasing stress in two ways at once – by participating in an enjoyable hobby and by getting moderate exercise. See the exercise appendix on pages 265 to 268 for more about moderate exercise as a fat-burner and how to differentiate it from more strenuous aerobic exercise.

Excessive exercise or exercise without food can actually be stressful and increase cortisol production, thus undermining efforts to reduce body fat. This is counter-intuitive to the "calories in with food, fat out with exercise" diet model you may have been living by, but nevertheless, it is true. When you engage in strenuous exercise before breakfast or after work but before dinner (or at least a good snack), your body pumps out adrenal hormones to cause the breakdown of glycogen in the liver so you have sufficient fuel for your exercise.[18] A release of insulin follows, which can, if excessive, results in fat storage. Prolonged strenuous exercise causes the same hormonal responses as exercise without food. After your glycogen stores are used up, fat is not mobilized to be burned for energy, but rather muscle mass is broken down for fuel. Since muscle has a higher metabolic rate than fat, if you lose muscle mass due to over-exercise, your overall resting metabolic rate will decrease, making it more difficult to lose weight.

Along with this to-do list of relaxation, sleep and moderate exercise, there are also things you should avoid in order to control your cortisol level. Avoid foods to which you are allergic. Our bodies cope with allergic reactions by secreting adrenal hormones, so avoid anything that causes you allergy problems. Cortisone-type medications also make weight loss extremely difficult and should be avoided if possible.

The glycemic-control diet books I consulted give varying advice about other foods and beverages which may increase your cortisol levels and about how strict you need to be in avoiding them. All restrict high glycemic index starches and sugars to varying

[15] Galland, Leo, MD, *The Fat Resistance Diet,* (New York: Broadway Books, 2005), 136.

[16] Hart, Cheryle R., MD and Mary Kay Grossman, RD, *The Insulin Resistance Diet,* (New York: McGraw-Hill, 2001, 2007), 189.

[17] Galland, Leo, MD, *The Fat Resistance Diet,* (New York: Broadway Books, 2005), 122.

[18] This is why exercise made me feel less hungry in the story on page 12 about using a low-calorie diet. Exercise without food was boosting my adrenal hormones and burning muscle mass and was, ironically, a part of why I could not lose weight. See page 267 for more about exercise done without food.

degrees and recommend keeping the total amount of carbohydrate eaten at one time to a moderate level. Caffeine can also be an adrenal stimulant, so all advised using caffeinated beverages with food and in moderation as described on pages 66 to 67. However, because green tea is low in caffeine and very potently anti-inflammatory, in *The Fat Resistance Diet,* Dr. Leo Galland recommends drinking green tea with chai spices (which are also anti-inflammatory) several times a day with a meal or snack.

A final way to moderate cortisol levels is with supplements. Relora™, which is an extract of magnolia bark and philodendron, was recommended by a holistic M.D. whom I feel successfully combines conventional and alternative medical approaches. I'm certain he was thinking of the cortisol connection to apple-shaped bodies when he recommended it because that body type is a visible indicator of the overproduction of cortisol. In addition to Relora™, *The Complete Idiot's Guide to Glycemic Index Weight Loss* recommends other cortisol-moderating supplements such as theanine (from green tea), the herb epimedium, and phytosterols.[19] For more about supplements for weight loss, see pages 90.

LEPTIN

Although insulin is the central player when it comes to weight loss and controlling and stabilizing insulin levels is the key to flipping your fat switch from "store" to "burn," leptin is probably the master hormone for long-term weight control. Leptin resistance (a state of having plenty of leptin but the body does not respond to its signal) may be the reason that maintaining weight loss is sometimes so difficult. Very low carbohydrate diets and the yo-yo dieting that tends to occur with attempts to lose weight by counting calories have both been found to increase leptin resistance.[20]

In an optimally healthy person, the body's fat regulates itself. When weight is gained, the fat produces leptin which suppresses appetite and increases resting metabolic rate, thus causing automatic weight loss.[21] When President Obama said in a television news interview that his weight had only fluctuated within a 5-pound range for years, this indicated that he has a properly functioning leptin control system.

Overweight people have abundant leptin being produced by their body fat, but their body does not respond to it as the president's body does. (But think of it this way – you aren't expected to solve all the problems of the country and the world either!) According to Dr. Galland, this insensitivity of the body's cells to the signals of the leptin, or leptin resistance, is caused by inflammation and excessive levels of cortisol and other anti-in-

---

[19] Beale, Lucy and Joan Clark, RD, CDE, *The Complete Idiot's Guide to Glycemic Index Weight Loss,* (New York: Alpha, 2005), 228-229.

[20] Galland, Leo, MD, *The Fat Resistance Diet,* (New York: Broadway Books, 2005), 71.

[21] "Leptin," *Vitamin Research News,* 24:2 (February 2010), 1-5.

flammatory substances our bodies make in response to inflammation.[22] This is how the anti-inflammatory foods which are the core of Dr. Galland's diet in *The Fat Resistance Diet* decrease leptin resistance and promote weight loss. See pages 262 to 264 for a list of these foods.

Along with other factors, inflammation is controlled by pro-inflammatory and anti-inflammatory **PROSTAGLANDINS** (one class of Barry Sears' favorite eicosanoids). The balance of pro-inflammatory to anti-inflammatory prostaglandins which we produce is determined by the types of fats we eat as well as by our state of insulin control. By consuming omega-3 fatty acids in the form our body uses best (such as EPA and DHA which are found in fish oil[23]) and moderate amounts of healthy polyunsaturated and monounsaturated fats, as well as by controlling insulin surges, this balance can be shifted to tone down chronic inflammation. Other foods, such as those listed on pages 262 to 264, also have anti-inflammatory effects. Including these foods in your diet regularly and generously can help reverse leptin resistance. In addition, your level of inflammation will be automatically be reduced as you lose weight, because your fat cells will become smaller and less leaky. (See page 33 for more about this). When you reach a healthy weight, you may find that you have a self-regulating leptin system such as President Obama has.

ADIPONECTIN is another hormone produced by our body fat. It reduces inflammation, increases insulin sensitivity, prevents high blood pressure, and helps us burn fat for energy. However, unlike leptin, as the body fat amount increases, the amount of adiponectin produced decreases.[24] There is an easy and tasty way to boost its level though – by eating foods high in anthocyanins. These are pigments found in deep red, blue, and purple foods such as dark cherries, blackberries, raspberries, blueberries, and pomegranates.[25] (For more about how these and other superfoods reduce inflammation, see pages 262). As you lose weight and your percentage of body fat decreases, your adiponectin level will rise, helping you to lose more weight and maintain the loss more easily than before. Eventually this should result in a self-regulating healthy weight.

---

[22] Galland, Leo, MD, *The Fat Resistance Diet,* (New York: Broadway Books, 2005), 27.

[23] Do not consume any food or supplement that you are allergic to, even fish oil. An allergy to the fish it is derived from can make fish oil pro-inflammatory for you. However, fish oil comes from a variety of species, so hopefully you can find a hypoallergenic source that you can tolerate. If you tolerate shellfish, krill oil, which comes from small marine crustaceans, is also a high EPA and DHA supplement.

[24] Galland, Leo, MD, *The Fat Resistance Diet,* (New York: Broadway Books, 2005), 29.

[25] Ibid., 8.

BRAIN NEUROTRANSMITTERS

Comfort foods, which are usually high in carbohydrates, encourage the production of brain chemicals such as serotonin[26] and endorphins. These chemicals make us feel calmer and better mentally, which is why we crave comfort foods when things are not going well for us. Barry Sears suggests that rather than resorting to comfort foods, one should double his daily dose of fish oil instead.[27] This is definitely an approach that I do not find myself inclined to follow when I am distressed! So if you succumb to comfort foods, you're normal. Just pick yourself up without self-recrimination and return to your healthy eating plan with your next meal. Indeed, after you've been eating healthily for a while, you may feel less well a few hours after eating more carbohydrates than usual, although you probably felt comforted mentally very quickly. This may help motivate you to control quantities the next time you need comfort foods. If you plan ahead for a controlled carbohydrate splurge when things are not going well, such as the one or two ounces of chocolate as discussed on pages 64 to 65 (only if you are not allergic to chocolate) or a hypoallergenic treat kept in your freezer for this purpose, this may satisfy your need for comfort without eating a very large amount of carbohydrate.

In *The Complete Idiot's Guide Glycemic Index Cookbook,* authors Lucy Beale and Joan Clark, RD, advise, "If a taste of chocolate within your allowed carbohydrate levels is more soothing than enervating, go ahead and luxuriate in its taste." They also include a chapter of chocolate dessert recipes.[28] Dr. Hart promotes chocolate for its positive effect on neurotransmitters.[29] Again, it is an individual matter. Some people may react adversely to the caffeine in the chocolate or to that amount of sugar. (If the sugar is the problem, see the recipe for stevia-sweetened chocolate on page 198). If you are allergic to chocolate, avoid it, or it will stimulate a cortisol response due to the allergic reaction that will destabilize your blood sugar. But for those who are non-allergic and non-caffeine-sensitive, you may be able to indulge in an occasional ounce or two of chocolate to help your neurotransmitter levels and balance your emotional need for pleasure with your physical needs. Listen to your body if you eat chocolate or drink anything containing caffeine, and take note of variations in your appetite and sleep patterns. For more about chocolate, see pages 64 to 65.

---

[26] Protein is essential to making the neurotransmitters serotonin and dopamine. For serotonin to be made, there must also be adequate carbohydrate consumed. Hart, Cheryle R., MD and Mary Kay Grossman, RD, *The Insulin Resistance Diet,* (New York: McGraw-Hill, 2001, 2007), 32.

[27] Sears, Barry, PhD, *The Anti-Inflammation Zone,* (New York, Regan Books, 2005), 141-142.

[28] Beale, Lucy and Joan Clark, MS, RD, CDE, *The Complete Idiot's Guide Glycemic Index Cookbook,* (New York: Alpha, 2009), 299.

[29] Hart, Cheryle R., MD and Mary Kay Grossman, RD, *The Insulin Resistance Diet,* (New York: McGraw-Hill, 2001, 2007), 107.

If you are allergic to chocolate, you need to be diligent about planning ahead for controlled splurges. Study the dessert and sweet snack recipes in this book, and select one or two that sound good. Make them and freeze most of what you made. It is important for you to keep some safe treats in your freezer at all times so you are prepared if the need for a controlled splurge arises. If you can't find a treat recipe that you can eat in this book, email us using the contact form on the www.food-allergy.org or www.foodallergyandglutenfreeweightloss.com websites. We may be able to suggest recipes from the books listed on the last few pages of this book or help you with a new recipe.

Moderate exercise also increases endorphin levels in the brain, and can be used as an alternative to comfort foods as a coping strategy. Have a nutritious snack before you exercise if you haven't eaten in a while to avoid the hormonal cascade described on page 42.

Another alternative to having high-carbohydrate food to increase your comfort level is to have a nutritious snack and treat yourself to some quiet time with relaxing music that you enjoy. Listening to music can increase endorphin levels in the brain. Go to the mall or go online and shop for a new CD by your favorite artist, or get two CDs and keep one in reserve for the next time you might be tempted by comfort foods.

A FINAL WORD

Make your hormones your allies. They will work for you more readily than against you if you know how to control them. With the information in this chapter, you CAN lose weight and gain control of inflammation. When you reach a healthy weight, your leptin resistance should decrease and your adiponectin increase so that your body fat is self-regulating. Your retrained palate and improved health will have taught you to appreciate "real" foods over processed foods most of the time. Thus, weight maintenance will not be the struggle it is now (assuming this is your first reading of this book). Your hormones will influence your appetite and metabolic rate, and your body will do most of the work of maintenance for you as you reach optimal health.

About Carbohydrates
Glycemic Index and Glycemic Load

All carbohydrates are not created equal. The same amount of carbohydrate from different foods can affect blood sugar and insulin levels very differently. This has been proven by glycemic index testing of thousands of carbohydrate-containing foods on human volunteers from many parts of the world. However, in the United States, information is sometimes controlled by a profit-oriented establishment, so we have been slow to accept the empirical proof that not all carbohydrates have the same effect on our bodies.

Because of this suppression of evidence, many conventional doctors believe untruths about carbohydrates and treat diabetics based on this misinformation. These doctors prescribe a standard diabetic exchange system diet for their diabetic patients, and conventional dieticians help the patients implement these diets. They define one exchange of a carbohydrate food as the amount of that food which contains approximately 15 grams of carbohydrate. For insulin-dependent diabetics, the number of carbohydrate exchanges in their diets is balanced with their insulin dosages. However, because the carbohydrate in an exchange of, for example, white rice has a greater and more rapid effect on blood sugar levels than the same amount of carbohydrate eaten in thick-rolled oats or stone ground whole wheat bread, the amount and timing of the patient's need for insulin differs. It's no wonder so many diabetics have difficulty maintaining stable blood sugar levels!

Another false assumption is that all complex carbohydrates such as starches are "good" and have a gradual impact on blood sugar levels, but simple carbohydrates such as sugars cause a higher blood sugar spike very rapidly. This also has been proven false by the reproducible testing of thousands of foods on human volunteers world-wide.

These assumptions were first challenged in the 1980s by Dr. David Jenkins at the University of Toronto in Canada. He measured the effects of a large number of foods on blood sugar levels of human volunteers. This testing became standardized and led to the development of the glycemic index, a system of scoring foods according to the effect they have on blood sugar levels of real people.

Glycemic index scores are based on the testing of pure glucose as a reference food. (However, some of the early testing used white bread as a reference food, which is obviously not as easy to standardize as pure glucose). For standard glycemic index testing, eight to ten volunteers are given a dose of 50 grams of pure glucose. Their blood is drawn and blood sugar levels are measured periodically over the next two hours. For each patient, these blood test results are plotted on a graph of blood sugar level versus time, and the area under the curve of the graph is calculated. The test is repeated on two or three occasions and the results are averaged. Then, at another time, the volunteers eat a portion of the test food which contains 50 grams of carbohydrate. For example, if bread is the test food, they will each eat about 3½ slices of bread. Their blood sugar levels are again tested over a two-hour period, plotted on a graph, and the area under the curve of the graph is calculated. This area is divided by that volunteer's average result when glucose was tested and the result of the division is multiplied by 100. The number obtained is the approximate glycemic index score (GI score or GI value) for the test food. This number is averaged with the result obtained for the other volunteers to calculate the GI score for the food tested. These GI tests for various foods have been shown to be reproducible in testing done in many countries around the world. The values obtained are reproducibly the same for both healthy volunteers and diabetics; however, diabetics have their blood drawn for a 3 hour period after the test meal rather than for two hours.

The GI score reflects what really happens to our blood sugar when we consume a certain food. The surprising thing is that some complex carbohydrates have a higher glycemic index scores than pure sugar. The GI score of a food cannot be predicted from whether it contains simple or complex carbohydrates or from the scores of foods in the same food category. (For example, fruits have a wide range of GI scores; grains have a similar wide range). In order to determine the glycemic index of a food, it must be tested[1] using real people. Based on these test results, foods are classified as being high GI if their score is 70 or higher, intermediate or medium if their score is 56 to 69, or low on the GI scale if their score is 55 or less.[2] Sandra Woodruff, MS, RD proposed a four-tier ranking for GI scores, which seems so sensible that I have used it in the tables on pages 250 to 261 of this book. She divides the "low" score range into very low if a food's score is 39 or less and low if it is between 40 and 55. Using her system of scoring, we can differentiate foods or recipes that are very good in their expected affect on blood sugar levels from those that are fantastic.[3]

---

[1] Testing is not needed for combination dishes or meals, such as a turkey sandwich; the GI can be calculated from the GI scores of the component ingredients and the amount of each used.

[2] Although most authorities use these ranges for low, intermediate and high GI scores, one internet source suggests that the ranges are based on political correctness rather than physiology and are motivated the desire to not alienate large food companies by declaring most of their products high GI. It defines the ranges as high if the score is above 50, intermediate in the 35 to 50 range and low if the score is below 35. (Foods with scores of less than 35 are called extra-low in the table in this book). This source is: www.montignac.com/en/ig_tableau_avertissement.php .

My suggestion is that you listen to your body rather about what foods are good for *you* as described on page 53 rather than being solely focused on the numbers. Your body, not the experts, knows what is best for you. The lower ranges may restrict your food choices more than is necessary. Limited choices are already a problem for those of use with food allergies, so if you feel you must use numbers, use the standard ranges.

[3] Woodruff, Sandra, MS, RD, *The Good Carb Cookbook: Secrets of Eating Low on the Glycemic Index,* (New York, Penguin Group, 2001), 8.

Foods are tested in the form in which they are eaten and many factors, such as cooking time and other ingredients included in the recipe, affect how rapidly the food is digested and absorbed. Therefore, how quickly and how much the food affects blood sugar levels depends on these factors. Because some foods such as flour are never eaten raw, without being combined and cooked with other ingredients, there are no published GI scores for these foods. For example, there are GI scores for many types of bread and cereal made with various flours, but no GI values for the flours themselves. One problem encountered in producing this book is the dearth of GI score data on foods made with grains other than wheat. (For more about how to get around this problem, see pages 52 to 53 at the end of this chapter). Because human testing data is needed to determine the GI of a food, the recipes in this book do not contain actual GI or GL (glycemic load) values. The principles of low-GI eating, such as using high-fiber ingredients that are not overly processed or over-cooked, using flours which come from grains that have low glycemic index scores in their whole-grain form, etc. are incorporated into the recipes, however.

One of the many factors that influences the glycemic index score of a food and determines the effect it has on our blood sugar and insulin levels is the foods that accompany it. Other foods that are eaten with the carbohydrate in a meal make a difference in how quickly the carbohydrate is digested and absorbed. For example, chocolate and high-fat ice cream have lower GI scores than white bread does because the fat they contain slows down their digestion and the absorption of the sugar they contain. This phenomenon allows us to occasionally enjoy these foods as a pleasure-boosting treat without destabilizing our blood sugar and insulin levels too much. To insure blood sugar stability, they are best eaten with a protein-containing meal or a protein food, however.

The amount and kind of fiber a food or meal contains affects the glycemic index of the food by slowing down the rate of digestion and absorption of the sugar or starch in the food. However, the fiber is not the only determining factor. The GI score is also dependent on the amount and type of processing the food has undergone. If the insoluble fiber coat of a grain is still intact (as in whole grain kernels), it adds considerably to the time and effort the body expends to digest the starch. Viscous soluble fiber in a grain such as oats forms a gel in the digestive system and slows down the rate of absorption. On the other hand, more highly processed oats, such as instant oatmeal, have a higher GI score than old-fashioned thick-rolled oatmeal.

The effect of insoluble fiber on the GI score of a food is very dependent on the processing. As mentioned above, a grain cooked whole with an intact fiber coat will have the lowest GI score of any way of eating that grain. If it is milled into very fine flour using metal rollers, the GI score will be high. The fiber will do very little to reduce the GI score of a food made with finely ground whole grain flour. For example, bread made from very finely ground whole wheat flour has about the same GI score as white bread. However, if bread is made from 100% stone-ground whole wheat flour, which is coarser flour, the GI score will be considerably lower than if it is made from refined white flour that has had the fiber removed or whole wheat flour that is finely ground.[4]

The acid level of a meal or food also influences its GI score.[5] Sourdough bread produces blood sugar and insulin levels that are 30% lower than other types of yeast bread because lactic and proprionic acids are produced by the sourdough fermentation process. Also, studies have show that a generous amount of vinegar in salad dressing (i.e. 4 teaspoons of vinegar with 2 teaspoons of oil) can lower the glycemic index value of a meal by 30%.[6] Lemon juice has a similar effect. If you do not wish to have a tangy salad with a meal, you may want to try the sugar-free lemonade recipe on page 231 instead. Acid foods lower the GI of a meal because the acid slows the rate at which food passes from the stomach and begins to be absorbed in the small intestine.

For starch-containing foods, the type of starch and physical state of the starch profoundly affect the GI score of the food. Starchy foods that contain mostly the starch amylose are slowly digested because amylose is composed of long chains of glucose molecules. These long chains line up to form a solid grid, which makes less of the glucose molecules open to digestion at one time. Starchy foods containing mostly amylopectin are digested more rapidly because short chains of a few glucose molecules branch off from the starch in many places. This leaves a large part of the starch open to contact with digestive enzymes, resulting in fast digestion and absorption of the glucose. Jasmine rice contains mostly amylopectin and is one of the few foods that has a higher GI score than pure glucose. The only grains with a high GI score in their whole grain form are some varieties of rice, including jasmine rice.[7]

The physical state of the starch in a food also greatly affects its GI value. If the particle size in the food is small, such as in finely milled flour, it is easy for digestive enzymes and water to penetrate the food, and it will be quickly digested. If the starch is cooked or prepared in a way that allows it to absorb a lot of water, it will be more "gelatinized" (basically wet and soluble all the way through) thus resulting in quick digestion. Pasta which is cooked briefly to be *al dente* (giving resistance to the bite) rather than being cooked to mushiness has a lower GI score than overcooked pasta.

Table sugar refined from sugar cane or beets (sucrose) has a GI score of 60 which is in the medium range. This surprises us because sugar is supposed to be THE "bad" food! It has a medium score because each sucrose molecule is composed of two simple sugars, glucose and fructose. Digestion breaks the two molecules apart and the glucose

---

[4] Brand-Miller, Jennie, PhD, Thomas Wolever, MD, Kay Foster-Powell. MND, and Stephen Colaguiri, MD., *The New Glucose Revolution,* (New York: Marlowe and Company, 2003), 45.

[5] Ibid., 47.

[6] Ibid., 42.

[7] Jasmine rice probably has a higher GI than glucose because the stomach must warm up a cold glucose solution before beginning digestion but gets right to work on warm rice.
Brand-Miller, Jennie, PhD, Thomas Wolever, MD, Kay Foster-Powell. MND, and Stephen Colaguiri, MD., *The New Glucose Revolution,* (New York: Marlowe and Company, 2003), 42-43.

molecule from each sucrose molecule (half of the carbohydrate) is absorbed rapidly. However, the fructose molecule (the other half of the carbohydrate) must go to the liver and be converted into glucose before it can enter the general circulation and impact blood sugar levels. This delay makes the GI score of table sugar considerably lower than that of pure glucose at 100.

In addition to the glycemic index score of a meal or food, the quantity eaten also determines the impact the meal or food has on blood sugar and insulin levels. How much carbohydrate is eaten is critically important. If you eat two cups of cooked pasta, it will have about twice the effect of eating one cup of pasta. The **GLYCEMIC LOAD** of a meal or snack is a measure of the impact of that meal or snack that accounts for both the GI score and the amount eaten. To calculate GL (glycemic load), the GI of a food is multiplied by the number of grams of carbohydrate in the serving and that number is divided by 100.

The concepts of glycemic load and the glycemic index of foods can be used to develop an eating plan that does not over-stimulate the pancreas to produce a spike of insulin after any meal or snack. This keeps insulin levels stable and low throughout the course of the day. As described on pages 27 and 38, stable and low insulin levels promote the burning of stored fat rather than the formation and storage of new fat from foods recently eaten. Instead, recently eaten food is used for the immediate energy needs of daily activities. Thus, if your insulin is low and stable, you should be using both fat stores and your last meal to produce energy and may notice that you have more energy and are less hungry that you were before you began an eating plan based on glycemic control.

In *The Complete Idiot's Guide to Glycemic Index Weight Loss,* Lucy Beale and Joan Clark, RD propose two diet variations.[8] One is a very simple diet that involves no calculations or record-keeping but which also offers little variety to satisfy the psyche. The second is an almost infinitely variable diet based on calculating the glycemic load of each meal and snack and controlling the number of GL units eaten per day. Because there are no GI values available for many foods used by those on gluten-free and food allergy diets, the recipes in this book do not include glycemic load numbers. However, the concept of glycemic load is built into the recommended serving sizes for the recipes in this book.

---

[8] Beale, Lucy and Joan Clark, MS, RD, CDE, *The Complete Idiot's Guide Glycemic Index Cookbook,* (New York: Alpha, 2009), 92-99.

OVERCOMING THE CHALLENGE OF USING THE GLYCEMIC INDEX ON FOOD ALLERGY AND GLUTEN-FREE DIETS

Using the glycemic index to plan your eating is not especially easy for anyone in the United States, even those on "normal" diets, because GI testing has not been done on uniquely American foods. In Australia and New Zealand, commercially made foods containing carbohydrates bear a Glycemic Index Foundation symbol which indicates if the food is low, medium, or high GI, and the nutrition label gives the food's glycemic score. Other countries are beginning to implement this food labeling concept but the United States is lagging behind because here most people, even among diabetics, have no idea of how useful glycemic index scores can be in controlling blood sugar and weight. Thus, there is very little demand for GI values on food labels in the United States. The books and online databases we have access to that contain the GI values for foods are based on brands of bread, crackers, and cookies made in other countries and unavailable to Americans. However, an apple or almond is the same here as in Australia, so we do have GI information we can use for basic foods such as meat, dairy products, cooked whole grains, and produce.

Along with the dearth of GI information because of lack of interest in the United States, there are some foods for which no one has information because foods are tested after preparation in the form that they are eaten. Uncooked flour of all kinds – wheat and special-diet flours alike – and other such ingredients have not been tested anywhere because they are not in the form in which they are eaten. In addition, cooking changes the GI of a food. Therefore, we cannot calculate the glycemic index or glycemic load of many of our meals and snacks or of most of the recipes in this book.

The more complex diet option presented in *The Complete Idiot's Guide to Glycemic Index Weigh Loss* gives almost infinite choice because you are calculating the glycemic load of each meal and snack and limit the GL units. For "independent thinkers," I would really like to offer an option similar to that diet in this book. Unfortunately, because we do not have GI values for most commercially made gluten-free or allergy foods, this is not possible. In this book the link and balance units for carbohydrate foods are based on 15 grams of carbohydrate for each carbohydrate unit without taking into account the GI of the food; thus, if the GI is actually quite low, the GL of that food may be lower than physiologically balances with one unit of protein. However, when you are linking and balancing foods, having extra protein compared to the carbohydrate you eat is all right.

In spite of the lack of GI date for many allergy and gluten-free foods, there is a method that can be individualized for YOU. It works as well or better than calculating the glycemic load of your meals and snacks and helps you determine how to link-and-balance your foods and what you should do with your diet. Listen to your body! If a certain food or combination of foods leaves you hungry in an hour or two, it may have had a higher GI score than you expected or you may have an undiagnosed mild allergy to the food. The next time you eat this carbohydrate food, try eating less of it per serving and linking it with more protein. If this does not help, listen to your body to detect other mild symptoms or delayed symptoms that may indicate you are allergic to one of the foods. Try balancing the carbohydrate with a different protein to rule in or out an allergy to the protein food. If you find that you cannot eat this carbohydrate food as part of a meal or snack and be satisfied for at least two hours, eliminate it for the time being. In a few months, your blood sugar control will be better and improving your inflammation status may have allowed a mild allergy to diminish to the point that you can again enjoy this food.

If you're not accustomed to listening to your body, you may wonder how it is done. Here are some personal link-and-balance anecdotes that might help you listen to your own body: I often eat fruit with nuts for between-meal snacks. If I eat a medium to high GI fruit, it takes more than an ounce of nuts eaten with it to keep me satisfied for 2½ to 3 hours. With a low GI fruit, I only need about ½ ounce of nuts. I can eat an apple or pear for a snack without any protein and be satisfied for 2 to 2½ hours. (The fruits that Dr. Hart allows her patients to eat without balancing with protein include apples, pears, peaches, plums, and grapefruit, but you must watch the quantity. No giant apples!) By noting how long it is until I get hungry after a snack, I can figure out how many nuts I need to balance certain kinds of fruits. This would tell me whether the fruit was high GI or low GI if I was unable to determine the GI values using a table such as those on pages 250 to 261.

Another personal observation about food preparation came when I first began experimenting with chana dal. (See page 127 for a recipe made with this very low GI bean). The first time I prepared it, I cooked it on the stove with some carrots and celery. I removed a little of the vegetable mixture and pureed them to give the soup a more traditional bean soup consistency and then reheated the soup to a simmer for a minute or so before eating it. After eating a single, not-overly-large bowl of the soup, I felt so extremely satisfied that I emailed a friend that I was convinced that what I'd heard about the GI of chana dal being 8 (which is extremely low) was true. The next time I cooked the beans in the crock pot on high starting at 6 a.m. because I didn't know how long it would take them to cook. They were very well done by early afternoon, so I pureed some of the soup, added it back to the pot, and turned the pot down to low until dinner time. That time the soup didn't seem as satisfying or "hold" me as long. I suspect that overcooking the chana dal, and especially overcooking the pureed starch, may have raised the GI of the soup. Therefore, the chana dal recipes in this book use other pureed vegetables (fennel, celery, etc.) to thicken soups or specify NOT cooking the dish any longer than it takes to reheat it after pureed chana dal is added back to the pot. This was an informal GI test of briefly cooked vs. overcooked chana dal with one human volunteer.

You can learn about the GI of foods by comparing your results with various foods by listening to your body in this way. Your body is different than mine, and you may need to be more or less "strict" to achieve good blood sugar and insulin balance. Since YOUR body is what counts for controlling your blood sugar and insulin levels, once you learn to do it, listening to your body is just as good as having GI value tables for the foods eaten by people with food allergies or gluten intolerance.

IN SUMMARY

In *The Insulin Resistance Diet,* Dr. Cheryle Hart, MD and Mary Kay Grossman, RD develop an eating plan that links and balances carbohydrate intake with a sufficient quantity of protein in each meal and snack to keep insulin and blood sugar levels stable. This is a very practical, easy-to-use system where hunger is controlled and hormonal balance favors burning rather than storing fat, thus leading to weight loss. The eating plan in this book is patterned after this "link and balance" system while making your eating plan compatible with your food allergy or gluten-free diet.

Carbohydrate foods are vital to our health. Without sufficient carbohydrates, we miss getting enough vital nutrients such as vitamins, minerals, phytonutrients and fiber. Furthermore, if we're short on carbohydrates, we cannot make neurotransmitters such as serotonin, and this produces a mental state that makes it more difficult to stick with a healthy eating plan. By using the information about carbohydrates in this chapter, we can eat an amount of carbohydrate sufficient to satisfy both our nutritional requirements and our need for enjoyment without causing blood sugar and insulin spikes. Thus, we can enjoy carbohydrate foods while achieving weight loss and better health.

ABOUT FATS
PRO-INFLAMMATORY, ANTI-INFLAMMATORY, AND THEIR USE IN COOKING

Although we have repeatedly heard that fats are "the bad guys" and should be avoided almost completely, natural fats are essential to good health. Without fats our cell membranes would fall apart, we would not be able to make hormones, and the absorption of fat-soluble vitamins would be impaired. However, like carbohydrates, fats are not all created equal. Some are "essential" meaning that we need them for body processes but cannot make them from other foods and therefore must get them in sufficient quantities from our diets. Other fats, such as unnatural trans fats, are harmful and we really should avoid them completely.

The kind of fats we eat is more important than the quantity of fat we eat if our goal is optimal health. Indeed, some weight loss diets result in fat malnutrition. In *The Fat Resistance Diet*, Dr. Leo Galland, MD describes patients who attempted to lose weight on both high-carbohydrate low-fat diets and high-protein high-fat diets presenting with symptoms of omega-3[1] fatty acid deficiency such as low resistance to infections, inflammatory conditions, brain fog, dry skin, brittle nails, and limp hair.[2]

There are several types of fats. Two of them are essential fats that we cannot make and therefore must consume in our diets: the linolenic or omega-3 fatty acid family and the linoleic or omega-6 fatty acid family. Omega-3 fatty acids have anti-inflammatory effects and are the cornerstone of most anti-inflammatory diet plans.[3] Oils which contain high levels of omega-3 fatty acids include flax oil, fish oil, canola oil, and walnut oil.

Omega-6 fatty acids are usually considered pro-inflammatory. Indeed, the over-consumption of highly processed soy or corn oil will promote inflammation. However, some sources of omega-6 fatty acids such as borage and evening primrose oil can have anti-inflammatory effects. The key to health in the consumption of essential fatty acids is balance. Omega-3 and omega-6 fatty acids should be consumed in approximately equal amounts. However, those who eat a standard American diet containing many processed foods usually consume about twenty times as much omega-6 fat as omega-3 fat.

---

[1] Fatty acids are classified by the position of the double bonds in the fatty acid molecules. Omega-3 fatty acids have a double bond three carbon atoms from the end of the molecule.

[2] Galland, Leo, MD, *The Fat Resistance Diet,* (New York: Broadway Books, 2005), 70, 76.

[3] Black, Jessica K., ND, *The Anti-Inflammation Diet and Recipe Book,* (Alameda, CA: Hunter House Publishers, 2006); Cannon, Christopher P., MD and Elizabeth Vierck, *The Complete Idiot's Guide to The Anti-Inflammation Diet*, (New York: Alpha, 2006); and Galland, Leo, MD, *The Fat Resistance Diet,* (New York: Broadway Books, 2005).

Omega-9 fatty acids such as are found in olives, macadamia nuts, and avocadoes do not promote inflammation. Olive oil is associated with decreased risk of cardiovascular disease and possibly might have anti-inflammatory benefits.

Saturated fats are the final category of fat in our diets. There is considerable debate about the "healthiness" of naturally saturated fats such as the fat in meat, dairy products, coconut oil, and palm oil. Some claim that all saturated fat is unhealthy. Other say that coconut oil helps promote weigh loss and can reduce the risk of heart disease[4] and that meat and milk from range-fed cattle is not detrimental to health because it is low in the most inflammatory fat, arachidonic acid.[5] Game meat is actually a good source of omega-3 fatty acids.[6] In contrast, feedlot-fattened grain-fed beef is high in arachidonic acid and low in omega-3 fatty acids. However, the fatty acid composition of grass-fed beef is very similar to that of wild game.[7]

Trans fats are unnatural saturated fats made from vegetable oils by the chemical process of hydrogenation, or the addition of hydrogen molecules to the fat to change double bonds to single bonds. These fats are not completely devoid of double bonds, however, and the ones that remain are in an unnatural (trans) configuration that our bodies cannot use to build functional cell membranes, etc. A 2001 report from the Harvard School of Public Health reports that, although most fats have no or a minimal correlation with negative health consequences, trans fats may promote insulin resistance as well as raising LDL (low density lipoprotein or " bad") cholesterol and lowering HDL (high density lipoprotein or "good") cholesterol.[8]

Unnatural fats should be completely avoided in a healthy diet. Do not be deceived by the new cans of shortening that say "No trans fat." The only difference between this new shortening and the shortening of a few years ago is that the vegetable oils are completely hydrogenated. No double bonds remain, so there are no trans-configuration bonds, but the shortening is still unnatural and may contain traces of the chemicals which were used to produce it. Most margarine is also composed of hydrogenated fats and should be avoided. Exceptions to this are margarine and shortening made by Spec-

---

[4] Bowden, Jonny, PhD, CNS, "Break Out of Your Shell," *Better Nutrition,* March 2010, 24. A study started in the 1960s has shown that residents of the Pacific islands of Pukapuka and Tokelau, who get 35 to 60% of their calories from fat coming mostly from coconut, are lean and healthy and have almost no heart disease, atherosclerosis, high cholesterol, kidney disease, or colon cancer. Former Surgeon General C. Everett Koop, MD, called the vilification of tropical oils "foolishness."

[5] Challem, Jack, "The Omega Factor: Figuring Out Fats," *Better Nutrition,* October 2009, 44.

[6] Braly, James, MD, *Dr. Braly's Food Allergy and Nutrition Revolution,* (New Caanan, CT: Keats Publishing, 1998), 143.

[7] Michael Pollan, Michael, *In Defense of Food: An Eater's Manifesto,* (New York: The Penguin Press, 2008), 171.

[8] Michael Pollan, Michael, *In Defense of Food: An Eater's Manifesto,* (New York: The Penguin Press, 2008), 44, from Frank B. Hu et al, "Types of Dietary Fat and Risk or Coronary Heart Disease: A Critical Review," *Journal of the American College of Nutrition* 20 (2001): 1, 5-19.

trum Naturals™. Rather than being made solid by chemically manipulating liquid vegetable oils, these products get their consistency from natural organic palm oil which is saturated and therefore solid at room temperature, yet it does not contain trans bonds or traces of chemicals.

Why is the type of fat we consume so important to good health and weight control? It is because the type of fat we eat in part determines whether our bodies make pro- or anti-inflammatory prostaglandins. A high intake of omega-3 fatty acids promotes the production of anti-inflammatory prostaglandins. However, people with allergies often cannot convert the alpha-linolenic acid in flax oil or green leafy vegetables to the omega-3 fatty acids our bodies use, DHA (docosahexaenoic acid) and EPA (eicosapentaenoic acid). Therefore, these fats must be consumed pre-formed; we must get them from our diets in fish or from supplements such as fish or krill oil.

Our bodies convert the linoleic acid (an omega-6 fatty acid) found in corn and soy oil to either GLA (gamma-linolenic acid), which is anti-inflammatory, or arachidonic acid, which has pro-inflammatory effects and results in the formation of pro-inflammatory prostaglandins. Massive consumption of omega-6 fatty acids pushes this conversion towards more arachidonic acid. Trans fats inhibit the formation of GLA. And finally, high levels of insulin shift the conversion of omega-6 fats toward the production of arachidonic acid and away from GLA.[9] Thus, a high insulin level in and of itself can promote inflammation.

So what can we do? Those who have food allergies or celiac disease are quite often low in the nutrients needed to convert omega-3 fatty acids to their active forms, EPA and DHA. These nutrients include zinc, magnesium, and vitamin B-6, and they are decreased due to malabsorption from a compromised intestine. Therefore, we must consume omega-3 fatty acids in their active, pre-formed state as DHA and EPA. Unless you eat a lot of fatty fish, this means taking fish oil, which has a reputation for unpleasant flavor. However, the Eskimo 3 brand fish oil I take as oil contains lemon and rosemary and tastes all right. The advantage of capsules is that you don't have to taste the fish oil at all. Whether GLA supplements are also needed or helpful is a matter of opinion. Barry Sears, PhD recommends taking GLA in a 4 to 1 ratio of DHA and EPA to GLA.[10] How much fish oil you need is also a matter of opinion. Dr. Leo Galland, MD recommends 2000 mg per day and recommends taking more only under a doctor's supervision because it can disrupt digestion, lead to easy bleeding, or cause other problems.[11] Dr. Sears' recommendations of 5 to 10 grams pre day are much higher and probably should be taken only under a doctor's supervision.

---

[9] Sears, Barry, PhD, *The Anti-Inflammation Zone,* (New York, Regan Books, 2005), 215.

[10] Ibid, 215.

[11] Galland, Leo, MD, *The Fat Resistance Diet,* (New York: Broadway Books, 2005), 102.

In addition, maintaining low and stable insulin levels through diet will shift the conversion of omega-6 fatty acids toward anti-inflammatory GLA instead of toward pro-inflammatory arachidonic acid. Therefore, following a healthy eating plan which controls your insulin levels should result in the production of less pro-inflammatory and more anti-inflammatory prostaglandins.

COOKING WITH OILS AND FATS

Polyunsaturated oils are fragile and easily damaged by high heat. This can result in the formation of a few trans bonds in the fat, but this is not as detrimental as the intentional creation of damaged fats to make shortening or margarine. However, because this change can occur, when you will be using high heat to sauté vegetables or brown meat, it is wise to use fat that is heat-stable such as monounsaturated olive or nut oils or naturally saturated fat such as butter, coconut oil, or palm oil.

However, you do not have to avoid polyunsaturated oils in low-heat cooking. It is good to get them into your diet as much as possible because they are the plant oils highest in omega-3 fatty acids. It is acceptable to use canola and walnut oil in baking because the inside of your baked goods can never exceed the boiling point of water (212 °F at sea level).[12] And the temperature which damages these oils is frying temperature, about 375°F. The temperature of baked goods such as bread and muffins is only 190 to 195°F when you remove them from the oven. Flax oil, which is the most fragile of the high omega-3 oils, should not be heated for long but is best used to dress cooked vegetables before serving and in salad dressings.

If you have food allergies, your allergies, along with the heat considerations above, will determine what types of oil you use in cooking. Use only the types of oil to which you are not allergic. The best omega-3 oils will not be anti-inflammatory for you if they cause an allergic reaction! Any allergic reaction increases inflammation, especially in the parts of your body that are most affected by the reaction. If your food allergies are severe enough to necessitate a rotation diet, be sure to rotate the oils you use also. You will probably have to rotate some oils that are higher in omega-6 fatty acids as part of your diet to get enough oils for all of the rotation days. Strictly following a rotation diet will decrease inflammation due to food allergies.

Chose expeller cold pressed unrefined oils when you shop. The heat and chemicals used to produce cheaper types of oil can damage the fatty acids they contain. If you have oil that smells rancid, throw it away. That smell means that the oil has been oxidized, or changed chemically by oxygen.

Canola oil is high in omega-3 fatty acids and is a good choice for most people's diets. However, it has received a "bad rap" in the past due to rumors not based on fact. Here

---

[12] Energy in the form of heat put into anything that contains water will be dissipated by evaporation of the water until the water is totally burned off.

is a brief history of canola oil. The original canola plants were not genetically engineered but were produced from rapeseed by conventional breeding 20 years before genetic engineering came into being. Although rapeseed is in the mustard (cabbage) family, it is not the plant from which mustard gas is made. Naturally produced canola oil contains no trans fats. As with many plants, there are some strains of genetically engineered canola. To avoid them, purchase organic canola oil, canola oil labeled "non-GMO," or oil made by a reputable producer such as Spectrum Naturals.™ Canola is not allergenic for most people, unlike corn and soy oils. However, if you have food allergies you may not be able to convert the omega-3 fatty acids in canola, walnut, or other cooking oils into the forms our bodies use (DHA and EPA) as discussed on page 57.

Olive oil is another good choice for a cooking oil. Few people are allergic to olives, so it is usually well tolerated allergy-wise. It is mono-unsaturated and is therefore more heat stable and resists rancidity better than polyunsaturated oils. It is ideal for sautéing vegetables, browning meats, and other high-heat cooking applications.

Other good cooking oil choices include nut oils and grapeseed oil. Grapeseed oil, although polyunsaturated, is more heat stable than many oils. Nut oils such as almond, macadamia, and hazelnut are high in monounsaturated fatty acids and are therefore heat stable and good for high-heat cooking applications as well as for baking, salads, and dressing vegetables. Monounsaturated oils are not pro-inflammatory and may have anti-inflammatory effects.

Walnut oil is high in omega-3 fatty acids and is therefore a useful addition to our diets. Use it for no-heat or low-heat cooking applications such as dressing salads and cooked vegetables or baking.

Corn and soy oil are from highly allergenic plants and are also high in omega-6 fatty acids so they are pro-inflammatory if they are eaten in large quantities. They are also most often made from genetically engineered strains of corn and soy, as are most corn and soy products produced in the United States. You will probably want to avoid these oils.

Other oils that are high in omega-6 fatty acids but are less allergenic than corn and soy oils include sunflower and safflower oil. These may have a part in your rotation diet if you cannot find enough monounsaturated or high-omega-3 oils to use on each rotation day.

IN SUMMARY

Natural fats are your friends, not your enemies. They hold our cell membranes together and make it possible for us to absorb fat soluble vitamins. With the right fats eaten in the right balance, they can increase satiety, reduce inflammation and help you lose weight.

DO IT YOUR BODY'S WAY

The fourth chapter of this book said "Do it your way." This is essential if you hope to follow a healthy eating plan for more than just a short time without feeling deprived. We must satisfy our psychological and emotional needs for pleasure as well as satisfying our physical needs for nutrients and fuel. Your own body's individual physiological needs are also crucial. For an eating plan to be optimally effective, it must be in tune with what your body needs as well as with what your psyche needs. You must do it your body's way. This means listening to your body and avoiding hunger. It also means avoiding foods to which you are allergic in order to avoid triggering the fat storage-promoting hormonal cascade described below.

AVOID YOUR ALLERGENIC FOODS

If you have food allergies, the first and most important principle of "doing it your body's way" is to avoid your food allergens strictly and, if needed due to multiple food allergies, rotate your foods to minimize the reactions to borderline food allergens. Eating foods to which you are allergic causes inflammation. This makes your adrenal glands secrete hormones which destabilize your insulin and blood sugar levels. The high level of insulin you then experience affects the activity of enzymes that control your fat metabolism (see pages 27 and 38 for more details) thus causing your body to hold on to and deposit fat rather than allowing you to burn it for energy. You must individualize your eating plan so that it fits your food allergies. There is no diet book or plan that you can follow "as is" if you have food intolerance or allergies. Although this book is written for people on food allergy and gluten-free diets, some of you still will be unable to use quite a few of the recipes in this book. (I don't eat most of them). Having to customize an eating plan if you have food allergies is to be expected because the list of problem foods varies from person to person. This is true even if the author of the diet understands food allergies. For example, Dr. Galland has been treating food allergies for over 30 years and is quite allergy-aware; yet there are allergenic foods on his list of 40 superfoods in *The Fat Resistance Diet.* I can eat less than one-third of the foods on his list. The bottom line is, if you have food allergies or gluten intolerance, you should expect to have to adapt any eating plan to your allergies or intolerances.

However, no one, even those with no food intolerances of any kind, should blindly follow any eating plan "as is." You should understand the principles behind the eating plan, determine whether or not they fit you and how well they fit, and customize the plan. YOUR BODY is the ultimate authority on what is good for it. Listen to it! Consider how any eating plan or any food affects you and then individualize what you eat.

AVOID HUNGER

In addition to avoiding allergic reactions, you should also avoid hunger that is prolonged or excessive. Like allergic reactions, hunger can trigger a fat deposit-promoting hormonal cascade. When you have tried to lose weight in the past, you probably experienced hunger between meals and summoned all of your willpower to resist eating. By the time the clock said it was time to eat, you were so famished that a normal portion of food was not enough to satisfy you. This is obviously not a good way to reduce how much you eat. It also inhibits fat burning and is not a pleasant way to live. Listen to your body! If you feel physical hunger, weakness, or irritability that is relieved by your next meal, your body is telling you that your blood sugar may be dropping and you need food. Hunger cannot be controlled by applying mind-over-matter willpower. It can be controlled by stabilizing your blood sugar and insulin levels. This is accomplished by eating the right types of food in the right combination at the right time. Listen to your body, apply the principles in this book, and you will be able to control your hormones and hunger, keep your body in the fat-burning mode, and lose weight.

In the *Anti-Inflammatory Zone,* Barry Sears, PhD advises keeping hardboiled eggs, cooked chicken and other prepared protein foods in your refrigerator at all times so a meal can be put together and eaten within a few minutes of experiencing hunger.[1] While this may not always be practical, especially for those who work away from home or have a family they want to eat with, I hope that you can carry some nuts, a linked-and-balanced snack (such as crackers and some nut butter or cheese) or an apple with you at all times and have a small snack when hunger hits. This will keep your blood sugar and insulin levels stable, thus preventing the fat-depositing hormonal cascade and allowing you to stay in the "burn fat" mode. It will also make it possible for you to eat moderately and yet be satisfied at your next meal.

Prolonged or extreme hunger means that your blood sugar is dropping or low; adrenal hormones will kick in to bring it back up eventually. These surges of adrenal hormones followed by fluctuations in insulin levels are counterproductive to losing weight and controlling inflammation.

There are times when it is difficult to avoid these hormonal surges because we don't know we are hungry, such as when we are asleep. Sleep can be a problem! In the study[2] discussed on pages 36 to 37, there was an exaggerated insulin response to breakfast, resulting in lower blood sugar levels than after other meals. There are steps to take to minimize this, however, Have a small protein or linked-and-balanced snack before bedtime. This is especially important when you first start the healthy eating plan in

---

[1] Sears, Barry, PhD, *The Anti-Inflammation Zone,* (New York, Regan Books, 2005), 70. Perhaps the lack of variety and strictly utilitarian approach to meals in *The Zone* diet books is part of the reason why people find this diet hard to follow long term.

[2] www.montignac.com/en/etude_scient_sur_meth_mont.php

this book and are trying to achieve hormonal control. In addition, always eat a proper linked-and-balanced breakfast within an hour of rising. These two practices will minimize the hormonal swings associated with sleep and help keep your body in the fat burning mode most of the time.

AVOID THIRST

Although the practice of forcing oneself to drink eight glasses of water per day has fallen from favor, be aware of when you may be getting thirsty. Thirst can masquerade as hunger. If you feel hungry soon after eating or when you don't expect to be hungry yet, try drinking some water first. If this doesn't satisfy you, then have a snack as discussed above. In addition, I personally find that thirst sometimes masquerades as fatigue. Listen to your body. Under some circumstances, you may need less than eight glasses of water per day. If the weather is hot and/or you are exercising heavily, you will need more water.

SATISFY YOUR NEED FOR PLEASURE

We are not physical creatures only. We have a physical need for food, but food also satisfies our need for pleasure in a very basic way. Be sure to enjoy what you eat. Pay attention to your food as you are eating it. Eat slowly, concentrate on the taste of the food, and savor every bite. Do not watch TV or read the newspaper or mail during meals. If you do, your physical need for food might be fulfilled before you meet your need for emotional satisfaction and pleasure, which can lead to overeating.

There will be some times when your emotional and pleasure needs may be exceptionally high. This can happen when you are under stress or need comfort. Stress can also result in physical hunger by causing fluctuations in cortisol and insulin levels which destabilize blood sugar. Therefore, exercising willpower to not eat when stressed may not be the best thing to do. Controlled eating is a better way to cope with the urge to eat comfort foods under stress. Try to stay on your healthy eating plan – meaning link and balance – but choose your favorite foods. If you are not allergic to chocolate, this may be the time for a controlled splurge such as one or two ounces of dark chocolate, eaten slowly and savored. Eat some nuts or other protein before or with the chocolate to balance the sugar it contains or enjoy stevia-sweetened chocolate. (See the recipe on page 198).

Be good to yourself in other ways and seek comfort and pleasure from other experiences in addition to food. Buy yourself a new music CD and listen to it, or enjoy – really listening – to some favorite music that you already have. Music can cause your brain to release endorphins, and low levels of endorphins can cause food cravings.[3] Listening to

---

[3] www.ehow.com/how_2063616_release-endorphins.html

a favorite piece of music for a half hour can produce a relaxation response and reduce stress.[4]

Exercise can also induce positive brain chemicals and hormonal changes. If you can exercise outdoors and enjoy the beauty of nature, that is an ideal way to help relieve stress. If it's raining, exercise inside while listening to your favorite music or watching an enjoyable DVD. A stationery bicycle is ideal for rainy days, or you may even purchase a stand that you can use to pedal your regular bike indoors when repetitive pedaling would be soothing but the weather is bad. Just remember to exercise after a meal or snack, not when you are hungry. Especially if you are exercising to release stress, if it has been two hours since you last ate, have a small linked-and-balanced snack before you exercise.

Don't despair if you end up eating something with a high glycemic index or that is high in fat during a stressful time. You are only human! Have some protein to balance your splurge and move on. Tomorrow will be another day. Re-read your reasons for embarking on a healthy eating plan and get back to it.

Holidays and special occasions can also increase our need for pleasure. Just seeing a spread of favorite foods and watching those around you stuff themselves will boost your appetite. Although you may end up eating more than you normally would, you will do better at keeping your body in the fat burning mode if you plan ahead for these situations.

Planning ahead does not mean skipping breakfast on Thanksgiving morning! (That is the calorie counter's definition of planning ahead). Skipping breakfast will flip your fat switch to the "save" mode and increase fat storage when you eat a big meal later in the day. Planning ahead means controlled indulgence. It does not mean receiving strange looks from the relatives as you painstakingly measure portions or starve yourself. Eat more turkey and less potatoes and gravy. Don't skip the potatoes and gravy if you enjoy them, however, or you will feel deprived! Pay attention to what you are eating and savor every bite. If possible, eat a salad with at least four teaspoons of vinegar or lemon juice in the dressing or have some stevia-sweetened lemonade with your meal. (See this recipe on page 231). The acid in these foods will lower the glycemic impact of the meal. Take a brisk walk with family members within two hours of eating and you will burn at least some of the fat and excess carbohydrate in your meal if you overindulged.

Sitting in front of the TV after Thanksgiving dinner is part of the problem! Consider breaking with that tradition. Instead, build some memories of a pleasant walk and good conversation with your relatives. If you must see the football game, tape it for later. One of my most cherished Thanksgiving memories is of the first year I cooked the family meal and, giving me a wonderful gift, my mother said, "I'll take over on the clean-up." I was then able to enjoy an after-meal walk with the men and our nieces who were, at that age, unable to sit still for long.

---

4 http://stress.about.com/od/tensiontamers/a/music_therapy.htm; www.holisticonline.com/stress/stress_music-therapy.htm

When you do indulge, pay attention to how you feel after a large, carbohydrate-heavy meal. Listen to your body. It may become very tired or sleepy and thus tell you that your healthy eating plan keeps you more energetic and clear-minded than you used to be. Knowing this will help you get back to your healthy eating plan and to follow it consistently more easily.

WHAT TO DO ABOUT "CAN'T LIVE WITHOUT IT" FOODS

For some people, a certain favorite food or beverage offers pleasure and satisfaction not possible from a substitute. You may have a food like this – chocolate, pizza, pasta, ice cream, coffee, etc. It can be a part of your healthy eating plan *if you are not allergic to it nor sensitive to it* in any other way (such as being caffeine sensitive; see pages 66 to 67 for more about this) and *if you can eat it in a controlled fashion.* However, if it is almost an addictive food for you, this may indicate food allergy. If you cannot eat it with control and always end up eating excessively, consider the possibility of allergy or another addictive process and avoid it totally for six months. After your inflammation and body fat levels have decreased, give it another try. You then might be able to eat the food occasionally without problems and in a controlled fashion.

You might also consider the possibility that your favorite food has a chemically addictive effect on you. As described on pages 20 to 21, many highly processed commercially prepared foods are formulated to be addictive. Look for homemade recipes[5] for such foods and make them yourself. Thus, you can satisfy your need for pleasure without eating your favorite food in a highly-processed, additive saturated, nutrient depleted, blood sugar spiking form and without destabilizing your insulin levels.

In *The Insulin Resistance Diet,* Dr. Cheryle Hart, MD recommends occasional planned, controlled splurges on favorite foods. If you are not allergic to chocolate, she especially recommends this for those who have low neurotransmitter levels.[6] (These people may suffer depression or anxiety on very low carbohydrate diets as a result of decreased neurotransmitter synthesis[7]). High quality dark chocolate is high in antioxidants, magnesium, tryptophan, and other nutrients[8] and is an ideal food for boosting neurotransmitter levels. Many of Dr. Hart's patients crave it for this reason. Because of their greater muscle mass, men are less likely to experience serotonin deficiency to

[5] If you can't find your favorite recipe made allergen or gluten-free, email us so we can develop and include the recipe in the next book. We may already have the recipe you are looking for and can email it to you. Please email us using the contact form on the food-allergy.org or foodallergyandglutenfreeweightloss.com websites.

[6] Hart, Cheryle R., MD and Mary Kay Grossman, RD, *The Insulin Resistance Diet,* (New York: McGraw-Hill, 2001, 2007), 210-211.

[7] The risk of decreased serotonin levels is one of the reasons that healthy eating plans with long-term success such as the one in this book are not extremely low in carbohydrates.

[8] "Five Best Snacks to Boost Your Mood,"*Care2 Newsletter,* February 26, 1010, www.care2.com/greenliving/5-best-snacks-for-mood.html?&page=4 .

the degree that women do. However, if you crave chocolate, there might be a physical reason; indulging in some chocolate may balance your serotonin level and allow you to continue on and succeed with your healthy eating plan. Dr. Hart recommends eating dark chocolate that contains at least 70% cocoa solids.

Authors Lucy Beale and Joan Clark-Warner, RD have both learned to enjoy chocolate in a healthy way on their eating plans. Their book, *The Glycemic Control Cookbook,* contains an entire chapter of chocolate desserts. Yet, these women have stayed slim on a glycemic control diet for years without being deprived of their favorite food – chocolate – prepared in low-GI ways. Because their recipes are designed to satisfy pleasure needs above all, they use butter, cream, and whole eggs in the recipes. (This differs from their cooking approach in the other chapters of their book). They advise, "Use real dairy butter [to] deliver the flavor and excellence you want" and "Use whole eggs [or] the dessert won't deliver full flavor and satisfaction."[9] If you have non-allergic family members or friends participating in the healthy eating plan with you, they may want to explore the recipes in *The Glycemic Control Cookbook.* Because their chocolate recipes are not hypoallergenic, a few chocolate recipes are included in this book. If you have candidiasis and should eliminate sugar, see the recipe for stevia-sweetened chocolate candy or chips or chocolate almond candy bars on pages 198 to 199. See also the gluten-free carob and chocolate brownie recipes on pages 200 and 201.

If you are not allergic to dairy products, commercially-made premium ice cream is an ideal food for a controlled splurge. Its high fat content decreases its glycemic index score. If you cannot have dairy products or the sugar in this ice cream due to candidiasis, see the dairy and sugar free ice cream recipes on pages 220 to 221.

If eaten in moderate quantities, pizza and pasta can be enjoyed as part of your eating plan. Pasta actually has a lower glycemic index score than rice if cooked *al dente.* For a wheat-free or gluten-free pizza recipe, see pages 153 to 155.

Listen to your body after you have a controlled splurge with one of your favorite foods. If you feel fine after eating it and also the next day, you can probably indulge in it occasionally. Enjoy! However, if you feel as if you might be having an allergic reaction, however mild (i.e. cravings, fatigue, aches and pains, headaches, bloating, etc.) seek another recipe that would also satisfy your pleasure needs. With the right recipes, you need not be deprived unless the range of your food allergies is very wide.

If you cannot find a recipe which you can eat for a favorite "can't live without it" food in this book, please email us using the contact form or contact information on the food-allergy.org or foodallergyandglutenfreeweightloss.com websites. This book is a basic book and as such includes a moderate number of recipes. I plan to have the next book in this series contain a full complement of recipes of all kinds. Hopefully your suggestions can be used to develop new recipes that will help you and others be satisfied and stay on a healthy eating plan.

---

[9] Beale, Lucy and Joan Clark, MS, RD, CDE, *The Complete Idiot's Guide Glycemic Index Cookbook,* (New York: Alpha, 2009), 300.

WHAT ABOUT "CAN'T LIVE WITHOUT IT" BEVERAGES?

For some people, a favorite "can't live without it" food is a beverage, and they usually consume it daily or several times a day. An occasional splurge just won't do! I've spoken to people who need to be on a special diet but absolutely must have some caffeine to get started in the morning, and they cannot stick with any eating plan that tells them they must eliminate all caffeine.

The various glycemic control and anti-inflammatory diet books I consulted while researching this book differ greatly in their advice about caffeine and artificial sweeteners. Some of the books absolutely prohibit **caffeine.** If you are sensitive to it, as about half of the population is, it may spike your insulin level. You may have to cut your caffeine intake down to a low amount or eliminate it to be able to lose weight on your healthy eating plan. Listen to your body when you consume caffeine. If it makes you hyper, jittery, causes excessive hunger, or produces sleep disturbances even when consumed early in the day, you should decrease your consumption to a level which eliminates these symptoms. If eliminating the symptoms is not possible, try switching sources (as from coffee to tea) or possibly giving caffeine up altogether. Since sensitivity is dose-dependent, coffee or black tea may give you the jitters or make you excessively hungry, but green, white, or twig tea, with their lower caffeine content (about 35 to 40%, 5 to 15%, and 10% of the caffeine in black tea, respectively) may not cause problems. Better yet, try decaffeinated coffee or tea and listen to your body after you drink them. Some brands are quite low in caffeine and others still contain enough to cause symptoms in those who are very sensitive to caffeine. In addition, some individuals may react to chemicals in conventionally produced coffee and may wish to try organic coffee to see if this eliminates their symptoms.

Dr. Galland includes green tea as one of the most potent of his 40 anti-inflammatory foods and recommends that patients drink his anti-inflammatory green chai tea with meals and snacks several times a day. If you would like to have green tea regularly as an anti-inflammatory food but are sensitive to the low level of caffeine it contains, try decaffeinated green tea. You can also easily remove caffeine from any tea at home.[10]

The glycemic control diet books I read which allow the consumption of **caffeine** all specify that it should be used **in moderation** and **with food.** In *The GI Diet,* Rick Gallop says that many have successfully lost weight on his diet while drinking one cup of full-caffeine coffee or black tea with breakfast every day. If you are doing this, not experiencing symptoms of caffeine sensitivity or blood sugar instability, and are able to lose weight without a struggle, enjoy your morning beverage! If, however, you cannot lose weight, you may want to eliminate caffeine for a week or a few weeks and see if you lose more easily.

---

[10] I like to enjoy my favorite green teas which are not available decaffeinated by brewing them using the method given in the "Caffeine-Controlled Green Tea" recipe on page 229.

Listen to your body if you eat or drink anything containing caffeine, and take note of variations in your appetite and sleep patterns. I find that coffee, even decaffeinated, will make me tired within an hour or two and more hungry than usual for the rest of the day. Very low-caffeine types of tea such as white or twig tea do not have this effect; they do give me more energy but without subsequent fatigue. Listen to your body! It is the final authority on whether and how much caffeine is right for you. If you tolerate it at a low level, see the recipe on page 229 for making tea at the caffeine level which is right for you.

A study recently published in the *Archives of Internal Medicine* has given us even more to think about when deciding whether to consume coffee or tea.[11] Using data analyzed from over 450,000 participants in 18 studies, it was found that there was an inverse relationship between the amount of coffee or tea consumed and the risk of developing diabetes. Each cup consumed daily decreased the risk by 7%. Even decaffeinated coffee had a protective effect with three to four cups associated with a 33% lower risk of diabetes, indicating that the caffeine is not the protective factor, but rather the nutrients contained in the beverages. Therefore, those who are caffeine sensitive but not allergic to coffee or tea may want to try decaffeinated varieties of these beverages. If you are not sensitive to the traces of caffeine they may contain, you might reduce your risk of diabetes and other problems by enjoying decaffeinated coffee or tea.

The use of **artificial sweeteners** on a glycemic control diet also can be controversial. In *The GI Diet,* Rick Gallup uses them freely in his recipes and promotes diet sodas as acceptable pleasures. Several of the other books I consulted prohibit their use completely. Artificial sweeteners are unnatural food additives made in a laboratory, and as such, are difficult for many of us to trust. Cyclamates were removed from the market many years ago due to a cancer link, saccharin causes kidney cancer in mice if consumed in extraordinarily high amounts, and there has been an increase in brain cancer since aspartame was introduced into our foods.[12] Sucralose causes unhealthy changes in intestinal flora, and intestinal dysbiosis from any cause can lead to a worsening of food allergies. Aspartame often causes headaches in those with food allergies. In the *Yeast Connection* books, Dr. William Crook, MD considers saccharin the least problematic artificial sweetener[13] and the one to use if you have difficulty avoiding them altogether. If you crave a diet soda and want to avoid aspartame and sucralose, fountain diet sodas are sweetened with saccharin. The snack bars in Target stores, movie theaters, and some gas stations even offer caffeine-free saccharin-sweetened diet Coke™ or Pepsi™ which allows you to also avoid caffeine.

---

[11] *Archives of Internal Medicine,* 2009; 169(22): 2053-2063, http://archinte.ama-assn.org/cgi/content/abstract/169/22/2053 .

[12] "A Poisonous Sweetener,"*Care2 Newsletter,* October 13, 2009, www.care2.com/greenliving/a-poisonous-sweetener.html .

[13] Crook, William G., MD, *The Yeast Connection,* (Jackson, TN: Professional Books, 1985), 124.

A middle ground position on artificial sweeteners is found in *The Insulin Resistance Diet*. Authors Cheryle Hart, MD and Mary Kay Grossman, RD allow the controlled use of artificial sweeteners in a way that does not destabilize blood sugar and insulin levels. They say that the sweet taste of a diet soda causes the release of a small amount of insulin[14] and advise consuming diet sodas only with food so that the insulin has something to act on. A diet soda between meals when you are hungry, taken without food, can make your blood sugar go down due to the insulin release, and then your adrenal glands may release adrenaline and cortisol to raise your blood sugar levels. Although you may feel less hungry after drinking a diet soda, it is due to a hormonal roller coaster raising your blood sugar, and the rise in insulin and adrenaline levels this causes may interfere with the fat-burning enzyme and thus interfere with weight loss. However, in *The Insulin Resistance Diet* Dr. Hart does allow diet sodas in moderation with food.[15] As with caffeine, if you are drinking them with food and losing weight easily, enjoy! If not, try giving them up for a week or a few weeks and see if you lose more easily. Substitute iced or hot herbal tea or decaffeinated black or green tea, stevia-sweetened lemonade, page 231, or the new stevia-sweetened soda, Zevia,™ for diet sodas if you want something to drink instead of water. (Beware of Zevia™ if you are allergic to corn, however, because it contains corn-source erythritol).

Although I personally agree with those who say artificial sweeteners are unnatural chemicals, not having them can make it impossible for some people to stay on a diet. For those who are just starting a food allergy diet, beverages can be more problematic than a long list of must-avoid allergenic foods that are found in almost everything. A few years ago I talked to a young woman who was literally in a panic over her recently-diagnosed food allergies and diet. Although she was struggling to eliminate several major food allergens and rotate all foods, her worst problem – which was causing her panic – was that she could not get through more than a several hours without a diet Coke.™ Eliminating it for any longer made her feel so terrible that she literally could not function. I suggested that she follow the rotation diet in *The Ultimate Food Allergy Cookbook and Survival Guide* (see the last few pages of this book for more information) for the rotation

---

[14] In addition to Dr. Hart in *The Insulin Resistance Diet*, other authorities believe that the sweet taste of artificial sweeteners causes the release or insulin. This position is also presented by Lucy Beale and Joan Clark, MS, RD, CDE, *The Complete Idiot's Guide Glycemic Index Cookbook*, (New York: Alpha, 2009), 139. Hart, Cheryle R., MD and Mary Kay Grossman, RD, *The Insulin Resistance Diet*, (New York: McGraw-Hill, 2001, 2007), 96.

[15] Grossman, Mary Kay, RD, *Foods by Chance or by Choice*, (Free download form irdiet.com, 2008), 12. In this download from Dr. Hart's website, irdiet.com, which is more recent than her book *The Insulin Resistance Diet*, patients are allowed to drink diet sodas without balancing them with a protein food. I suspect that how much insulin response one experiences after drinking a diet soda without food is an individual matter and that some people can do this and still lose weight while others will destabilize their insulin levels enough to interfere with weight loss, especially in the early weeks of their healthy eating plan. As blood sugar and insulin control improve with more time on the plan, diet sodas may become less likely to destabilize them and thus interfere with weight loss if they are consumed without food.

of foods and add a rotation of four different caffeinated beverages to that diet – coffee, tea, yerba maté, and her beloved diet Coke.™ A few weeks later I received a postcard from her telling me that her symptoms had been eliminated, she felt as if her life had been restored to her, and that she had been able to cut down on the amounts of the beverages. I suspect that she could not have begun taking the steps necessary to improve her health without continuing to consume some aspartame and caffeine. Possibly, as her health continued to improve, she might have been able to reduce her dependence on highly caffeinated beverages; even if that was not the case, she was certainly better off than she had been when she first called me. So in my opinion, when it comes to caffeine and artificial sweeteners, you should "do it your way," whatever that happens to be, but also do it your body's way (i.e. use caffeine and artificial sweeteners with food only) and listen to your body.

YOUR BODY'S WAY IS BEST

If you have tried to lose weight in the past and not been able to lose or to keep the weight off without a struggle, it may have been because you were working against rather than with your body and dieting in a way that raised your insulin level. In *The Insulin Resistance Diet,* Cheryle Hart, MD asks and then answers this question: "If high insulin levels make you fat, then would *lower* insulin levels make you thin? The answer is yes. Keeping insulin levels from spiking is the key to your weight loss solution and is the basis of our Link-and-Balance Eating Method. This unique method teaches you ways to eat every kind of food, even carbohydrates, while keeping your insulin at fat-losing levels."[16] The one qualification I would make to her statement is that you cannot eat foods you are allergic to without producing a hormonal cascade that will raise your insulin levels and thus interfere with weight loss. Therefore, you must also avoid your allergenic foods if you have food allergies, in addition to linking and balancing your foods. In other words, do it your body's way for both insulin control and allergy control, and you will be able to lose and maintain weight loss.

Your body is wise and will help you control your weight if you work with it using the knowledge and recipes in this book. Keep your insulin levels low and stable on this healthy eating plan individualized for your allergies. Control inflammation by stabilizing your insulin levels, eating anti-inflammatory foods, and gradually reducing your level of body fat. You CAN reach and maintain a healthy weight! Just listen to and work with your body.

---

[16] Hart, Cheryle R., MD and Mary Kay Grossman, RD, *The Insulin Resistance Diet,* (New York: McGraw-Hill, 2001, 2007), 5.

PUTTING PRINCIPLES INTO PRACTICE
YOUR CUSTOMIZED
HEALTHY EATING PLAN

You have read about carbohydrates, fats, factors that influence inflammation, and factors that affect your level of insulin, cortisol, leptin, and other hormones and regulate body fat. Now it is time to translate the principles in the previous chapters into practice. This will allow you to lose weight, control inflammation and improve your health without being hungry or deprived. Listen to your body and individualize the healthy eating plan in this chapter to fit YOU as you read about what to eat, when to eat, and how to combine foods to achieve your goals on the next few pages.

As previously mentioned, when I was preparing to write this book I studied a number of glycemic control and anti-inflammation diet books and evaluated them for their suitability for those with food allergies and gluten intolerance. I looked for diets that provided sufficient food to keep from setting your metabolism at a lower rate than before you started (thus making it harder to lose weight and keep it off), provided enough carbohydrate to support the synthesis of neurotransmitters, and were simple and easy to follow yet offered possibilities for variety and enjoyment to satisfy the psyche as well as the body. I tried the diets myself to the degree that I could within the boundaries of my own food allergies. Unfortunately for the purposes of this book, I am not overweight, but my arthritis gives me an easy barometer with which to gauge how effective diets are at reducing inflammation.

Because I'm not a good weight loss "guinea pig" myself (although I am eating this way for arthritis), I can't speak from recent personal experience on how this system works for weight loss. However, (1) the physiology of this eating plan makes sense, (2) I did lose weight easily and comfortably on a similar eating plan 33 years ago and have kept it off for over three decades, (3) I have some human volunteer "guinea pigs" who I am advising and observing (see pages 269 to 271) and (4) the glycemic control weight loss books on which this book is based say that their diets are effective at helping people reduce their weight permanently and boast hundreds or thousands of satisfied users of the diets. In the near future I plan to revise and expand this book to include a full complement of recipes of all kinds for a wide range of allergy and celiac dietary needs. I'm hoping that before then those of you who use the eating plan in this chapter will give me some feedback on how it works for you and what additional recipes would help you. Please send feedback using the contact form on the www.food-allergy.org or www.foodallergyandglutenfreeweighloss.com websites.

What To Eat and When To Eat It
on Your Healthy Eating Plan

This section is an outline of meals and snacks that will help you control your blood sugar and insulin levels, thus leading to hunger-free weight loss and decreased inflammation. This outline is not set in stone. Read the principles behind this outline on pages 74 to 83 to understand more details of this eating plan and thus know how to modify it to fit YOU. If you have read or will read the previous chapters, they explain the physiology behind how and why this eating plan works. In the interests of simplicity and clarity, however, here is a short didactic outline.

THE PLAN

FOOD UNITS: Use the tables (pages 250 to 261) and recipes in this book to determine how much of each kind of food constitutes one unit of carbohydrate or protein. If you are reading labels and calculating how much food is one unit, use the number of grams per unit given below for your calculations.

Carbohydrate: Choose carbohydrate foods that are low or moderate on the GI scale most of the time. Each unit of carbohydrate contains about 15 grams of carbohydrate, not counting fiber. Thus, if a label says a serving contains 20 total grams of carbohydrate and 5 grams of fiber, that serving is one unit. **TWO UNITS (30 grams) is the maximum amount of carbohydrate that should be eaten at any meal or snack.** Fruits, grain-based foods, and a few starchy vegetables[1] count as carbohydrates. See pages 251 to 256 for a list of foods that count as carbohydrate units and the amount that is one unit. A few people may need to pair each unit of protein with a smaller amount of carbohydrate than 15 grams. However, do start with 15 grams of carbohydrate balanced with each protein unit and see you how do. See pages 31, 75, 91, and footnote 1 on page 36 for more about this individual variation in balancing foods.

Protein: Each unit contains 7 grams of protein and is the amount in one ounce of lean meat, poultry, fish, low-fat cheese, or one egg. Legumes are included in the protein food category rather than being counted as vegetables, with ⅓ cup of legumes being one unit. See pages 257 to 260 for a list of foods that count as protein units. If your meal or snack does not satisfy you with the number of units specified under "Meals and Snacks" below, you can eat more protein to satisfy your hunger. Two to three units of protein per meal may be enough for women and older people, but men and younger women may need more.

---

[1] Do not miss the vegetable section at the end of the carbohydrate foods on page 256. The vegetables that are concentrated sources of carbohydrate and must be counted as carbohydrate units include corn, potatoes, sweet potatoes, plantains, taro roots, and true yam.

Fat: Eat 4 to 5 tablespoons (45 to 55 grams) per day, counting the amount in foods such as meat and cheese and being sure to get ⅙ of your fat intake as omega-3 containing fats over the course of a week. See pages 257 to 261 for a listing of foods that contain a significant amount of fat that must be counted. Fat may be eaten with any meal or snack. Including fat-containing foods in each meal or snack will keep you satisfied longer. If you are using commercially made foods and reading the amount of fat from the nutrition labels, your daily intake of fat should be 45 to 55 grams.

Other foods: Most vegetables are not counted in the categories above and can be eaten in any quantity at any meal or snack. The exceptions among commonly eaten vegetables[2] are corn and potatoes, which count as carbohydrates and must be balanced with protein. See the listing of vegetables on page 256 to determine what serving size of starchy vegetables is one carbohydrate unit. Be sure to eat 5 to 9 servings of fruits and vegetables per day.

MEALS AND SNACKS

EAT FOR BREAKFAST:

> 1 to 2 units of carbohydrate (starch and/or fruit)
> 1 to 2 units of protein or more to satiety

The number of units of protein must be the same as or greater than the number of units of carbohydrate. If this is not enough food to satisfy your hunger, add more protein or vegetables to the point of satiety. Eat breakfast within one hour of arising. If you are on a rotation or very restricted allergy diet, you may wish to eat your dinner menu for breakfast, such as meat and vegetables dressed with oil, adding some carbohydrate if possible. See pages 102 to 114 for breakfast ideas.

EAT FOR SNACKS, 3 snacks per day (or more if needed) 2 to 3 hours after meals. Have snacks at mid-morning, mid-afternoon, bedtime, and at other times if you are hungry[3]:

> 1 to 2 units of protein (unless eating an apple or similar fruit for between meal
>   snacks only; see details in the next paragraph)
> 0 to 2 units of carbohydrate (fruit and/or starch)
> Vegetables if desired, as much as you want

---

[2] Some less commonly eaten vegetables that are concentrated sources of carbohydrate are plantains, sweet potatoes, taro root, yucca (cassava) and true yam.

[3] For more about how often and when snacks should be eaten to control hunger, blood sugar, and insulin levels, see page 61 and the next page.

The number of units of carbohydrate in your snack must be the same or less than the number of units of protein. Dr. Hart advises usually including two types of food in each meal or snack.[4] Therefore, unless you're eating nuts or string cheese while working just because it is snack time, not out of hunger, you might want to include a vegetable if you skip the carbohydrate. An exception to the "protein with each meal and snack" rule is, for between-meal snacks, to eat a moderately sized high-fiber fruit (apple, pear, peach, two plums, or a grapefruit half[5]) from which the carbohydrate is absorbed so slowly that it does not need to be balanced with protein. For the bedtime snack or if you are stressed or especially hungry, don't skip the protein – eat protein even with these fruits.

Snacks are at the core of this healthy eating plan because they make it possible to keep your insulin level low and stable. Hunger means that your blood sugar is low or falling. A snack eaten soon after getting hungry will prevent the release of adrenal hormones that raise insulin levels and make it impossible for you to burn fat. Thus, a small snack eaten in time will keep you in the "burn fat" mode. Snacks also keep you from getting too hungry to be satisfied with moderate-sized portions at your next meal. Be sure to have a snack at least every three hours, especially when you are just starting this eating plan and trying to get your hormone levels stabilized.

See pages 115 to 119 for snack ideas.

EAT FOR LUNCH AND DINNER:

1 to preferably 2 units of protein or more to satiety
0 to 2 units of carbohydrate (starch and/or fruit)
Vegetables if desired, as much as you want

The units of protein must be the same as or greater than the units of carbohydrate. If this is not enough food to satisfy your hunger, add more protein or vegetables to the point of satiety. If you wish to, or must due to allergies, it is all right to eat a meal of only protein and vegetables, but some carbohydrate rounds out the meal and helps you make the serotonin needed for sleep. For lunch and dinner ideas, see pages 120 and 158.

---

[4] If your non-allergic eating plan companions have a cup of sugar-free fruit yogurt for a snack, that is two foods – yogurt and fruit.

[5] This is an updated list of fruits that do not need to be balanced with protein with portion sizes from *The Feel Good Diet*. The fruits currently allowed without protein balancing are 1 apple, pear, peach or nectarine, 4 apricots, 14 cherries, 2 small plums, or ½ grapefruit. Hart, Cheryle R., MD and Mary Kay Grossman, RD, *The Feel-Good Diet,* (New York: McGraw-Hill, 2007), 74, 105.

Principles of Your Individualized
Healthy Eating Plan

The meal and snack outline above should have variety and be individualized to YOU and your food allergies or intolerances. As you follow the principles below in choosing what you will eat, pay attention to how you feel. Then, based on how YOUR body responds, individualize and tweak your eating plan until is works well for you.

PRINCIPLE #1: CONTROL YOUR FOOD ALLERGIES AND/OR GLUTEN INTOLERANCE.

Eating foods you are allergic to causes inflammation which interferes with hormonal stability, good blood sugar control, and weight loss. If your levels of adrenal hormones and insulin are raised by an allergic reaction, that has the same effect as eating too much of a high GI carbohydrate in encouraging your body to deposit fat. Therefore, the most important principle of your healthy eating plan is to avoid gluten if you are gluten intolerant and to avoid all foods to which you are allergic. If your allergies are widespread among foods and/or severe enough to require a rotation diet, rotate all of your foods. (For more about how to use a rotation diet, see *The Ultimate Food Allergy Cookbook and Survival Guide* as described on the last pages of this book). Keep the members of the food families together on the same day of your rotation diet. Rotate oils even if this means you are using an omega-6 oil as your "oil of the day" on some rotation day(s). Spread out whatever anti-inflammatory foods from Dr. Galland's anti-inflammatory superfoods list (pages 262 to 264) you tolerate over your rotation days, placing them with other members of the same food families, so you hopefully get at least some anti-inflammatory foods in your diet each day and in as much variety as your allergies allow.

PRINCIPLE #2: WHEN YOU EAT MATTERS ALMOST AS MUCH AS WHAT YOU EAT.

Do not prolong the overnight fast of sleep unnecessarily. Eat a good protein and carbohydrate and/or vegetable containing breakfast within an hour of arising. Eat three meals and three snacks per day, or more snacks if needed. You may need snacks more often and more than three snacks per day if your blood sugar and insulin levels are fluctuating wildly when you first start this eating plan, or if you are under stress, are having an allergic reaction, or you have a major high-GI dietary slip-up. Ideally, each meal or snack should keep you from being hungry for 2½ to 3 hours. During the day, especially when you first start this eating plan, do not let more than three hours elapse between meals and snacks. Since dinner tends to be the most satisfying meal of the day,[6] if you are not hungry three hours after dinner you can postpone having a bedtime snack until a convenient time before bedtime.

If you become hungry less than two hours after a meal or snack, try to determine why. The first thing to consider is thirst, which can masquerade as hunger. This is not the time to reach for a diet soda, though! It could send you on a hormonal roller coaster, which will make you feel less hungry, but is counterproductive for weight loss. Have a drink that does not contain caffeine or artificial sweeteners such as water or herbal tea, hot or iced.

If you are still hungry several minutes after your drink, the problem is probably hunger rather than thirst. Have a protein-containing snack with some vegetables without further delay to stabilize your blood sugar and keep your insulin level low. (Add a small amount of carbohydrate ONLY if it has been more than two hours since your last meal or snack). Then try to figure out why you got hungry early. Are you under stress or having an allergic reaction? If so, it is affecting your hormones and you may need snacks more often until the situation causing the stress is resolved or the allergic reaction has cleared. Read more about stress on pages 41 to 42 and if possible try to relax using the methods suggested on page 42.

Was your last meal or snack too high in carbohydrate or too low in protein? The balance needed is an individual thing. While Dr. Cheryle Hart, MD recommends linking 15 grams of carbohydrate with 7 grams of protein for most of her patients, she says that a few patients require a lower amount of carbohydrate to balance with each protein unit in order to become and stay satisfied and to lose weight. Barry Sears, PhD recommends eating 9 grams of carbohydrate with each 7 grams of protein, but Dr. Hart maintains this lower amount of carbohydrate can be insufficient for proper neurotransmitter production in some people. It is an individual matter, so again listen to your body and try changing the proportions of the foods the next time you eat the same foods together as a snack. In addition, if you have a previously undetected food allergy to one of the foods, this can cause a hormonal response that results in early hunger. With a little experimentation and by listening to your body, you will be able to keep yourself in better balance.

You may be thinking, "I don't have time for all of these meals and snacks. This is going to disrupt my work schedule!" Indeed, people who get very involved and busy with their work often work through hunger and unintentionally ignore it, thus unbalancing their blood sugar and insulin levels and thereby leading to excessive hunger by the next time they stop for a meal. EAT YOUR SNACKS! They don't have to take long.

---

[6] In the Canadian study discussed on pages 36 to 37, on the glycemic control diet the participants' blood sugar and insulin levels were quite stable after dinner and during the evening hours. This data may a demonstrate why evening can be a less-hungry time of day if you have eaten to control blood sugar and insulin earlier in the day. For the study, see www.montignac.com/en/etude_scient_sur_meth_mont.php

If you are busy and not apparently hungry between meals, just munch on 8 or 10 nuts while you are working for a between-meal snack.[7] If you are aware that you are hungry between meals, take the time to eat an ounce of protein with a little carbohydrate (one 15-gram unit or less) and/or vegetables. Be prepared! Carry along some nuts, an apple or pear, and/or a link-and-balanced snack for between-meal snacks every day. Although between-meal breaks from work are mandated by law, they do not occur in some jobs. You need to find a way to eat between-meal snacks anyway. A friend of mine who is a librarian carries along cheese sticks which are crumbless and can be discretely eaten between clients while she is working at the reference desk.

Make time to eat a protein-containing breakfast every morning within an hour of arising. Get rid of your preconceived ideas about breakfast having to be cereal, pancakes or eggs. For the allergic, meat and vegetables make a good, satisfying breakfast. If you run out of energy mid-morning, you might try a breakfast burrito (recipes on pages 102 to 105) to be sure you get something that will really sustain you. Prepare the burritos in advance and take them with you in the morning if you're short on time. Non-allergic family members or friends who are following this healthy eating plan with you might appreciate the additional meal and snack ideas containing commercially prepared foods in *The Insulin Resistance Diet.*

PRINCIPLE #3: PROTEIN IS ESSENTIAL.

Protein plays a crucial role in a link-and-balance glycemic control eating plan because it is vital to maintaining low and stable insulin levels. Protein promotes satiety that lasts long after a meal. However, if you have kidney disease or have ever been told to limit your protein intake for another reason, do not follow this program. If you need to lose weight, consult your doctor for how to do it.

A Canadian study [8] demonstrated the controlling influence of protein in the diet on hunger. The overweight study participants ate three diets, each for a six day period, with two weeks "off" between the diets. On the first diet they were allowed to eat until satisfied on a low-glycemic diet. The second diet was a standard American Heart Association approved low-fat diet on which they ate until satisfied. While on the low-glycemic index diet they automatically ate 25% less calories than when on the low-fat diet. For the third diet they ate an AHA approved low fat diet with the amount of food restricted to the lower calorie level they had automatically eaten on the glycemic index controlled

---

[7] Consider carrying a small Ziploc™ bag containing a few nuts in your pocket if you are finding it difficult to eat your snacks.

[8] Dumesnil, Jean G, "Effect of a Low-Glycemic Index, Low Fat, High Protein Diet on the Atherogenic Metabolic Risk Profile of Abdominally Obese Men," *British Journal of Nutrition,* 86(2001): 557-568; www.montignac.com/en/etude_scient_sur_meth_mont.php .

diet. The results were that they gained weight on the unrestricted low fat diet. They lost weight on both the low-GI diet and the calorie-controlled low fat diet, but they lost about 50% more weight and almost twice the waist circumference on the glycemic index controlled diet as they did eating the same number of calories of a low-fat diet. Their blood fat, blood sugar and insulin levels were measured on the last day of each diet. On the glycemic index controlled diet their blood sugar and insulin levels showed less pronounced spikes and their triglycerides decreased by about one third. On both AHA diets, their triglycerides increased by about one fourth. To read more details about the study, visit this webpage: www.montignac.com/en/etude_scient_sur_meth_mont.php.

The results of this study showed that by linking protein foods with carbohydrate foods, we can moderate the effect the carbohydrates have on insulin levels and thus lose weight while eating enough food to be satisfied. We can enjoy our favorite foods and consume enough carbohydrates to allow adequate neurotransmitter production. In addition, we reap the health benefits of the vitamins, antioxidants, anti-inflammatory phytonutrients, and fiber found in carbohydrate-containing foods.

With a very few exceptions (i.e. between meal snacks of very high-fiber fruits such as a moderately sized apple, pear, plum, peach, or grapefruit half as listed under "Snacks"), protein foods should be a part of every meal and snack. Here are some good choices:

Lean meat, poultry, and **fish,** and also **eggs** if you are not allergic to them. It is important that the meat be lean because the fat in conventionally raised beef is high in arachidonic acid which leads to the production of pro-inflammatory prostaglandins. (Eat range-fed beef or game meat for a less inflammatory fat profile in your meat). You should eat two or more ounces of meat, poultry or fish or two eggs per meal. Eat one to two ounces per snack or enough to satisfy your hunger. Meat does not have to be eaten plain but rather can be an ingredient in your favorite entrées. See the main dish recipes on pages 137 to 158 and lunch dish recipes on pages 120 to 136 for creative ideas to liven up your meals.

Legumes, or cooked dried beans and peas, are an excellent choice for protein foods because they are also very high in fiber. Although they do contain carbohydrates, a large amount of it is indigestible (fiber) and the remainder comes automatically balanced with protein. In *The Insulin Resistance Diet* Dr. Hart recommends consuming at least ⅔ cup of cooked legumes per meal, ⅓ cup for a snack, or enough to satisfy your hunger if you are still hungry after eating the recommended amounts. By listening to your body's hunger signals after a meal at which you ate slowly enough to take time to experience and enjoy your food, you will individualize your protein intake to your body's needs. Canned legumes prepared without sugar are an ideal quick and easy protein source for meals and snacks.

Low-fat dairy foods are excellent protein sources and can be eaten if you are not allergic to them. If you are allergic to cow's milk, check your allergy testing results with your doctor and see if you can try goat or soy dairy products. As with meat, low-fat dairy products are preferable because they minimize your consumption of pro-inflammatory arachidonic acid and help you stay within the recommended 45 to 55 grams of fat per day. If you are allergic to cow's milk products but can eat goat or soy products, a good choice is plain goat or soy yogurt mixed with fresh or unsweetened canned or frozen fruit and, if you prefer your yogurt sweeter, with a pinch of Protocol for Life Balance™ stevia. (This next generation stevia has very little of the licorice aftertaste that stevia used to have). For non-allergic eating plan companions who can have cow's milk, Dr. Hart recommends fat-free or low-fat no-sugar-added cups of yogurt. (See page 68 for more about the artificial sweeteners in this yogurt. Since the sweeteners come with food – high quality milk protein – they should not destabilize blood sugar and insulin levels). Although some dairy products such as milk contain lactose, this is not a high GI sugar and comes automatically balanced with milk protein. The one-protein-unit serving sizes for the most common dairy foods are 8 ounces of milk, 1 cup of yogurt, or 1 ounce of low-fat cheese. For other dairy products, see the tables on pages 257 to 258. As with the other protein foods above, if you are still hungry after consuming these sizes of servings, eat enough to satisfy your hunger.

Nuts. seeds, and no-sugar-added nut butters are handy and portable protein snack foods that, with the exception of peanuts, are often tolerated by those with food allergies. However, they should be "clean" nuts. Be careful to avoid nuts with gluten-containing flavors and additives if you are gluten-intolerant or have food allergies and to avoid nuts with sugar in their coating. Purists usually eat raw nuts for their perfectly undamaged fat profile. The normal serving size for nuts is one ounce. If you are using this eating plan to control inflammation rather than for weight loss and one ounce doesn't satisfy you, eat more – enough nuts to satisfy your hunger. For weight loss, Dr. Hart recommends eating no more than two ounces of nuts per day because of their high fat content. However, although they do contain more fat than many of the protein foods above, the fat in nuts is anti-inflammatory fat. It is better for your weight to consume a little extra fat in a snack of easily portable nuts than it is to miss the snack and destabilize your insulin level, thus promoting fat storage.

The thing to remember about **the amount of protein eaten** is that it **must be enough to balance the amount of carbohydrate eaten** at the same meal or snack. Satisfy your hunger with more protein if needed but stop eating when you are satisfied rather than stuffed. Whatever you haven't finished can be saved for the next meal or snack and you will enjoy it just as much or more then.

PRINCIPLE #4: CARBOHYDRATES ARE ALSO ESSENTIAL, BUT THE QUANTITY OF CONCENTRATED CARBOHYDRATE FOODS MUST BE CONTROLLED AND BE BALANCED WITH SUFFICIENT PROTEIN AT EACH MEAL OR SNACK.

Carbohydrate foods are essential for good health. They provide a quick source of fuel for our brains which cannot derive energy from other types of food. Plant foods are our only source of fiber, and insufficient fiber in the diet has been associated with insulin resistance.[9] Most of the foods on Dr. Galland's anti-inflammatory food list on pages 262 to 264 come from plants. Thus, very-low carbohydrate, high protein diets deprive us of the foods which are our best sources of vitamins, minerals, bioflavanoids, carotenoids, anti-oxidants and other nutrients vital for good heath.

However, carbohydrate-dense foods such as **breads and grain products** eaten alone can cause spikes in insulin levels, especially if they are high on the GI scale. Therefore, all carbohydrate-dense foods need to be eaten with protein, and most of the time they should be chosen from foods low or intermediate on the glycemic index. To achieve balance, for every 15 grams of carbohydrate in a meal or snack, you should consume 7 grams of protein at the same time. This is the core principle of the link-and-balance method of controlling blood sugar and blood insulin levels. On pages 251 to 256 you will find a listing of serving sizes for carbohydrate foods (with one unit approximately equaling 15 grams of carbohydrate) and on pages 257 to 260 you will find a similar list for protein foods (with one unit approximately equaling 7 grams of protein), Use these lists to make food choices for balanced meals and snacks. **Do not eat more than 2 units (30 grams) of carbohydrate-dense foods per meal or snack.** More than 30 grams of carbohydrate eaten at once and not used for physical activity within two hours will result in the deposition of fat. If you get hungry in less than two hours after a meal, you should have a protein snack with vegetables but do not consume more concentrated carbohydrate foods.

Although **vegetables** contain carbohydrates, with a few exceptions, they are not carbohydrate dense. They contain fiber which moderates the absorption of the carbohydrates and they also contain a fair amount of water. Therefore, most of them need not be balanced with protein. There are few carbohydrate-dense vegetables which are exceptions to this rule (**corn, plantains, potatoes, sweet potatoes, taro root and true yams**) and they **must be balanced with sufficient protein.** You may eat the other, non-carbohydrate-dense vegetables in unlimited amounts to satisfy hunger. Be sure to eat enough fruits and vegetables – at least five servings per day according to Dr. Hart and nine servings per day according to Dr. Galland – for the anti-inflammatory weight loss-promoting nutrients they contain.

---

[9] Hart, Cheryle R., MD and Mary Kay Grossman, RD, *The Insulin Resistance Diet,* (New York: McGraw-Hill, 2001, 2007), 75.

Some **fruits** are so high in fiber that, according to Dr. Hart, they may be eaten alone for a snack without balancing them with protein. This is because the fiber slows down the absorption of the carbohydrates which they contain. These fruits include apples, pears, peaches, plums and grapefruit; they must be eaten raw, not juiced, not cooked. If you eat them alone, do not eat more than one moderate serving for a snack. If you want a larger serving of these fruits or if you are eating any other kind of fruit, balance the carbohydrate in them with protein as you do for carbohydrate-dense foods. To determine how to balance various fruits with one serving of protein, see the table on pages 251 to 252. Each serving of fruit containing 15 grams of carbohydrate should be balanced with 7 grams of protein. Do not eat more than 30 grams of carbohydrate from all sources combined at any meal or snack.

PRINCIPLE #5: FAT IS ESSENTIAL AND SHOULD NOT BE OVERLY RESTRICTED.

Our bodies cannot make essential fatty acids so we must consume them in the fats we eat every day. How much fat we need can be controversial. Standard American weight loss diets (Weight Watchers,™ American Heart Association recommended diets, etc.) drastically restrict the amount of fat consumed. Even among the glycemic control and anti-inflammatory diet books I consulted there is a wide range of recommendations. Barry Sears, PhD is on the high end of fat recommendations. He recommends that if you have lost all the weight you need to lose and are into a weight maintaining mode, or if you are still hungry after consuming his balanced meals, rather than eating more protein, you should eat monounsaturated fats.[10] (Personally, I doubt that more fat would adequately satisfy me, and there are people who have trouble digesting much fat). At the other extreme, in *The GI Diet,* Rick Gallup limits fat consumption to about two teaspoons per day. He warns that after losing weight on his diet, one's metabolism may have reset to a lower level, and less food may be needed to maintain one's weight than before dieting.[11] In my opinion, this might be the case because his diet, with its strictly controlled portion sizes for all foods (not just carbohydrates) can be lower in fat and calories than is ideal.

The middle-ground recommendations for fat consumption of Dr. Leo Galland, MD are moderate and sensible. He recommends 2 grams of omega-3 fatty acids per day to insure an adequate supply of anti-inflammatory fat in the diet. (This may need to be taken in supplement form such as fish oil by those who are allergic and cannot convert omega-3 oils to their active forms). He instructs that no trans-fats should be eaten and that our dietary fat intake should be about 25 to 30% of our total caloric intake. This translates into about four to five tablespoons of fat per day (or 45 to 55 grams), some of

---

[10] Sears, Barry, PhD, *Mastering the Zone,* (New York, Regan Books, 1997), 37.

[11] Gallop, Rick, *The GI [Glycemic Index] Diet,* (New York: Workman Publishing, 2002), 97.

which occurs naturally in protein foods such as meat and dairy products. In the course of a week's time, dietary fat intake should consist of:

About ⅓ saturated fats eaten in meat and dairy products

About ⅓ monounsaturated fats such as that from heart-healthy olive oil, olives, avocados, almonds, cashews, pistachios, macadamias, hazelnuts and pine nuts, or oils from these nuts and

About ⅓ polyunsaturated fats such as omega-3 fats from fish, fish oil, canola oil, walnuts or walnut oil, and flax seed or flax oil or omega-6 fats such as from sesame seeds and oil, Brazil nuts, grapeseed oil, sunflower seeds or oil, and safflower oil. For those who are not allergic to corn and soy, cold-pressed corn and soy oils are also acceptable omega-6 oils. Omega-3 and omega-6 fats should be consumed in about equal amounts.[12]

Because Dr. Galland says that these proportions are based on a weekly fat intake, do not worry if you must rotate your food oils and consume grapeseed oil or safflower oil on a day or two of your rotation and walnut, canola, avocado, or olive oil on the other days. Rotation and control of your food allergies must take precedence over strictly meeting the ideal percentage of various oils in your diet. Note that his recommendations are for approximate amounts.

Not only are fats essential because you must consume them to get essential fatty acids, but also because we cannot absorb fat soluble vitamins such as vitamins A, D, E, and K without sufficient fats in our diets. Our brains and nerves are sheathed in a layer of tissue that contains about 60% fat and will not function properly if this sheath breaks down. Our cell membranes also depend on fat to give them structural integrity.[13] Although unnatural fats (chemically saturated fats such as trans fats) are unhealthy, natural fat is not our enemy; it is essential for health. Imbalance in the natural fats we consume or the amount we consume is the only problem.

PRINCIPLE #6: FIBER AND PHYTONUTRIENTS ARE ESSENTIAL. EAT PLENTY OF THEM.

In *The Fat Resistance Diet*, Dr. Leo Galland gives one rule for choosing which carbohydrate foods to eat. He says, "When choosing carbs, make sure you get the most fiber and phytonutrients for the calories you consume."[14] Fiber is essential because it slows down the absorption of food from the intestinal tract (thus lowering its glycemic impact), absorbs toxins, and prevents constipation. When my husband greatly boosted his fiber intake by eating two to three bowls of multi-bean soup for dinner every night for over a week when he had a tooth break recently, he felt incredibly stable blood-sugar

---

[12] Galland, Leo, MD, *The Fat Resistance Diet,* (New York: Broadway Books, 2005), 43-45.

[13] Michael Pollan, *In Defense of Food: An Eater's Manifesto,* (New York: The Penguin Press, 2008), 49.

[14] Galland, Leo, MD, The Fat Resistance Diet, (New York: Broadway Books, 2005), 63.

wise. Phytonutrients such as bioflavanoids and carotenoids reduce inflammation and have numerous other health benefits.[15] For a list of foods high in anti-inflammatory phytonutrients, see pages 262 to 264.

PRINCIPLE #7: EAT FREQUENTLY AND IN MODERATE AMOUNTS TO KEEP YOUR BODY FROM USING THE TWO HOUR WINDOW AFTER MEALS TO STORE FAT.

Frequent meals and snacks are essential to controlling insulin levels. Additionally, if you eat frequently, you will naturally be less hungry at each meal or snack, especially after you have followed this eating plan for a while and your insulin levels have become consistently stable. Your body has a 2-hour window after meals in which it determines whether or not to deposit fat.[16] Any carbohydrates from the meal that are not used as fuel during these two hours will be converted to fat for storage. By not exceeding 30 grams (two units) of carbohydrate per meal or snack, you will avoid converting excess carbohydrate into fat for storage. Excess protein and fat above what you use in that two hours can also be deposited as fat within these two hours, but protein is not converted to fat as readily as carbohydrate, and neither of these create a high insulin response which promotes depositing fat by activating the fat storage enzyme lipoprotein lipase.

If you go for long periods of time without eating, your metabolism slows down and your body enters a starvation mode. Then when you do eat, the high insulin levels you have will cause more of what you eat to be stored as fat. After all, your hormones think you are living in a land of famine! Studies show that people who eat at least five times a day are the most successful at achieving and maintaining a healthy weight.

PRINCIPLE #8: STAY WELL HYDRATED.

Thirst can masquerade as hunger. Although the practice of forcing oneself to drink eight glasses of water per day has fallen from favor, be aware of when you may be getting thirsty. If you feel hungry soon after eating, try drinking some water first. I also find that thirst sometimes masquerades as fatigue.

[15] Galland, Leo, MD, The Fat Resistance Diet, (New York: Broadway Books, 2005), 61-63.
[16] Hart, Cheryle R., MD and Mary Kay Grossman, RD, *The Insulin Resistance Diet,* (New York: McGraw-Hill, 2001, 2007), 66.

PRINCIPLE #9: LISTEN TO YOUR BODY

Take note of how long various foods and combinations of foods in meals and snacks keep you from becoming hungry; judge what works best for YOU from these observations. By making adjustments in what you eat based on these observations, you can discover and eliminate previously undetected food allergens, keep yourself from getting hungry early and stabilize your insulin levels. See page 53 for more about how to listen to your body.

GO FOR IT!

See pages 102 to 158 for ideas and recipes to get you started on meals and snacks that implement the healthy eating principles in this chapter. Then be creative, do things your own way, and use the tables on pages 250 to 261 to incorporate your favorite foods into linked-and-balanced meals and snacks. Listen to your body and modify what you eat if it tells you that something is not right. Enjoy eating while you slim down, reduce inflammation, and improve your health on your own individualized healthy eating plan.

PRACTICAL TIPS FOR SUCCESS

If you're read this far, you know what to do to begin and stay on a healthy eating plan. However, a few practical tips may help you further in implementing the plan. This chapter contains information to help you start, persist, and succeed.

The first practical issues you will face when starting this plan are questions like these: "What should I eat for breakfast?" and "It's 10:30 a.m. and I'm getting hungry. What would be a good link-and-balanced snack?" Before you start your healthy eating plan and about once a week thereafter, you must **get organized and plan ahead for what you will eat.** Those of us with multiple food allergies are already accustomed to planning ahead and carrying our own meals and snacks along with us wherever we go. With the wide variety of gluten-free foods now on the market, perhaps gluten-intolerant readers are more like mainstream Americans, buying whatever food they need throughout the day as they go along. This is probably not the ideal way to get good nutrition for anyone, especially with the dubious quality of most processed commercially prepared foods. For those on this healthy eating plan, remember that food processing raises the glycemic index values of carbohydrate foods. Therefore, it is best to chose minimally processed whole foods instead. Optimal nutrition and economy are found in well planned grocery shopping trips, home-prepared meals, and brown-bagged lunches and snacks.

Before you start on this eating plan, take time to look at the meal and snack ideas and recipes in this book. Plan what you are going to eat for the next week, make a grocery list, and shop for what you need. Prepare the foods you will be taking in your lunches and having for snacks. Take nuts and other quick snacks to work and stash them in your desk. If you will be leaving home the next day for more than an hour or two, every evening pack your snack(s) and/or lunch for the next day and put it in the refrigerator, possibly in a brown bag ready to grab and go. That way if anything slows you in the morning, you will still have your safe food with you. Carry non-perishable snacks such as nuts, dried apples or apricots (the lowest GI dried fruits), single-serve packs of nut butter, and medium GI crackers in your car or backpack so you will be ready for a snack at any time. (For blood sugar stabilizing gluten-free cracker recipes see the almond flour crackers on pages 184 to 185 or "Quinoa Sesame Crackers" on page 183). Fresh fruit and vegetables are wonderful accompaniments to the protein foods in your snacks. However, they can't stay in your car or backpack at room temperature forever, so set an apple and small bag of carrots (or whatever fruits and vegetables you prefer or which fit your rotation diet) next to your lunch in the fridge so they're ready to go too.

If you use any commercially prepared foods, you will need to roughly translate the nutrition labels on those foods into link-and-balance units. To calculate carbohydrate units, subtract the grams of fiber from the total grams of carbohydrate for a serving and divide this number by 15. Divide the number of grams of protein by 7 to get the number of units of protein in a serving. Keep in mind that these foods may not be as good for weight loss as home prepared foods because the carbohydrates in them are likely to be highly processed and come from high GI foods such as rice. Even if they are whole grain, the flour may not be stone ground (and thus these may have as high a GI score as their white flour-containing counterparts) and may have been processed in other ways as well.

Your non-allergic eating plan companions may not be used to the constraints of an allergy or gluten-free diet and thus be less inclined to spend time cooking and preparing brown-bag lunches. If they are willing to cook with you, it will give them the best nutrition, but if they elect not to cook (a luxury those with food allergies don't have), tell them to read the "Real World Strategies" chapter of *The Insulin Resistance Diet* by Cheryle Hart, MD and Mary Kay Grossman RD for information about eating out and using convenience foods at home. Although they may not have to do much cooking, they should still prepare for snacks by stocking their desks, cars, and backpacks with non-perishable snacks of protein and low- to medium- GI carbohydrate foods and by having fresh fruits and vegetables ready to take along when they leave.

Motivation is crucial to success in any endeavor. By now you probably have created a list of your reasons and motivations for following a healthy eating plan. After you have been on the eating plan for a short time, in addition to those reasons on your list, **your body may also offer you motivation.** A few months ago I began this eating plan motivated by a desire to help my arthritis. If you have problems with any kind of non-silent inflammation, you will probably find it easy to follow this diet fairly consistently after you've been on it a while. When I stray off course in a major way, my joints tell me loudly and clearly that I should have followed the eating plan instead!

If your main motivation is to lose weight, following the plan consistently could be more challenging because no part of your body tells you to get back in line when you've gone astray. There may be delicious prepared foods and favorite restaurants calling to you instead. Keep that list of reasons why you decided to embark on a healthy eating plan handy and refer to it often! Although you should not weigh yourself or measure your waist often enough to get daily motivation from your body in that way, if you take note of how you feel after eating certain foods, listen to your body, and achieve balance in your blood sugar and insulin levels on this eating plan, you should start feeling more energetic or noticing other changes. If you fall off the plan and eat too much high-GI carbohydrate, you may notice being tired or having other symptoms. Hopefully, remembering how it feels to have stable blood sugar and insulin levels vs. how you feel after eating too much carbohydrate will help you get back on track more easily.

Other people can help or hinder you as you strive to follow your eating plan consistently. If you encounter or live with nay-sayers, summon your "determination" (an advantage of the Savioli personality) and tell them that you have decided this is the way for YOU to slim down, and that it is important for your health. Although I don't favor the type of diet promoted by Weight Watchers,™ their **social support system** is very helpful. If you have a friend or family member who will join you in a health eating plan, the companionship involved in following it together will be enjoyable and a reward that will keep you going. You can congratulate each other on buying smaller clothes and encourage each other to get back on track quickly when you fall off.

Many of us live with non-allergic people or have wheat-eating friends who might join us on a healthy eating plan. Therefore, this book contains a few wheat and milk containing recipes for "normal" eating plan companions on pages 238 to 249. I also recommend that they read *The Insulin Resistance Diet* by Cheryle Hart, MD and Mary Kay Grossman, RD for more meal and snack ideas and for the tables which contain foods not included in this book.

Moderation is important. Counting calories does not work for weight loss; what is important is whether your body burns food (and body fat) for energy or deposits what you eat as fat. However, even if you have low and stable insulin levels and are in the "burn" mode, if you eat much more than you can burn in the next two hours, the excess will be stored as fat. Therefore, do pay attention to how much you eat, especially to eating **not more than 2 units of carbohydrates at any meal or snack.** If you get hungry in less than two hours after a meal or snack, you may need another snack to stabilize your blood sugar (see page 61 for more about this) but it should be a protein snack (possibly with vegetables) and should not contain more concentrated carbohydrate. In addition, hidden fat in foods can fool you! Stick to 4 to 5 tablespoons (or 45 to 55 grams) of fat per day from all sources as recommended by Dr. Galland. (See page 81 for more about this). Don't be paranoid about fat, but be sure to count the fat hiding in foods such as full-fat dairy products and fatty meats. Control portion sizes of these foods to **keep your fat intake at the right level** (4 to 5 tablespoons or 45 to 55 grams total per day). The fat in conventionally-produced animal foods contains a high level of arachidonic acid, so be moderate with these fats. Although nuts are also high in fat, their fat is "good" anti-inflammatory fat. From an energy-in vs. energy-out standpoint, the fat in nuts should be controlled too, but from an inflammation and blood sugar/insulin-control standpoint, if you need nuts for a non-perishable, portable snack, don't miss your snack because you are stressing the amount of fat too much. Becoming so excessively hungry that you enter a hormonal cascade which triggers insulin release will cause more fat to be deposited more readily than eating a few nuts will.

Once your blood sugar and insulin levels are consistently in good control, your hunger level will be a good indicator of how much food you really need, and exercising moderation in how much you eat will come naturally.

Be your own best friend. Even if you have a supportive family and friends and/ or a companion who also is following the eating plan, you can benefit from some TLC from yourself. Be kind to yourself. If you go off the diet for a meal or a day, don't think you have failed or beat yourself up over it. There is nothing sinful about eating several cookies or a half-bag of potato chips! Just pick yourself up, eat some protein to start rebalancing your insulin and blood sugar levels, re-read the list of reasons you started on the eating plan, and go back to it.

Cut yourself some slack. If you will be in a social situation where you will find it difficult to stay on the eating plan, give yourself permission to indulge in moderation in whatever is served that your food allergies or intolerances allow. If you are feeling deprived, plan a controlled splurge on a favorite food (see pages 61 to 62 for more about this) and enjoy it to the hilt. You will go back to the eating plan with renewed determination and optimism especially if the feelings of deprivation resulted from low neurotransmitter levels in your brain which have just been boosted by chocolate.

Part of being your own best friend might be removing that judgmental bathroom scale from your life. Weight fluctuates with water retention, menstrual periods, etc. and even though you may be doing everything right, your scale might not reflect this, leading to discouragement. Although "to weigh or not to weigh" is a personal decision and something you should do your own way, I'd encourage you to weigh yourself infrequently (as in once a month at the most) or never. If you want something to measure to monitor your progress, use a tape measure instead. On this eating plan, the goal is to decrease body fat and build muscle instead. Muscle is heavier than fat, so there may be times when you notice little or no change in your weight while you really ARE slimming down. Your waist measurement is a much better indicator of real progress of losing fat than your weight. But again, measure your waist only once a month or once very two months. Patience is a virtue for healthy (slow and steady) slimming down. Or better yet, just notice how your clothes are fitting. When they loosen up, you're making progress!

One of the most practical tips for succeeding on your eating plan is to **eat a substantial protein-containing breakfast within an hour of arising in the morning.** Your mother was right. Breakfast really is the most important meal of the day. After preaching this to my family for years, as mothers tend to do, I recently discovered just how important breakfast is myself. I have always eaten breakfast, but not always in the first hour after getting up. My husband likes to eat about 9 a.m. on the weekend, so on weekends I'd have a good link-and-balanced pre-breakfast snack and then eat my normal meal with him. On weekdays, my habit was to get up early and email my sons at school, return emails from friends and those who had visited my website, fill orders that had come in since the previous day, and spend the first couple of hours of the day on the computer. I usually would get an apple or other fruit plus nuts to eat while working on the computer but I didn't have a REAL breakfast until I'd been up for a couple of hours.

While I was typing this book, I began to wonder about some connections between what I was writing and my own health. While talking to a friend who is a nutritionist with a PhD in biochemistry about new supplements to treat intestinal dysbiosis, I mentioned that I had just gotten my first bottle of Penzey's Vietnamese cinnamon and loved it so much that I'd eaten it generously sprinkled on fresh fruit three days in a row. Then, thinking that I ought to rotate cinnamon, I had taken a few days off from it and not felt as well. I asked her what she thought about it having anti-microbial properties in addition to its ability to improve insulin resistance. She told me that when some of her clients got their blood sugar under control, it would often lead to an improvement in intestinal yeast, and that maybe I should consider consuming the cinnamon every day for a while, which I began doing. Two days later, while working in the kitchen after writing most of the day, I realized that I had typed "eat breakfast within one hour of arising" in more than one place since I had spoken to my friend, and that I wasn't doing it myself! I wondered if perhaps my blood sugar isn't as stable as I assumed and, if so, a change in my breakfast time might have the same effect as cinnamon on dysbiosis by stabilizing my blood sugar. In addition, I don't have to worry about sensitizing to "eat breakfast early" like I might to cinnamon. The next morning I ate my usual breakfast of game meat and vegetables a half hour after getting up and had an energetic day. Now I'm trying to make early breakfast a habit. Whether this will "cure" intestinal dysbiosis[1] for me remains to be seen, but it certainly can do me no harm.

Breakfast can seem like a problem for people with food allergies in general. I frequently receive calls from people who have recently been diagnosed with food allergies and can no longer eat Wheaties™, Cheerios™, pancakes, eggs, or bacon. They feel like there's nothing left to eat for breakfast. When these people call in the future, if they are convinced they don't have blood sugar issues, I may continue to tell them about rotating buckwheat pancakes, quinoa granola, millet mush, etc. However, an all-carbohydrate breakfast is not what readers of this book need. **Put aside your preconceived ideas about breakfast being composed of only traditional breakfast foods and all others foods being only for lunch and dinner.** If you are on a rotation diet, it will save work to begin your rotation day at dinnertime and eat leftovers for breakfast the next day. I eat game meat and vegetables every morning, and I enjoy them. They energize me and give me the strength I need to start my day. See pages 102 to 114 for new breakfast ideas. If you are looking for a substantial breakfast that can be made ahead and eaten on the run, try the breakfast burritos recipes on pages 102 to 105.

I know some people feel that they just can't face food first thing in the morning, but I hope that you will try to eat a small link-and-balanced snack or meal an hour or so after you get up. Perhaps as your health improves due to being on the healthy eating plan, your morning appetite will improve. I admit that it's easier to eat breakfast when you've been awake long enough to be really hungry for it, but try doing it "on schedule" for a week or two and see if you notice a difference. Eating meals before you're starved helps with portion control as well.

---

[1] See *The Ultimate Food Allergy Cookbook and Survival Guide* as described on the last pages of this book for more about food allergies and dysbiosis.

Exercise, properly employed, can be of great value for slimming down. Choose types of exercise that you enjoy, and if possible, do them in an enjoyable place. If you are under stress, exercise can help you relax and moderate the effect of stress hormones that otherwise might lead to depositing fat. (For more about stress, see pages 41 and 42). However, conventional weight loss math notwithstanding, more exercise is not always better. If you are sedentary, do begin a moderate exercise program such as regular walks as described on page 266. However, if you are already exercising more than a few hours a week, you may need to exercise less and in a way that encourages your body to burn fat.

Exercise before breakfast or when you are hungry right before dinnertime encourages the burning of muscle for fuel. Decreasing muscle mass in this way decreases your metabolic rate and makes weight loss more difficult. Therefore, always exercise after a carbohydrate and protein containing meal or snack. (Carbohydrate is the only food that gives quick energy so it should be included in what you eat before exercise). Too much aerobic exercise is also counterproductive. Do not do more than 25 minutes of aerobic exercise at a time. That is because we use up our glycogen stores in the first 25 minutes; and then if we keep exercising, we will break down muscle protein to use for fuel. Doing 25 minutes of aerobic exercise three days a week will keep your metabolic rate up at a higher level all week, and that should be your limit for aerobic exercise. If you want to burn more fat, participate in moderate exercise on the other days of the week. Examples of moderate exercise include gardening, housecleaning, brisk walking, and moderately paced bicycling or swimming. Monitor your pulse to differentiate what is aerobic activity from what is moderate exercise. (To calculate your target pulse rate for aerobic activity, see page 265). Exercise that produces a rise in pulse that is lower than your target rate and allows you to carry on a conversation is moderate exercise. Even when intermittent, moderate exercise is the best kind of exercise for burning fat.[2] See pages 42 and 265 to 268 for more about exercise.

Foods and supplements are other factors that can help you succeed at slimming down. **Cinnamon** helps to decrease insulin resistance and stabilize insulin levels.[3] Use ¼ to ½ teaspoon per day on or in your food. The studies done on cinnamon and insulin all used the cassia variety of cinnamon, which is the most common variety in the United States. However, if you want something delicious as well as to know exactly what variety of cinnamon you are using, try Penzey's extra-fancy Vietnamese cinnamon, which is a cassia cinnamon, for a real treat. Other types of cinnamon also have a moderating effect on insulin, so if you like a milder, fruity cinnamon, you may enjoy Penzey's Ceylon cin-

---

[2] Hart, Cheryle R., MD and Mary Kay Grossman, RD, *The Insulin Resistance Diet*, (New York: McGraw-Hill, 2001, 2007), 191-197.

[3] Campbell, Amy, "Can Cinnamon Help You Control Your Diabetes?" *Diabetes Self-Management Blog*, October 10, 2006.

namon instead. Ceylon cinnamon is preferable for those taking anticoagulant medications. To get Penzey's cinnamon, see "Sources," page 282.

If you have an apple-shaped body type, you are genetically predisposed to producing a high level of cortisol. Under a doctor's supervision, you might want to try **cortisol moderating supplements.** Our allergy doctor, who is a nutritionally-oriented MD, recommends Relora™, a magnolia bark supplement, to moderate cortisol levels. Additional supplements that may be used for cortisol control include epimidium and phytosterols.[4] Ask your doctor before taking these as well. Phytosterols are also found in plant foods, so you can improve your status on them by eating more fruits and vegetables.

5-hydroxy-tryptophan (5-HTP) is a form of the amino acid tryptophan which leads to the synthesis of the neurotransmitter serotonin and helps to control appetite and improve mood and sleep. Take 30 to 50 mg of 5-HTP on an empty stomach one half to one hour before dinner. 5-HTP is not effective if taken with food.[5]

Supplements for general nutritional support may also be helpful when you are trying to slim down because they give your body the tools it needs to process food properly, use insulin effectively, etc. People with food allergies or celiac disease often have compromised intestinal absorption and therefore may be low on nutrients needed for insulin function such as chromium, vitamin D, and vanadium, or omega-3 fatty acids which are needed to control inflammation, and other vitamins and minerals that help with weight loss. Dr. Galland has developed a supplement called Metabolic Co-Factors™ to help his patients who are following his "fat resistance diet" to lose weight. (See "Sources," pages 281 to 282, for more on how to get this supplement, which is very "clean" allergy-wise). In addition to the nutrients in Metabolic Co-Factors™, he and the authors of almost all the books I studied recommend fish oil supplements to control inflammation, thus promoting weight loss. If you don't want to take several or many pills each day, a supplement that provides all of the nutrients mentioned above in only two capsules is Carlson Lab's Nutra-Support Diabetes Formula™. (See "Sources," pages 281 to 282, for information about getting this supplement also).

TROUBLESHOOTING YOUR HEALTHY EATING PLAN

The best way to know if your healthy eating plan is right for you and is working well is to listen to your body. Paying attention to how you feel in relation to when and what you eat is the best way to evaluate and fine tune the balance of your eating plan and your insulin and blood sugar levels. When your insulin is stable, you should not be experiencing excessive or early hunger. If you feel more energetic and have also noticed improvement in inflammatory health conditions, your body is telling you, "This eating

[4] Beale, Lucy and Joan Clark, RD, CDE, *The Complete Idiot's Guide to Glycemic Index Weight Loss,* (New York: Alpha, 2005), 228-229.

[5] Ibid., 229.

plan is good for me!" If your goal is weight loss, occasionally take note of whether your clothes are beginning to fit more loosely or use a tape measure to monitor your waist measurement.

If your blood sugar and insulin levels are stable, you should not be having cravings for sweets or rich foods. Of course, if someone presents you with a plate of freshly baked cookies, normal appetite will make you want to sample them! However, craving sweets without this type of external stimulus indicates a problem. Either your blood sugar and insulin levels are not stable or you are having cravings due to food allergies or candidiasis. Try to remedy this by eating a link-and-balanced snack as often as you are hungry, or at least every three hours, and always having protein with each meal or snack, even if it is something like an apple that does not usually require protein balancing. Dr. Cheryl Hart reports that chromium deficiency is often associated with sugar cravings, so recommends 200 to 400 mcg per day of chromium polynicotinate.[6] If you are taking one of the general nutritional support supplements listed on the previous page, you will get enough chromium plus other nutrients that have been shown to help stabilize blood sugar. Make sure the carbohydrates you eat have low or moderate scores on the glycemic index. Finally, try eating one unit of carbohydrate with meals or snacks rather than two. If these changes do not help the cravings, a consultation with a doctor who treats food allergies and candidiasis may be in order. (To find the right doctor who "believes in" food allergies and treats candidiasis, visit the AAEM website at www.aaemonline.org and also see the advice on the next page).

In *The Insulin Resistance Diet* Dr. Cheryle Hart, MD gives some advice for troubleshooting your healthy eating plan that many would find surprising.[7] Ironically, she describes having patients who cannot lose weight because they are not eating enough! They skip breakfast and the between-meal snacks she advises. Therefore, although they are eating what most low-calorie dieters would consider ideal for weight loss, their bodies are in the "starvation mode" of holding on to whatever they eat. Their insulin levels are high, their bodies conserve fat stores, and if much energy is needed for exercise or other physical exertion, they burn muscle protein for energy. The advice she gives them is to eat a link-and-balanced breakfast shortly after arising every day, eat more frequently, having a snack or meal every two to three hours, and to link and balance protein and carbohydrate at each meal and snack. Thus, their bodies will be liberated from "starvation" and burn the food they are eating, as well as stored fat, for energy.

In *The Fat Resistance Diet,* Dr. Leo Galland, MD also describes patients who came to him eating 1200 calories a day and not able to lose weight. They were invariably poorly nourished and as he improved their diets, they began losing weight and improving their health problems while eating more food.

---

[6] Hart, Cheryle R., MD and Mary Kay Grossman, RD, *The Insulin Resistance Diet,* (New York: McGraw-Hill, 2001, 2007), 94.

[7] Ibid., 221.

Of course, the opposite – eating too much – can also interfere with weight loss. This can happen when a person is impelled by appetite rather than by physical hunger to eat more than their body really needs. If you are not overweight and are following this healthy eating plan to control inflammation, by all means, eat enough to satisfy your appetite, but if you need to lose weight and are not losing after a few months on the diet, begin to keep careful tabs on how much fat you are eating and limit your fat intake to the recommended 45 grams per day, being sure to count the less-obvious fat you may not be aware of in foods such as dairy products and meats. Consider that you might be one of the people described three paragraphs above who require a lower carbohydrate intake to achieve balance, and reduce your carbohydrate intake to one unit of low or moderate GI carbohydrate per meal or snack if eating too much fat is not the problem. Also keep in mind that for everyone, hormones are in control of whether you store or burn fat, so do not ignore actual physical hunger, which is a signal that your blood sugar is low or falling which may cause the release of adrenal hormones followed by a fat-depositing insulin spike. For a personal look at eating for appetite, see *A Tale of Two Dieters,* on pages 269 to 273.

If you are listening to your body and following its cues for eating neither too much nor too little and at the right time, yet you are not feeling more energetic, nor experiencing improvement your inflammatory health problems or finding that your clothes are looser after a few months on your healthy eating plan, I suggest reading the "Appetite vs. Hunger" and "Troubleshooting" sections of *The Insulin Resistance Diet* by Dr. Cheryle Hart, MD and Mary Kay Grossman, RD. If you are still not able to figure out what the problem is, you may have medical issues that are interfering with weight loss such as thyroid dysfunction[8] or undiagnosed food allergies. A visit to a holistic, nutritionally-oriented doctor may be in order. Avoid doctors who are very "conventional" and do not believe in food allergies, are not aware of the glycemic index, or are likely to recommend a standard low-fat low-calorie diet. If you don't already have a good primary health care provider, I would recommend visiting the AAEM website (http://www.aaemonline.org/) and calling the offices of the doctors in your area to research them and/or anyone else they might recommend for a general check-up and advice on weight issues.

---

[8] Not all thyroid dysfunction will show up on simple blood tests for thyroid hormones such as T3 and T4. In cases of Wilson's syndrome, the test results may be normal but the thyroid hormone is not properly active. This is another good reason to see a more holistic doctor such as those you will hopefully find on the AAEM website.

IN SUMMARY

If we make good nutrition and optimal health our primary goals, normal weight should follow. It will not happen overnight, so be patient and remain optimistic. To achieve ideal health we need to control our blood sugar and hormone levels by eating balanced meals and snacks often enough. It is also essential to reduce inflammation by eating anti-inflammatory foods (see the list on pages 262 to 264) and taking supplements such as omega-3 fatty acids, as well as by controlling insulin levels. As our health improves, we can achieve and maintain normal weight and gain new energy and enthusiasm for life.

The Key is in the Kitchen
Cooking for Success

The previous chapters explained how to eat to control blood sugar, hormone levels and inflammation and thus how to achieve and maintain normal weight and optimum health. This chapter offers practical advice for eating this way when we must superimpose the requirements of our food allergy or gluten-free diets. Because of our allergies or intolerances, our diets must be individualized. This means you probably must do some cooking, but with knowledge and organization, it can be easier than you imagine. What happens in the kitchen is crucial to good health.

The first step in taking charge of your eating is planning. Review the recipe ideas on pages 102 to 158 and decide what you want to eat for meals and snacks for the next week. When you begin, keep your meals and snacks simple to make things easier; expand your repertoire after you are well organized and accustomed to your healthy eating plan.

After you have decided what you will eat, use your chosen menus for meals and snacks to make a grocery shopping list. Be sure to list the foods you will need for snacks. They are just as important – or more so – as meals. (Perhaps the snack foods part of the list can be duplicated from week to week, thus saving you effort the next time you plan your shopping). Add the ingredients necessary for your meals to the list. Initially, you may be stocking your kitchen with flours and other non-perishable items needed for the recipes. As you become established in cooking for your healthy eating plan, the foods on your weekly grocery shopping list will probably consist mostly of foods purchased for near-immediate use such as fresh produce, frozen vegetables, dairy products (or tolerated alternatives), meat, poultry, or fish. For maximum efficiency, grocery shop once a week right *after* a meal so you are not hungry and can stick to your list without being distracted by tempting displays of high GI foods.

Plan which meals to have on which days with your schedule in mind. If you regularly arrive home shortly before dinner, plan to cook on the weekend and stock your freezer with meals to eat during the week. Every weekend make a large batch or two of entrées or entire meals. Divide the leftovers into meal-sized portions and freeze them. After a few weekends of doing this, you will have an assortment of your favorite dishes frozen and will not have to eat the same thing two consecutive nights. Each evening remove an entrée or meal from the freezer and put it in the refrigerator to thaw. The following day when you arrive home, you just have to heat the meal and possibly cook a vegetable and prepare a salad.

When you will be away from home for more than a few hours, prepare ahead for the snacks and lunches you will need while you are gone. The evening before, make your lunch and organize the snacks you will need the next day. Put them in your refrigerator, ready to grab and go the next morning.

Special Ingredients for Low GI Baking

Most of the ingredients used in this book are staples in allergy and celiac diet cooking. However, there are a few ingredients that are uniquely and especially useful for low GI cooking which are discussed below. (For more about all of the ingredients used here, see *Allergy and Celiac Diets With Ease, Gluten-Free Without Rice,* or the other books described on the last few pages of this book). Becoming familiar with and using these special low GI ingredients will enable you to make delicious foods that you will help you lose weight on your healthy eating plan.

ALMOND FLOUR: Nuts are nutritious, low GI additions to your healthy eating plan. They are a good source of protein, healthy fat, vitamins and minerals. Almonds have the added advantage of being available in a flour form that can be used in baking. Not all almond flour is suitable for baking however. It must be made from blanched (skinless) almonds and be very finely ground.[1] In addition, most recipes made with almond flour require eggs, a problem for those allergic to eggs. However, a flaxseed egg substitute (see page 237 for the recipe) can be substituted in some of the almond flour recipes here. Almond flour should be stored in the refrigerator or freezer to keep the fat from becoming rancid. Of the several types of finely-ground blanched almond flour available online, I prefer Honeyville™ almond flour because it is most economical and also excellent for baking. See "Sources," page 281, to purchase this flour.

HIGH PROTEIN NON-GRAINS such as **BUCKWHEAT, QUINOA** and **AMARANTH** are especially versatile and used in many recipes in this book. They are gluten-free and have low GI scores[2] when eaten as cooked whole grains, unlike some of the more common gluten-free grains such as rice.[3] None of them are members of the botanical family of true grains, and although they are cooked as grains, they are technically seeds. Thus they are higher in protein than true grains. Allergies to quinoa and amaranth are uncommon; buckwheat allergies are slightly more prevalent because it is more commonly eaten.

Quinoa is one of the best protein sources among plant foods, containing 16 to 23 percent protein and all nine essential amino acids. It is also a good source of minerals such as magnesium, phosphorus, and manganese, B vitamins, vitamin E, antioxidants, and fiber. When preparing whole quinoa, be sure to rinse off the natural soap-like coating on the seeds before cooking it as directed in the recipe.

---

[1] Bob's Red Mill™ almond flour/meal is too coarse to work in most of the recipes in this book, which is unfortunate because it is widely available. See "Sources," page 281, to purchase almond flour that gives good results in baking recipes.

[2] The source of this information is www/mendosa.com/gilists.htm. The GI of cooked whole buckwheat groats is 45, quinoa is 53, and data is not available for amaranth, but it is similar in composition to quinoa, its botanical cousin.

[3] The source of this information is www/mendosa.com/gilists.htm. Several types of cooked brown (whole grain) rice listed on the table in this website have high GI scores.

Flours made from all three of these plants add superior nutritional value and variety to gluten-free diets. Quinoa and buckwheat make tasty high protein gluten-free yeast breads. (See the recipes on pages 189 to 192). All three flours are tasty and versatile in a wide variety of recipes for non-yeast baked goods and treats which are included in this book.

HIGH FIBER FLOURS such as **HI-MAIZE™ CORNSTARCH** and **SUSTA-GRAIN™ BARLEY** are helpful for blood sugar stability because their fiber slows the absorption of carbohydrates. Hi-maize™ cornstarch contains 6 grams of fiber in a mere 1½ tablespoons of starch; Sustagrain™ barley has three times the soluble fiber of oats. These ingredients can be purchased from the King Arthur Flour Baker's Catalogue. (See "Sources," page 278).

SWEETENERS such as **AGAVE** and **STEVIA** are two relatively new arrivals to the health food market that allow us to enjoy sweet treats without destabilizing our blood sugar levels (although agave should be eaten in moderation). Agave has a GI score of between 11 and 32, depending on the source. Since stevia is a natural non-nutritive sweetener, it has no impact on blood sugar. In fact, the herb it comes from is promoted as an aid for diabetes. This herb is *Stevia rebaudiana* and is a member of the composite (lettuce) family. It has been used in Japan, Paraguay, Brazil, and other parts of the world for hundreds of years. Furthermore, it is approved by the FDA for use as a supplement and as an "additive" in soda pop, although they have ruled against labeling it as a sweetener. It is available in several forms; the white powder is used in the recipes in this book because it is the purest form of the sweetening agent found in the plant. Most stevia has a slight licorice-like taste which may be noticeable in bland recipes but is almost undetectable in recipes containing strongly flavored ingredients. However, recently "next generation" white stevia powder has been introduced that is treated during production with an enzyme that reduces the licorice taste. The stevia recipes in this book were developed using the purest[4] of the new stevia powders which is made by Protocol for Life Balance.™ The amount of stevia in a recipe may be given as a range because the perception of how sweet stevia tastes varies from person to person. There is also variation between brands of stevia. See "Sources" pages 282 to 283 for information about obtaining Protocol for Life Balance.™ pure stevia powder and page 280 to order measuring spoons which you can use to measure ⅛, ¹⁄₁₆ and ¹⁄₃₂ teaspoon amounts of stevia.

Although the **LEAVENING INGREDIENTS** used in this book are not unique to glycemic control recipes, they are different from those used in most celiac cookbooks and allergy cookbooks. Because most baking powder contains cornstarch and corn is a common allergen, most of the baking recipes in this book contain a built-in baking powder of baking soda and **UNBUFFERED VITAMIN C POWDER OR CRYSTALS.**

---

[4] Many of the "next generation" stevia powders are cut with allergenic ingredients such as maltodextrin, which comes from corn. Protocol for Life Balance™ stevia is pure stevia extract with no additional ingredients added.

When purchasing vitamin C to use for leavening, be sure that the vitamin C powder or crystals that you use are unbuffered i.e., they do not contain minerals to moderate their acidity. Because the role of vitamin C in leavening is to provide acid, buffered vitamin C will not make your baked goods rise properly. If you are allergic to corn, also make sure your vitamin C is corn-free. See "Sources," page 280, for information about ordering cassava-source unbuffered vitamin C.

Stabilizers such as **GUAR GUM** and **XANTHAN GUM** are commonly used in gluten-free baking. They can be substituted for each other in the same amount. I use them only in recipes where they are absolutely essential for leavening, such as in yeast breads, because they are ingredients to which people often develop new allergies. In addition, xanthan gum is made from a bacteria, *Xanthamonas compestris*, which is grown on a corn-based medium. Therefore it is usually not tolerated by individuals who are allergic to corn. Guar gum comes from a bean and is often not tolerated by those who are allergic to soybeans or other beans.

I suspect that most readers of this book are on restricted diets and out of necessity have become experienced in allergy or gluten-free cooking. However, if you need a wider variety of recipes or more information about special ingredients or cooking, see the books listed on the last few pages of this book.

Techniques for Success in Baking

Baking is the area of allergy and gluten-free cooking which generates the most questions. Therefore, although this may be review for some readers, I am including some baking basics here:

The first basic for success in special diet baking is having the correct ingredients. High quality flour that is consistent from bag to bag will save you money, time and trouble in the long run. Arrowhead Mills™ and Bob's Red Mill™ are brands that I use and recommend for most types of alternative flour. If you are can tolerate spelt, always use Purity Food™ brand flour. I have encountered more variability in spelt flour than in other types of flour, and it is not worth it to save a few pennies by purchasing an unknown brand from a health food store bulk bin if you end up with bread that no one wants to eat. If you use other brands of spelt flour for non-yeast baked goods, you will have to add more flour than the recipes here call for and expect less satisfactory results. If you use them for yeast bread, don't be surprised by collapsed loaves. For baking with almond flour, use finely ground blanched flour such as Honeyville™ brand. The widely available almond flour/meal made by Bob's Red Mill™ is not finely ground enough to use in baking. See "Sources," pages 279 and 281 for information on ordering Purity Foods™ spelt flour and Honeyville™ almond flour.

Be careful about purchasing other ingredients also. As mentioned above, if you are leavening your baked goods with baking soda plus vitamin C, be certain that the vitamin C powder or crystals that you use are unbuffered and, if you are allergic to corn, are corn-free. (See "Sources," page 280, for information about ordering cassava-source unbuffered vitamin C). If you purchase gluten-free baking mixes, be sure to read the label carefully every time because the ingredients may have changed.

The second basic for success in baking is accurate measuring of ingredients. Use the correct measuring cups for the ingredient you are measuring – nested sets for flour and other solids ingredients and glass or clear plastic cups with markings for liquids. To measure flour, stir the flour to loosen it. Using a large spoon, lightly spoon the flour into the cup. Level it off with a straight edged knife or spatula. If you are measuring an amount of flour for which you do not have a measuring cup, such as ⅝ cup, use the table of measurements on page 275 to determine how to measure. In this case, measure by using ½ cup plus ⅛ cup.

To measure liquids, fill the cup with liquid until the meniscus (the bottom of the curve of the liquid) lines up with the line on the cup of the amount you want to measure. Move so you can read the cup at eye level as it sits on your counter. If your recipe calls for several liquids, you can save yourself the time of washing an extra bowl by measuring and mixing them all in the same measuring cup before adding them to the dry ingredients. For example, if you need 1 cup of water, ¼ cup of apple juice, and ¼ cup of oil, add water to the 1 cup line on the measuring cup, apple juice to the 1¼ cup line, and then add oil to the 1½ cup line. Then stir the liquids together thoroughly in the cup immediately before adding them to the dry ingredients.

To measure small amounts of flour, starch, salt, baking powder, spices, and other dry ingredients with measuring spoons, dip the spoon into the container, stir up the ingredient to loosen it, and fill the spoon generously. Pull it out and level it off with a straight edged knife or spatula, or level spices using the straight edge of the hole in the spice container. To measure small amounts of liquids, pour the liquid into the measuring spoon until it is level with the top of the spoon. Do not let it bead up over the top of the spoon.

At least the first time you make a recipe, follow the recipe exactly to insure success. Substitutions in baking often do not work on the first try or the first several tries if you are changing the flour. For more about ingredient substitutions, see pages 272 to 274.

The third baking technique crucial to success is proper mixing. Because the types of flour used in special diet baking produce a more fragile structure which must trap the gas produced by the leavening, how you mix non-yeast baked goods and how quickly you get them into the oven is very important. Before you begin baking, preheat your oven. Prepare the baking pans ahead of time; oil and flour them with the same oil and flour used in the recipe. Mix the dry ingredients together in a large bowl and the liquid ingredients together in your measuring cup or another bowl. Working quickly, stir the liquid ingredients into the dry ingredients until they are **just mixed.** It is critical that you do not mix for too long or the leavening will produce most of its gas in the mixing bowl rather than in the baking pan in the oven. Only stir until the dry ingredients are barely moistened; a few floury spots in your batter or dough are all right. As soon as you have mixed just enough, quickly put the batter or dough into the prepared baking pans and pop them into the preheated oven.

The recipes in this book made with almond flour involve stiffer batter than for the flours above and may contain flaxseed egg substitute, so the mixing technique is different. Stir together the dry ingredients as above. Use a hand blender to combine the flaxseed egg substitute (which is very thick) or egg with the other liquid ingredients. Then add the liquids to the dry ingredients. In addition to stirring, you may need to mash them together with the spoon if, for example, you are making stiff cracker dough.

To test quick breads, muffins, and cakes for doneness, insert a toothpick into the center of the pan. If it comes out dry, it is time to remove the pan from the oven. Most baked goods should be removed from the pan immediately after you take them from the oven, but some fragile cakes and cookies benefit from cooling in the pan for about 10 minutes. The recipe will tell you when to do this. Allow your baked goods to cool as directed in the recipe before you slice them or store them in a bag. While plastic bags and containers are great for storing most baked goods, crackers will stay crisp if you store them in a metal tin.

The final and best tip for cooking is to enjoy what you have made and the improved health that results from following your healthy eating plan.

About the Recipes

This portion of the book contains recipes and ideas for meals and snacks to help you get started doing it your way as you develop a repertoire of foods you enjoy eating on your healthy eating plan. These chapters do not contain an exhaustive list of things you might eat, they are just a sample. Do not limit yourself to these recipes and ideas; variety is the basis of good nutrition as well as the spice of life. I am planning future books which will offer you more recipes for your healthy eating plan. However, recipe development takes considerable time, and I did not want to delay this book until a comprehensive recipe collection was ready to be included. While you are waiting for more recipes, be creative. It is not difficult to adapt your favorite main and side dish recipes to fit the link-and-balance guidelines on page 71.

Readers who have cooked for gluten-free diets may find the style of the recipes in this book different from other recipes they have used. In traditional gluten-free cookbooks, it is common to see baking recipes that call for a dozen or even twenty ingredients. The goal of these recipes is to produce baked goods which are as much like conventional foods as possible; this is done by using several flours together and small amounts of many stabilizing ingredients. A celiac friend assures me that these recipes do taste better, but there are trade-offs in terms of both time and allergies. If you bake with simpler recipes and do not eat the same set of flours and stabilizers every day, you are less likely to develop an allergy to ingredients you use often. Furthermore, using recipes with fewer ingredients will save you time on measuring.

The ingredient lists for the recipes in this book are shorter than in some allergy and most gluten-free recipes books. Thus, it takes less time to measure and make the recipe. In addition, when the ingredient list contains only the items which are absolutely necessary, those with food allergies are more likely to be able to use the recipe without leaving something out or trying to make a substitution. (See pages 272 to 274 for more about making substitutions in baking). In addition, when an allergic reaction occurs after a meal and you only ate a few foods rather than a dozen or more, it is much easier to figure out which food was the problem.

Some recipes in this book contain ingredients which some readers do not tolerate. Rather than overly restricting the diet of less-sensitive readers to the level of the most allergic, a wide variety of recipes is given. Most recipes have options for ingredient choices that will allow more people to eat them. If you have severe food allergies and do not find a recipe that you can tolerate for a certain food in this book, you may be able to find one in *The Ultimate Food Allergy Cookbook and Survival Guide,* a book for the most allergic of people, which is described on the last pages of this book.

TAKE THE NUMBERS WITH A GRAIN OF SALT

At the end of each of the recipes in this book you will find a list of how many carbo-hydrate and/or protein units and how much fat a serving of the recipe contains. In spite of these numbers, you should **listen to your body** rather than falling back into the trap of counting and tallying points, calories, or grams. Nutritional information is offered at the end of each recipe because the units of carbohydrate and protein per serving, with the serving size, will help you to link and balance protein and carbohydrate in your meals and to keep the amount of carbohydrate at 2 units (30 grams), thus maintaining your body in a "burn fat" mode. The grams of fat per serving is given to help you keep your total fat intake per day at a moderate level.

The nutrition facts on commercially prepared foods can be used to link and balance protein with carbohydrate. To calculate the carbohydrate units from the nutrition facts, subtract the grams of fiber from the total grams of carbohydrate to get the grams of net carbohydrate. Then divide that number by 15 to get the number of carbohydrate units in one serving of the food. You may need to adjust the serving size to achieve proper balance with protein in your meal or snack. To calculate protein units from the nutrition facts, divide the grams of protein by 7 to get the number of protein units in one serving of the food. Again, you may need to adjust the serving size.

In addition, keep in mind that all nutritional analyses, including those on commer-cially prepared foods, are approximations. There may very well be variations between the ingredients used and those that were tested to reach the data on which the nutritional calculations were based. For example, a freshly picked carrot will contain much more vitamin A precursor (beta-carotene) than a carrot that has been sitting in cold storage for several months. Therefore, nutritional analyses should be taken with a grain of salt.

In some of the recipes here, the nutritional analyses are also approximate because you are given ingredient choices or because the ingredient amount is given as a range. When such choices exist in a recipe in this book, the grams of fat and carbohydrate and protein units were calculated[1] using the first ingredient given in a list where there is a choice and with any optional ingredients omitted. Where a range in the amount of an ingredient is given, the nutritional analysis was based on the first amount given.

Now it's time to cook and enjoy eating what you've cooked!

---

[1] The nutritional analyses of the recipes in this book were calculated using *Food Processor for Windows, Version 7.7,* by ESHA Research, Inc., P.O. Box 13028, Salem, OR 97309.

BREAKFASTS

Your mother was right – breakfast is the most important meal of the day. It is especially vital for those trying to control their blood sugar because breakfast breaks the fast of sleep and gives your body fuel for the first few hours of the day. Variety in your breakfasts provides good nutrition as well as helping prevent the development of new food allergies. When someone says to me, "I've eaten oatmeal every morning for years," I suspect oatmeal is an allergy problem for that person.

Break away from the idea that proper breakfast foods are only cereal, eggs, bacon, toast, etc. Leftovers from dinner the day before are a great high-protein breakfast that will get your day off to a good start. If you start your rotation day at dinner time and make enough food to have leftovers, you will have a rotated breakfast ready in the morning, and you will be well nourished and out the door in record time.

Although this book is written for those with food allergies – and eggs are a common food allergen – the recipes in this chapter include eggs and dairy products for those who can have them, such as gluten-intolerant but non-allergic individuals. Both eggs and dairy are good sources of protein and contribute many nutrients to the diets of those who tolerate them. If you are allergic to cow's milk, check your allergy testing results with your doctor and see if you might be able to try goat, soy, or other alternative milk products. (However, be aware that rice milk is low in protein and has a high GI score).

In addition to the recipes in this chapter, other breakfast menu ideas include:

Cooked grains such as quinoa or teff, recipes on pages 160 to 163, with some meat such as lean sausage (recipe on page 105) and fresh fruit

Muffins, crackers, or toasted yeast or non-yeast bread (recipes on pages186 to 196) with nut butter, cheese, or scrambled or hard-boiled eggs

And as mentioned above, leftover meat and vegetables or other entrées from the previous night's dinner make a great breakfast.

Use the recipes and ideas in this chapter to discover how delicious and satisfying breakfast can be!

TRADITIONAL BREAKFAST BURRITOS

**Gluten-Free IF
made with GF tortillas**

This recipe is for one burrito because some people do not like eggs re-warmed in the microwave oven. However, if you're not too fussy or on a rotation diet, you can make a large batch (such as a five to seven-times batch) and have a breakfast burrito waiting in the fridge, ready to microwave, every day of the week.

1 tablespoon chopped raw onion (optional)

1 teaspoon oil (optional)

¼ cup chopped cooked vegetable of your choice such as broccoli or asparagus

1 ounce, or about ¼ cup, chopped ham, Canadian bacon, or cooked sausage, recipe on page 105 (optional)

1 to 2 eggs

1 teaspoon milk (optional – may be omitted or you may substitute an alternative type of milk)

Dash of salt if you are not using a salty meat such as ham or bacon

1 ounce, or about ¼ cup, grated cheddar cheese (optional, any type such as goat, soy, or cow's milk cheese, preferably low fat)

1 or more whole-grain tortillas which are allowed on your allergy or gluten-free diet containing 30 grams or less of net carbohydrates (or for your non-allergic companions, try Tumaro's™ Low-in-Carbs tortillas)

If you are not using the onion, you can omit the oil and cook this recipe in a non-stick pan if desired. If you are using the onion, sauté it in the oil in a frying pan until it is soft and just beginning to brown. Add the cooked vegetables and meat to the pan and heat them through. In a bowl, beat the egg(s) with the milk and salt if you are using them. Pour the egg mixture into the frying pan and cook, stirring occasionally, until the eggs are set. Remove the pan from the heat and stir in the cheese. Warm the tortilla(s) for a few seconds in the microwave to soften and, if you are using an 8 or 10-inch tortilla, roll the filling in it to form a burrito. For 6-inch tortillas, pile the fillings on the tortilla(s) and eat it with a fork. Makes 1 serving. Before adding the tortilla, if made with one egg and no meat or cheese, this breakfast contains 1 protein unit, and 9 grams of fat; with two eggs and no meat or cheese it contains 2 protein units and 15 grams of fat. Adding one ounce of cheese adds 1 protein unit and as many grams of fat as nutrition label for the package indicates. Adding one ounce of meat adds 1 protein unit and as many grams of fat as nutrition label for the package indicates. Also add carbohydrate units from the package of the tortilla you use. With two thin or one thick 6-inch corn tortilla add 1 carbohydrate unit; with a Tumaro's™ Multi-Grain Low-in-Carbs tortilla add 1 protein unit and ⅓ carbohydrate unit. (This is net carbohydrate; you will also get 8 grams of fiber).

Note on corn tortillas: If you are not allergic to corn, you may want to use corn tortillas in this recipe because they are gluten-free. If you purchase the thin "frying" variety rather than the thicker "bread" variety of tortillas you will get less carbohydrate. Read the nutrition label on the back of the tortilla package to determine how many (2 or 4) tortillas contain 30 grams of net carbohydrate (total carbohydrate grams minus grams of fiber). I use Mission™ Extra Thin Yellow Corn Tortillas which contain 28 grams of net carbohydrate in 4 tortillas (about 2 carbohydrate units).

EASY EGG-FREE BREAKFAST BURRITOS

Gluten-Free IF
made with GF tortillas

You can make these burritos in large batches and store them in the freezer or refrigerator for a quick on-the-go breakfast. A triple batch will prepare you for an entire work week.

Italian style

2 ounces cooked ground beef (about ⅝ cup)
½ cup cannellini beans, drained (about ⅓ of a can)
3 tablespoons to ¼ cup spaghetti sauce or pizza sauce, recipe on page 233
Dash of sweet basil (Omit if you are using the pizza sauce).
½ teaspoon dry minced onion or a dash of garlic salt or to taste (optional)
2 ounces or about ½ cup grated mozzarella cheese (optional, any type such as goat, soy, or cow's milk cheese), preferably part-skim or low-fat
2 10-inch tortillas which are allowed on your allergy or gluten-free diet containing 30 grams or less of net carbohydrates, preferably whole grain (For your non-allergic companions, try Tumaro's™ Low-in-Carbs tortillas).

Mexican style

2 ounces cooked ground beef (about ⅝ cup)
⅓ to ½ cup cooked vegetables such as peppers (mild, hot, or a mixture) and onions
¼ cup salsa
Dash of sweet basil
½ teaspoon dry minced onion or a dash of garlic salt to taste (optional – Omit if onions are included in the vegetables you are using).
2 ounces or about ½ cup grated cheddar cheese (optional, any type such as goat, soy, or cow's milk cheese), preferably low-fat
2 10-inch tortillas which are allowed on your allergy or gluten-free diet containing 30 grams or less of net carbohydrates, preferably whole grain (For your non-allergic companions, try Tumaro's™ Low-in-Carbs tortillas).

In a bowl combine the cooked beef, vegetables, sauce or salsa, and seasonings. Stir in the cheese. Divide the mixture in half and roll each half in an 8 or 10-inch tortilla, or if you are using 6-inch tortillas, put the filling on the tortillas and eat with a fork. Heat briefly in the microwave oven before serving. Makes 2 servings each of which, without the tortilla and cheese, contains 2 protein units, and 8 grams of fat. With two thin or one thick 6-inch corn tortilla(s) add 1 carbohydrate unit to a serving; with a Tumaro's™ Multi-Grain Low-in-Carbs tortilla add 1 protein unit and ⅓ carbohydrate unit (net carbohydrates; you will also get 8 grams of fiber) to each serving. If you use the cheese add one protein unit and the number of grams of fat the package indicates for one ounce of cheese.

Note on corn tortillas: If you are not allergic to corn, you may want to use corn tortillas in this recipe because they are gluten-free. If you purchase the thin "frying" variety rather than the thicker "bread" variety of tortillas you will get less carbohydrate. Read the nutrition label on the back of the tortilla package to determine how many (2 or 4) tortillas contain 30 grams of net carbohydrate (total carbohydrate grams minus grams of fiber). I use Mission™ Extra Thin Yellow Corn Tortillas which contain 28 grams of net carbohydrate in 4 tortillas.

BREAKFAST SAUSAGE PATTIES

`Gluten-Free`

Although both types of sausage below are usually made with pork, and as such can be high fat, they are also delicious made with leaner meat such as turkey.

Traditional sausage

> 1 pound ground white-meat turkey, buffalo, or other lean meat
> 2 to 3 teaspoons fennel seed, or to taste
> ½ teaspoon salt
> ½ teaspoon pepper, to taste (or use more for more anti-inflammatory effect)

Chorizo sausage

> 1 pound ground white-meat turkey, buffalo, or other lean meat
> 1 to 2 teaspoons finely minced garlic, or to taste (optional)
> 2 to 3 teaspoons oregano
> ½ to 1 teaspoon cayenne pepper, or to taste (optional)
> ½ to 1 teaspoon salt
> ½ teaspoon pepper, to taste (or use more for more anti-inflammatory effect)

Chose one set of ingredients above. Mix the ingredients together thoroughly with your hands and shape them into four patties. If you are using a high-fat meat or a tender meat, turn the broiler on to 450°F. Put the patties on a broiler pan and broil them for ten minutes on each side, turning them halfway through the cooking process. (The total cooking time is 20 minutes).

If you are using a low-fat or less tender meat such as game meat, arrange the patties in a single layer in a large frying pan and brown them on both sides over medium heat. Add water to a depth of ¼ to ½ inch. Cover the frying pan with a lid. Cook the sausage patties over medium heat for about ½ hour or until the water has all evaporated. Uncover the pan and continue cooking the sausage until the patties are well browned. This cooking method yields exceptionally tender and delicious turkey sausage. Leftover sausage freezes well and can be re-warmed quickly and easily in the microwave. Makes 4 servings, each of which contains 3 protein units and 8 grams of fat if made with lean ground turkey.

ON THE GO SMOOTHIE

Yogurt smoothie

> 1 cup non-fat or low-fat plain yogurt of any type you tolerate (goat, sheep, cow, or soy yogurt)
>
> ½ to ⅔ cup of strawberries or other fruit to yield about ⅓ cup pureed fruit
>
> ¹⁄₁₆ teaspoon pure white stevia powder such as Protocol for Life Balance™ brand (optional, to taste) OR 1 tablespoon agave, Fruit Sweet™ or single-source honey, to taste (optional)

Cottage cheese smoothie

> ½ cup skim milk
>
> ½ cup 1% or 2% cottage cheese
>
> ½ to ⅔ cup of strawberries or other fruit to yield about ⅓ cup pureed fruit
>
> ¹⁄₁₆ teaspoon pure white stevia powder such as Protocol for Life Balance™ brand (optional, to taste) OR 1 tablespoon agave, Fruit Sweet™ or single-source honey, to taste (optional)

Choose one set of the above ingredients. Puree the fruit with a blender or hand blender. Add the yogurt or milk plus cottage cheese and optional sweetener and blend until smooth. Makes one serving. The yogurt smoothie contains ⅓ carbohydrate unit if strawberries are used, 2 protein units and 0 grams of fat if made with non-fat yogurt or 4 grams of fat if made with low-fat yogurt. The cottage cheese smoothie contains ⅓ carbohydrate unit if strawberries are used, 2½ protein units and 1 gram of fat.

BANANA BREAKFAST SMOOTHIE

This is a good way to use up those over-ripe bananas. Just peel them, break them into chunks, put the chunks in a plastic bag, and pop them into the freezer. They'll be ready for breakfast when you are.

> 1 6-ounce carton non-fat or low-fat plain or no-sugar fruit yogurt of any type you tolerate (goat, sheep, cow, or soy yogurt)
> ¼ to ½ frozen small banana, cut into chunks (Use the smaller amount if you are also using other fruit).
> ½ cup strawberries or other fruit (optional)
> ½ cup milk, preferably non-fat, of any type you tolerate (cow, goat, soy, etc.)
> $\frac{1}{16}$ teaspoon pure white stevia powder such as Protocol for Life Balance™ brand (optional, to taste) OR 1 to 2 tablespoons agave, Fruit Sweet™ or single-source honey, to taste (optional)
> 1 teaspoon vanilla (optional)

Put all of the ingredients into a 4-cup measuring cup or the cup that comes with a hand blender or into the bowl of a blender or food processor. Blend until smooth. Makes one serving which contains ⅔ to 1 carbohydrate unit, 2 protein units and 0 grams of fat if made with non-fat yogurt.

BERRY-ORANGE BREAKFAST SMOOTHIE

> 1 cup non-fat or low-fat plain yogurt of any type you tolerate (goat, sheep, cow, or soy yogurt)
> ½ to 1 cup frozen unsweetened strawberries or other berries
> ¼ cup orange juice
> $\frac{1}{16}$ to ⅛ teaspoon pure white stevia powder such as Protocol for Life Balance™ brand OR 2 to 3 tablespoons agave, Fruit Sweet™ or single source honey, to taste (optional)

Put all of the ingredients into a 4-cup measuring cup, the cup that comes with a hand blender, or the bowl of a blender or food processor. Blend until smooth. Makes one serving which contains ⅔ to 1 carbohydrate unit, 2 protein units and 0 grams of fat if made with non-fat yogurt.

Maple-Flavored Pancake Syrup

If you love maple syrup but want to avoid its unsettling effect on your blood sugar, here is an alternative that contains almost no carbohydrate. Enjoy the syrups in this and the following recipes on French toast (pages 110 to 111) or ice cream (pages 220 to 221).

2 tablespoons plus 1 teaspoon Signature Secrets Culinary Thickener™
    OR 1 teaspoon arrowroot OR 1½ teaspoons tapioca starch
1 cup water
Non-nutritive sweetener equivalent to 12 teaspoons of sugar – ⅛ to ¼ teaspoon
    pure white stevia powder such as Protocol for Life Balance™ brand, to
    taste, OR 1 to 1¼ teaspoons liquid saccharin, to taste, OR 6 packages
    Equal™ or an equivalent amount of any other non-nutritive sweetener**
½ teaspoon maple flavoring
½ teaspoon vanilla extract

If you are using the Signature Secrets™ thickener, combine it with the water in a 4-cup measuring cup, the cup that comes with a hand blender, or the bowl of a blender or food processor. Blend for a minute or two until thoroughly combined into a syrupy liquid. If you are using the arrowroot or tapioca starch, mix it with the water in a saucepan and bring it to a boil. Allow it to boil for a minute or so until it becomes clear and thickens.

Mix the sweetener and flavorings into the thickened water. Store any syrup you do not use immediately in a jar and refrigerate. Shake it thoroughly before serving it again. Makes about 1 cup of syrup, or 8 two-tablespoon servings each of which contain negligible carbohydrate (1 gram or less per serving) and no protein or fat.

* **Note on instant thickeners:** Signature Secrets™ thickener is made from a corn derivative similar to cornstarch but which does not need to be cooked. To order this thickener, see "Sources," page 280.

**Note on non-nutritive sweeteners: Most non-nutritive sweeteners do not taste like sugar, but those that taste the best have the most health drawbacks. Stevia is a potently sweet herb which has been used in Japan in diet foods for 40 years and for centuries in South America. It has a long track record of safety, but some brands have a licorice-like aftertaste. In some recipes such as the next for fruit syrup, this taste is masked by other ingredients. Saccharin has also been used for many years. Dr. William Crook, author of the well known series of *Yeast Connection* books, felt that saccharin is acceptable in moderation and has a place in a low-yeast diet. Aspartame (Nutrasweet,™ Equal™) has a history of causing headaches in many individuals, especially among the allergic, and is possibly implicated in even more serious problems when used in large amounts.

Fruit Pancake Syrup

Gluten-Free

The bright fruit flavor of this syrup makes the taste of stevia undetectable, especially if you use a "next generation" stevia such as Protocol for Life Balance™ brand.

½ pound fresh or frozen strawberries or blueberries (about 2 cups of fresh berries)

1 cup water, or ¾ cup if you are using tapioca or arrowroot and wish to serve the syrup immediately

⅛ to ¼ teaspoon pure white stevia powder such as Protocol for Life Balance™ brand, to taste*

1 to 2 tablespoons Signature Secrets Culinary Thickener™ OR 1 teaspoon arrowroot or tapioca starch

If you are using the arrowroot or tapioca starch, put the fruit, water, stevia, and starch in a saucepan. Mash or use a hand blender to partially puree some of the berries. Bring this to a boil and simmer one minute until it is thickened and clear. If you want to serve it immediately, use ¾ cup of water. Since this batch makes many servings, I make it ahead with 1 cup of water, which results in a good syrup consistency after refrigeration.

If you are using the Signature Secrets Culinary Thickener,™ add 1 tablespoon of the thickener to the water, blend it with a hand blender, blender or food processor and let it stand a couple of minutes. If it is not thick enough for you, add more of instant thickener and blend it. Add the fruit (thawed if you are using frozen fruit) and stevia and partially puree the fruit.

Serve the syrup immediately or store any syrup you do not use right away in a jar in the refrigerator. Stir it before serving it again. Makes about 1¾ to 2 cups of syrup or 14 to16 two-tablespoon servings, each of which contain negligible carbohydrate (about 1 gram per serving) and no protein or fat.

*Note on stevia:** Start with the smaller amount of stevia and taste the finished syrup. Thoroughly stir or blend in more stevia if needed. The amount needed will depend on the sweetness of the fruit.

Note on instant thickeners: Signature Secrets Culinary Thickener™ is made from a corn derivative similar to cornstarch but which does not need to be cooked. To order, it see "Sources," page 280.

MAKE AHEAD FRENCH TOAST

**Gluten-Free IF
made with GF bread**

4 to 5 1 to 1½-ounce slices of any bread which you tolerate on your diet,
    preferably whole grain

4 eggs

⅓ cup skim, whole, or goat milk

1 teaspoon agave, Fruit Sweet™, or single-source honey OR ⅟₃₂ teaspoon pure
    white stevia powder such as Protocol for Life Balance™ brand (optional)

1 teaspoon vanilla extract (optional)

Dash of salt

1 to 2 tablespoons butter, goat butter, or Earth Balance™ non-hydrogenated
    margarine for buttering the toast and greasing the baking dish

Toast the bread lightly, allow it to cool, and butter it on both sides. Lightly butter a
9 by 13 inch baking pan, preferably made of glass. Arrange the toast in the pan; if the
slices don't quite fit, piece in partial slices so the whole pan bottom is covered. Beat the
eggs lightly. Then add the milk, sweetener, vanilla, and salt to the beaten eggs and mix.
Pour this mixture over the toast in the baking pan and refrigerate for at least four hours,
or up to 36 hours. Preheat your oven to 350°F. Bake for 35 to 45 minutes, or until the
French toast is browned and puffed up. Makes 4 servings, each of which contains 1 carbohydrate unit, a little over 1 protein unit and 10 grams of fat.

NUTTY FRENCH TOAST

**Gluten-Free IF
made with GF bread**

4 eggs, lightly beaten

⅓ cup milk

2 teaspoons agave or 1 stevia spoon* of pure white stevia powder such as
    Protocol for Life Balance™ brand (optional)

¼ teaspoon salt

1 teaspoon cinnamon

1 teaspoon vanilla extract (optional)

½ cup almond, hazelnut or pecan meal or flour (more coarsely ground meal
    will work as well as finely ground nut flour)

1 to 2 tablespoons oil (preferably olive) or butter

4 slices of whole grain bread which you tolerate on your diet or of 100% stone
    ground whole wheat bread, pages 239 to 240, for your non-allergic
    companions**

In a flat bowl, lightly beat the eggs. Add the milk, sweetener, salt, cinnamon, and vanilla and beat again. Stir in the nut meal or flour thoroughly. (Either Bob's Red Mill™ coarse almond meal, the nut meals from King Arthur Flour™, or finely ground blanched almond flour will work in this recipe). The batter settles, so stir it between dipping slices so most of the nut meal or flour isn't left at the bottom of the bowl when you are finished.

Heat the oil or butter in a large skillet. Dip the slices of bread into the batter, turn them to coat the other side of the bread, and add them to the skillet. If it looks as if you will have more batter than you need, pour a little on the tops of the slices. When the bottom of the slices brown, turn them and cook the other side. Stir the batter each time before dipping more bread in it. Makes 4 servings each of which contains 1 carbohydrate unit, 2 protein units, and 12 grams of fat.

***Note on the amount of stevia:** The bottles of Protocol for Life Balance™ brand stevia and several other brands of white stevia powder come with a very small plastic measuring spoon that gives sweetness equivalent to 1 to 2 teaspoons of sugar. Use that spoon for this recipe

**Note on the bread: If you are cooking this for both a gluten-free or allergy diet and also for wheat-eating companions, first dip the special diet bread into the batter and cook it. Then dip the whole wheat bread and cook it in the same pan.

Eggs Benedict

**Gluten-Free IF
made with GF bread**

Preparing the light hollandaise sauce below in a microwave oven makes this gourmet breakfast recipe easy as well as lower in fat than using traditional hollandaise sauce.

> 2 whole grain English muffins or slices of any whole grain bread you tolerate on your diet
> 4 one-ounce slices of Canadian bacon
> About 1 teaspoon oil or butter
> 4 large eggs
> "Light and Easy Hollandaise Sauce" on the next page

If you are using English muffins, split them in half. If you are using bread and you wish to reduce the amount of carbohydrate per serving, use a large (3½ inch) biscuit cutter to cut rounds out of the bread slices. Toast the muffins or bread. Place the Canadian bacon on a dish to microwave or in a skillet to heat it. Oil or butter the cups of an egg poaching pan or four silicone egg poachers. (See "Sources," page 279, to order these from King Arthur Flour). Measure the ingredients for the hollandaise sauce into a bowl, except for the lemon juice and salt.

Bring water to a boil in the bottom of the poaching pan or in a sauce pan if you are using silicone egg poachers. Microwave or warm the Canadian bacon. Break the eggs into the cups of the pan or the silicone egg poachers. Gently place the silicone egg poachers in the boiling water in the saucepan. Cover the pan with its lid. While the eggs are poaching, prepare the sauce as directed in the recipe below.

While the sauce is microwaving, place the toasted muffins or bread on serving plates. Top each with one slice of Canadian bacon. When the eggs are cooked, loosen them from the cups with a spoon and place them on the Canadian bacon. Top with hollandaise sauce. Makes 4 servings each of which contains 1 carbohydrate unit, 2 protein units, and 11 grams of fat.

LIGHT AND EASY HOLLANDAISE SAUCE

Gluten-Free

Hollandaise sauce is low in fat when made with yogurt. Try this on broccoli or asparagus for a special treat!

> 2 teaspoons tapioca starch or arrowroot
> Pinch of white pepper, or black pepper if white is not available (optional)
> 1 tablespoon water
> 1 cup plain yogurt of any type you tolerate, preferably non-fat or low-fat
> 1 large egg, lightly beaten
> 1½ tablespoons butter, cut into pieces
> 1 tablespoon lemon juice
> Dash of salt

In a glass bowl, stir together the starch, pepper, and water. Add the yogurt and slightly beaten egg and whisk with a wire whisk. Put the bowl in the microwave oven and microwave on high power for three minutes, whisking well after each minute of cooking, or until the mixture is thickened. (Don't worry if the mixture looks curdled when you first remove it from the microwave before you have whisked it. It will become smooth as you whisk). Add the lemon juice and salt, whisk again, and microwave for an additional 30 seconds. Whisk and serve.

Makes about 1½ cups of hollandaise sauce, enough for about three recipes of "Eggs Benedict," above, or 12 2-tablespoon servings, each of which contains 2 grams of fat if made with nonfat yogurt or 3 grams of fat if made with whole milk yogurt. If you don't mind using half an egg for this sauce and having part of the egg left over, you can halve this sauce recipe. I prefer to make a whole batch and refrigerate the leftover sauce in a glass jar to serve with future meals. Re-warm leftover sauce in the microwave, beating it with a wire whisk to make it smooth.

Vegetable Frittata

Gluten-Free

Zucchini frittata was a Sunday night dinner staple during the summer when I was a child. However, this frittata is equally delicious made with other vegetables. Cheese adds a little more protein but is not essential. (Our summer dinners were cheese-free because my dad was allergic to milk). This quick dish is great for breakfast as well as for a light lunch or dinner.

> 1 small zucchini (5-6 ounces) OR one half of a 10-oz package of frozen
>   chopped broccoli OR about 1 cup of cooked asparagus
> If using the broccoli or asparagus, ⅓ cup chopped mushrooms (optional)
> 1 to 2 teaspoons olive oil or butter
> 4 large eggs
> 2 tablespoons milk (optional)
> 1 tablespoon grated Romano cheese (optional, with zucchini)
> Dash of salt (omit if you are using the Romano cheese)
> 1 to 1½ ounces or about ½ to ¾ cup shredded low-fat cheese – part-skim
>   mozzarella (good with zucchini) or low-fat cheddar, Swiss, or Monterey
>   Jack (optional, any type you tolerate such as goat, soy, or cow's milk cheese)

An hour or so before or the night before you plan to make this dish, remove the broccoli from the freezer. Put it in a strainer to thaw and drain. Put the strainer in the refrigerator if you thaw the broccoli the night before making this frittata.

Shortly before mealtime, beat the eggs. Add the optional milk, Romano cheese, or salt and beat again briefly. Set the eggs aside.

Thinly slice the zucchini or mushrooms if you are using them. Cut the asparagus into 1-inch pieces if you are using it. Put the oil or butter into an 8-inch skillet and add the zucchini or mushrooms. Cook the zucchini until it begins to brown, turning it to brown both sides, or sauté the mushrooms until they are tender. If you are making a broccoli-mushroom or asparagus-mushroom frittata, add the broccoli or asparagus to the pan after the mushrooms are cooked. Then stir, and heat through. If the oil or butter seems completely absorbed, add the second teaspoon of oil or butter. If you are using only the broccoli or asparagus, put the vegetables into the pan with the oil or butter and heat through.

Spread the vegetables evenly in the bottom of the skillet. Gently pour in the eggs and cover with the skillet's lid. Cook over medium heat for 2 to 3 minutes. Remove the cover and lightly stir the eggs so that the liquid egg reaches the bottom of the pan. This should result in the eggs being mostly cooked. Cover the pan again and cook just until the eggs are set. When the eggs are set, remove the pan from the heat, sprinkle with the grated cheese, re-cover the skillet, and set it aside for a minute or two until the cheese melts. Cut the frittata into two pieces to serve two. If you wish to serve four, double the recipe and cook it in a 10-inch skillet. For one serving, halve the recipe and cook it in a 6-inch skillet. If made with the cheese, each serving contains 2⅔ protein units and 19 grams of fat. Without the cheese, each serving contains 2 protein units and 15 grams of fat.

This recipe or a half batch of the recipe may also be cooked in an omelet pan. When the eggs are set, sprinkle the cheese on one side of the pan and fold it in half to melt the cheese.

HAM, CHEESE, AND POTATO FRITTATA

Gluten-Free

2 tablespoons chopped onion (optional)
2 tablespoons chopped bell pepper (optional)
1 to 2 teaspoons olive oil or butter
¾ cup cooked diced new red potatoes
⅓ to ½ cup diced ham
4 large eggs
2 tablespoons milk (optional)
1 to 1½ ounces or about ½ to ¾ cup shredded low-fat cheddar or Monterey
    Jack cheese (optional, any type you tolerate such as goat, soy, or cow's milk
    cheese)

Beat the eggs and milk and set them aside. Put 1 teaspoon of the oil or butter into an 8-inch skillet and add the onion and pepper. Sauté until they are tender. Add the potatoes and ham and heat through. If the oil or butter is absorbed, add the additional teaspoon of oil or butter. Spread the mixture evenly in the skillet. Gently pour in the eggs and cover with the skillet's lid. Cook over medium heat for about 2 to 4 minutes. Remove the cover and stir the eggs so that the liquid egg reaches the bottom of the pan. This should result in the eggs being mostly cooked. Cover the pan again and cook just until the eggs are set. When the eggs are set, remove the pan from the heat, sprinkle with the grated cheese, re-cover the skillet, and set it aside for a minute or two until the cheese melts. Cut the frittata into two pieces to serve two. If you wish to serve four, double the recipe and cook it in a 10-inch skillet. For one serving, halve the recipe and cook it in a 6-inch skillet. If made with the cheese, each serving contains 3½ protein units, 1 carbohydrate unit (if made with the potatoes) and 18 grams of fat. Without the cheese each serving contains 3 protein units, 1 carbohydrate unit (if made with the potatoes) and 17 grams of fat.

SNACKS

Snacks are a pillar of your healthy eating plan because they are vital to controlling your blood sugar and hormone levels. Eating often is essential on this plan, so easy ideas of what to have for a snack are welcome. Most of the time we want a quick snack that doesn't require much preparation. This chapter includes a list of quick and easy snack ideas below, plus recipes for snacks that are special enough for you to share with guests.

EASY SNACK IDEAS

Fresh fruits that may be eaten alone (not linked and balanced with protein) such as an apple, pear, peach, two plums or a half grapefruit. These must be eaten raw and unprocessed (i.e. not made into juice).

Raw apple or pear slices sprinkled with cinnamon, preferably Penzey's spicy Vietnamese cinnamon. (See "Sources," page 282, to purchase this special treat).

Nuts or seeds, alone or eaten with fruit. To get one protein unit, have ¼ cup of sunflower seeds, 1 ounce of peanuts or pumpkin seeds, 1½ ounces of cashews, almonds, shelled pistachios or walnuts, or 3 ounces of pecans or macadamia nuts,

Cheese of any kind. String cheese comes pre-packaged in the right size (one ounce) for a single serving, and one-ounce single-serving cheddar cheese sticks are also sold in larger grocery stores.

GORP – mixtures of nuts and raisins or other dried fruits. Mix the amounts of nuts given above with two tablespoons of raisins or other small or cut-up dried fruit. Use fruit dried without sugar.

A serving of any fruit with nut butter or cheese. The only limit on combinations is your imagination. Here are some examples:

> An apple with one or more ounces of cheddar cheese or string cheese
> A banana sliced lengthwise and spread with two tablespoons of peanut, cashew, or almond butter
> A small cantaloupe wedge (⅓ of a 5-inch cantaloupe) or canned peach half filled with ¼ cup of cottage cheese

One carbohydrate unit of crackers (15 grams of carbohydrate) balanced with two tablespoons of nut butter or one ounce of cheese. Suggestions for commercially made crackers which are higher in fiber than most include Mary's Gone Crackers™ gluten-free crackers and Ak-Mak™ stone ground whole wheat crackers. (See "Sources," page 283, to purchase these crackers). Cracker recipes are on pages 182 to 185.

Almond Sesame Crackers (page 184) or Choose-Your-Country Crackers (page 185) for a cracker-only snack. Because they are made with almond flour, these crackers do not have to be linked and balanced with a protein food. However, you can enjoy them with nut butter or cheese if you prefer!

Celery stuffed with nut butter or cheese

A 6 or 8-ounce cup of yogurt made from goat, sheep, soy or cow's milk (plain or no sugar added). Stir ¼ to ½ cup (or up to one unit – see pages 251 to 252) of chopped or mashed fresh berries or other fruit into plain yogurt and sweeten it with Protocol for Life Balance™ stevia if you prefer it sweeter. Your non-allergic companion(s) on the eating plan may appreciate the convenience of pre-mixed sugar-free fruit yogurt. My family enjoys Kroger™ Lite yogurt which is non-fat and artificially sweetened.

A hard boiled egg with crackers or toast. (See the bread and cracker recipes on pages 182 to 196. Have one carbohydrate unit of crackers or toast with one egg).

Fresh vegetable crudites (carrot, celery, broccoli, etc.) with garbanzo, lentil, or cottage cheese dip containing one protein unit if more. (See the dip recipes on pages 116 to 118).

One carbohydrate unit of crackers balanced with one protein unit of garbanzo, lentil, or cottage cheese dip. Suggestions for commercially made crackers are above, cracker recipes are on pages 182 to 185; and dip recipes with amounts that contain one protein unit are below.

GARBANZO DIP

Gluten-Free

This dip is great with crackers or fresh vegetable crudités.

> 1 16-ounce can of garbanzo beans, drained, or about 1½ to 1¾ cup of cooked garbanzo beans
> ⅓ cup water
> ¼ to ½ teaspoon salt or garlic salt, or to taste
> 2 teaspoons tart-tasting unbuffered vitamin C powder or 2 to 4 tablespoons lemon juice, to taste
> ⅛ teaspoon dry mustard (optional)
> ⅛ teaspoon pepper (optional)

Put the beans in a blender or food processor with the metal pureeing blade. Process them using a pulsing action until they are finely ground. Add all of the other ingredients and puree until smooth. (You may have to do this in small batches if you are using a blender). Refrigerate the dip. Serve on crackers or use it as a dip for raw vegetables. You can freeze any leftover dip in serving-sized portions. Makes about 1½ cups of dip or 4 servings which contain one protein unit each and 5 grams of fat if you use water-packed beans. The carbohydrates in cooked legumes are so high-fiber that Dr. Cheryle Hart does not count them.

LENTIL SPREAD

Gluten-Free

Serve this spread on crackers or in sandwiches. Its flavor reminds me of liverwurst or paté.

> 1 16-ounce can* of lentils, drained, or about 1½ cups of cooked lentils
> ½ to 1 onion, peeled and chopped, or 2 to 3 tablespoons dry chopped onions (optional, but the onion gives the spread most of its flavor)
> 1 tablespoon oil (only needed if using fresh onion)
> ½ cup walnuts or other mild tasting nuts or ¼ cup mild-tasting natural nut butter
> 1 to 1¼ teaspoons salt, to taste
> ½ teaspoon pepper, or more to taste

If using the fresh onion, sauté it in the oil until it is soft, or soak the dry onion in hot water for a few minutes until rehydrated and then drain off the excess water. Grind the walnuts with the pureeing blade of a food processor. (If you with to use a blender or hand-blender, you will have to make this recipe with nut butter. Since this mixture is thick, it is worth getting out the processor if you have one). Add the rest of the ingredients to the ground nuts or nut butter and puree until smooth. Taste and adjust the seasonings. Refrigerate the spread or freeze it in serving-sized portions. Makes about 2 to 2½ cups of spread or seven ⅓-cup servings which each contain 1 protein unit. If the oil is used to cook the onion, one serving contains 6 grams of fat; if not, it contains 5 grams of fat. The carbohydrates in cooked legumes are so high-fiber that Dr. Cheryle Hart does not count them.

*Note:** Canned lentils can be difficult to find. Your health food store may carry West-brae™ Organic Lentils which contain just lentils, water, and sea salt.

Cottage Cheese Dip

Gluten-Free

1 carrot
3 large radishes
1 cup low-fat cottage cheese
¼ cup plain non-fat or low-fat yogurt, sour cream, or mayonnaise
½ teaspoon salt
¼ teaspoon pepper
2 teaspoons caraway seeds (optional)

Peel the carrot and grate it by rubbing it over the largest holes of a cheese grater. Finely chop the radishes. Puree the cottage cheese with a hand blender, food processor or blender until smooth. Add the yogurt, sour cream or mayonnaise, salt, and pepper and puree the dip again briefly. Stir in the caraway seeds, carrot, and radishes. Refrigerate until serving time. Makes about 1¾ cups of dip or five ⅓-cup servings which each contain 1 protein unit and 1 gram of fat if made with low-fat cottage cheese and nonfat yogurt. Serve with raw vegetables for dipping.

Quesadillas

**Gluten-Free IF
made with GF tortillas**

These are great appetizers for occasions when you have guests, but you can enjoy them any time. Make the cheese mixture ahead of time and store it in your refrigerator or freezer for a quick snack.

8 ounces of sausage, preferably turkey chorizo, page 105, commercially made chorizo sausage, or other turkey sausage
4 ounces or about 1 cup of grated cheddar cheese (preferably low-fat, any type you tolerate such as goat, soy, or cow's milk cheese)
4 ounces or about 1 cup of grated part-skim mozzarella or Monterey jack cheese (preferably low-fat, any type you tolerate such as goat, soy, or cow's milk cheese)
1 poblano pepper or about 2 ounces of other peppers to suit your taste in hotness
¼ cup chopped onion (optional)
16 thin corn tortillas* or 8 Tumaro™ Low in Carbs tortillas for your wheat-eating companions
Vegetable oil spray or oil for brushing the tortillas

Cook the sausage in a frying pan, breaking it up and stirring it as it cooks, until it is thoroughly cooked and beginning to brown. Drain all the fat. Place the meat on paper towel to cool.

Seed and finely chop the pepper. Finely chop the onion if you are using it. In a bowl, mix together the cheeses, sausage, and chopped vegetables. Preheat your oven to 350°F. Oil three to four baking sheets.

Spray or brush one side of half of the tortillas with oil. Put them oiled-side down on the prepared baking sheets. Top the tortillas with the cheese mixture. Spray or brush one side of the rest of the tortillas with oil and put them on the cheese mixture oiled-side up. Bake them for 5 to 10 minutes or until the cheese is melted and the tortillas are beginning to crisp. Remove them from the oven and cut the corn quesadillas into halves or the wheat quesadillas into quarters to serve. Makes 16 servings, each of which contains ½ carbohydrate unit, 1 protein unit, and 5 grams of fat if made with lean (11% fat) turkey sausage, low fat cheese and the oil spray.

For a quick snack for one or two people, cut the tortillas to make 1-portion size quesadillas. (Cut them into halves for corn tortillas or into quarters for wheat tortillas). Assemble the quesadilla(s) as above. Heat them on an oiled tray in a toaster oven or microwave then on low to medium power for 1 to 2 minutes. Microwaved quesadillas will not be crisp.

*Note on corn tortillas: If you are not allergic to corn, you may want to use corn tortillas in this recipe because they are traditional in and go very well with Mexican food as well as being gluten-free. However, be careful to purchase the thin "frying" variety rather than the thicker "bread" variety of tortillas or you will be getting twice as much carbohydrate per serving as you expect. Read the nutrition label on the back of the tortilla package to determine whether the tortillas are the thin variety, i.e. whether 4 tortillas will contain 30 grams of net carbohydrate or less (total carbohydrate grams minus grams of fiber). I use Mission™ Extra Thin Yellow Corn Tortillas which contain 28 grams of net carbohydrate in 4 tortillas.

LUNCHES
LIGHT MEALS, SOUPS, AND SANDWICHES

The best way to control what you eat on an allergy or gluten-free diet, especially if you also want to achieve glycemic control through your eating habits, is to prepare your own food. Lunch can be the most challenging meal because it is often eaten away from home. However, with the information and recipes in this book, you can have delicious and nutritious take-along lunches to fit your healthy eating plan. As with breakfast, if you are on a rotation diet, the most efficient way to prepare your meals is to start your rotation day at dinnertime and have leftovers for breakfast and lunch.

This chapter contains ideas for lighter meals such as soups, sandwiches, and salads hearty enough to make an entire meal. These recipes provide a change from eating heavier dinner foods in the middle of the day. If you are allergic to yeast or cannot have vinegar due to gluten intolerance, you still can have salads. See page 177 for a recipe for "Basic Vinaigrette" which can be made with vitamin C or lemon juice instead of vinegar.

The soups in this chapter are highly nutritious and satisfying, and many are easy to make in your crock pot. Make a large batch of soup, freeze it in serving-sized portions, and you will always be prepared with a container of soup for a brown-bagged lunch or for whenever you need a quick lunch or dinner at home.

Although sandwiches are the mainstay of conventional lunches, bread can be a challenge on food allergy and gluten-free diets. Let's face it, gluten-free bread is most often not light and fluffy. If you are trying to control your weight, two normal-sized slices of gluten-free bread in a sandwich may contain two or three times as many grams of carbohydrate as an equivalent volume of wheat bread. If your special-diet bread is made with rice, those carbohydrates are also high on the glycemic scale. This is one reason that people who replace wheat breads in their diet with rice breads, in normal-looking amounts, often gain weight. This chapter offers suggestions for controlling the amount of carbohydrate you eat at lunch while still enjoying a sandwich, plus it provides a few family favorite sandwich recipes for you to try. Remember to include a salad or some carrot sticks in your sandwich lunch to supply extra fiber which will moderate the impact of the bread on your blood sugar level.

ITALIAN POWERHOUSE SALAD

**Gluten-Free IF
made with GF pasta**

With plenty of protein, some low-GI carbohydrate and a generous amount of fiber, this salad will keep you satisfied for a long time.

About ¾ pound raw chicken breast with bones and skin or 1½ cups cooked
    cubed roasted chicken (about 8 ounces)

Salt

3 ounces rotini, bow tie, or other pasta of a type you tolerate (about 1½ cups
    dry pasta)

About ½ to 1 teaspoon olive oil

¼ cup sliced black olives, about half of a 2.25 ounce can (dry weight)

⅝ cup bottled gluten- and allergen-free diet Italian salad dressing or "Basic
    Vinaigrette," page 277, divided

8 cups torn romaine lettuce

½ cup grape tomatoes

¼ cup grated Romano cheese, if tolerated (If you are allergic to cow's milk, try
    all-sheep milk Romano).

Put the chicken in a baking dish and sprinkle it lightly with salt. Bake at 400°F for about an hour, or until the skin is lightly browned and the chicken is cooked all the way through when you cut it with a knife. Cool the chicken in the refrigerator. Then remove the skin and bones and cut the chicken into ½ inch cubes. (Kitchen shears work well for this). The chicken may be prepared a day or two before you plan to serve this salad or you can use leftover chicken from a previous meal.

Cook the pasta as directed on page 163 until *al dente*. Do not overcook it. Drain it by holding the lid ajar on the pan, add cold water to the pan, and drain it again. Repeat if necessary to cool the pasta to room temperature. Toss it with just a little olive oil to coat the pasta and keep it from sticking together. Refrigerate the pasta.

In a medium bowl or storage container, stir together the cooked pasta, cooked chicken, and olives. Add ⅜ cup of the dressing and toss. Refrigerate for at least 2 hours or overnight.

If you have time and prefer to not eat your meat cold, remove the pasta mixture from the refrigerator about an hour before you plan to eat this salad. At mealtime, put the lettuce in a large bowl. Add the remaining ¼ cup of dressing and toss. Slice the grape tomatoes in half and add them to the lettuce. Add the pasta mixture and toss. Sprinkle with the cheese and toss again. Makes 4 servings, each of which contain 1 carbohydrate unit, 3 protein units, and 11 grams of fat if made with diet Italian salad dressing.

Note on brown-bagging this salad: For a take-along lunch, divide the mixtures and other ingredients used in this recipe into the desired number of portions. Add the extra salad dressing to the chicken mixture after it has marinated, and put a portion of the mixture into a small container. Carry portions of the lettuce, tomatoes, and cheese into a larger container that can serve as a bowl, and combine the contents of the two containers in it at lunchtime.

Mexican Powerhouse Salad

Gluten-Free IF
made with GF tortillas

Here is a similarly satisfying whole-meal salad with a Mexican theme.

About ½ pound raw chicken breast with bones and skin or 1⅛ cups cooked
    cubed roasted chicken (about 6 ounces)
Salt
1 15-ounce can black beans
½ cup bottled gluten- and allergen-free diet Italian salad dressing or "Basic
    Vinaigrette," page 177, divided
8 6-inch thin corn tortillas* OR other tortillas you tolerate which contain the
    same amount of net carbohydrate OR 4 8-inch wheat tortillas such as
    Tumaro's™ Low in Carbs Tortillas for your wheat-eating companions
Oil spray or about 1 teaspoon oil
1 15-ounce can non-fat or vegetarian refried beans
8 cups torn romaine lettuce
½ cup grape tomatoes
¼ cup finely diced poblano pepper or other pepper to your taste in hotness (optional)
⅓ cup shredded Monterey jack cheese, preferably low-fat, of any type tolerated
    (goat, soy, cow's milk, etc., optional)
⅓ cup shredded cheddar cheese, preferably low-fat, of any type tolerated (goat,
    soy, cow's milk, etc., optional)
Salsa (optional)

Several hours or even a day or two before you plan to serve this salad, cook and cube the chicken as in the recipe above. (Another option is saving leftover chicken from a previous meal to use in this salad). Drain and rinse the black beans. Combine the cubed chicken, black beans, and ¼ cup of the dressing and refrigerate for at least two hours or overnight.

If you have time, an hour or so before you wish to serve this salad, remove the chicken and bean mixture from the refrigerator and allow it to stand at room temperature to take the chill off it.

Preheat your oven to 375°F. Oil two baking sheets and both sides of the tortillas. Place the tortillas on the sheets and bake them, turning after about 4 minutes, for 7 to 10 minutes or until they are crisp and beginning to brown. Divide the tortillas between four serving dishes. Spread them with the refried beans.

In a large bowl, mix the lettuce, tomatoes, and the remaining ¼ cup of the dressing. Divide the lettuce mixture between the four serving dishes. Top the lettuce with the bean and chicken mixture, dividing it between the four dishes. Sprinkle each dish with

¼ of the optional chopped pepper. Sprinkle each salad with ¼ of both types of cheese. Serve with salsa if desired. Makes 4 servings, each of which contain 1 carbohydrate unit, 4 protein units, and 10 grams of fat if made with diet Italian salad dressing.

*Note on corn tortillas: If you are not allergic to corn, you may want to use corn tortillas in this recipe because they are traditional in and go very well with Mexican food as well as being gluten-free. If you purchase the thin "frying" variety rather than the thicker "bread" variety of tortillas you will get less carbohydrate. To tell thin from thick tortillas, read the nutrition label on the back of the tortilla package and determine how many (2 or 4) tortillas contain 30 grams of net carbohydrate (total carbohydrate grams minus grams of fiber). I use Mission™ Extra Thin Yellow Corn Tortillas which contain 28 grams of net carbohydrate in 4 tortillas.

VEGETARIAN MEAL SALAD

Gluten-Free IF
made with GF tortillas

This vegetarian salad or sandwich is loaded with nutrition.

2 cups coarsely chopped spinach, lightly packed into the measuring cup
1 medium-sized cucumber, peeled and cut into ½ inch cubes (about 1½ cups cubes)
1 large carrot, grated (about 1 cup grated)
1 large ripe avocado, cut into ½ inch cubes
1 cup cheddar or Monterey jack cheese, preferably low fat, of any type tolerated (goat, soy, cows; milk, etc.), cubed (about 4 ounces) OR ⅔ cup crumbled goat or sheep feta cheese (about 3 ounces)
½ cup sliced or coarsely chopped almonds or other nuts or sunflower seeds
1½ teaspoons tart-tasting unbuffered vitamin C crystals or 2 tablespoons of lemon juice or vinegar
Dash of salt (optional)
Dash of pepper (optional)
2 teaspoons water (only if you are using the vitamin C)
2 tablespoons oil
8 6-inch thin corn tortillas* OR other tortillas you tolerate which contain the same amount of net carbohydrate OR 4 8-inch wheat tortillas such as Tumaro's™ Low in Carbs Tortillas for your wheat-eating companions (optional)

Combine the spinach, cucumber, carrot, avocado cubes, cheese, and seeds or nuts in a large bowl. In a separate small bowl or glass jar, mix the vitamin C crystals plus water OR the lemon juice or vinegar with the salt and pepper. Add the oil and mix or shake it until it is thoroughly combined. Pour the dressing over the vegetable mixture and toss until all the ingredients are coated with the dressing. Serve the salad alone or serve it on top of tortillas to eat with a fork and knife. Makes 4 servings, each of which contains 1 carbohydrate unit if the types of tortillas above are used. If served as a salad without the tortillas, each serving contains no carbohydrate units 2 protein units, and 23 grams of fat. If you serve this on another type of tortillas, they should not exceed 2 carbohydrate units per serving.

***Note on corn tortillas:** If you are not allergic to corn, you may want to use corn tortillas which are gluten-free. If you purchase the thin "frying" variety rather than the thicker "bread" variety of tortillas you will get less carbohydrate. Read the nutrition label on the back of the tortilla package to determine how many (2 or 4) tortillas contain 30 grams of net carbohydrate (total carbohydrate grams minus grams of fiber). I use Mission™ Extra Thin Yellow Corn Tortillas which contain 28 grams of net carbohydrate in 4 tortillas.

Soups

Making your favorite soups from the recipes that follow and freezing them in individual servings will keep you prepared for lunch or dinner at all times. A few of these soups can be made quickly on the stove and several can cook in a crock pot all day while you are away. Many of them feature cooked dried legumes which are excellent for glycemic control with their high protein and fiber levels. In *The Insulin Resistance Diet,* Dr. Cheryl Hart counts dry legumes as a protein food and allow patients to eat legumes without balancing the carbohydrates they contain (mostly insoluble fiber) with another protein. The serving sizes for the soups below are calculated to contain two protein units per serving. If you are serving soup as a meal rather than a side dish, men and younger women may want to eat more than one bowl of soup.

QUICK AND EASY VEGETABLE SOUP

**Gluten-Free IF
made with a GF grain**

This large batch of soup makes a great meal plus plenty of delicious leftovers to put in your freezer.

> 6 cups of gluten-free beef broth (See "Sources," page 277).
> 1 15-ounce can diced tomatoes
> 1 10-ounce package of frozen peas and carrots
> ½ of a 10-ounce package of frozen baby lima beans

1 small stalk of celery, sliced
1 small onion, chopped, or 3 tablespoons dry chopped onion (optional)
¼ head of cabbage, chopped
½ cup cooked quinoa, brown rice, or other cooked grain (optional)
2 to 3 cups of cubed cooked beef, such as leftover roast

Combine the beef broth, tomatoes, frozen vegetables, celery and onion in a large pot and bring the soup to a boil over high heat. When it comes to a boil, reduce the heat to low and simmer the soup for 10 minutes. Add the cabbage, cooked grain, and beef and bring the soup back to a boil. Reduce the heat and boil gently for another 5 minutes. Makes 5 servings, each of which contains ¼ carbohydrate unit if made with quinoa or another grain, 2 protein units, and 4 grams of fat.

CAULIFLOWER AND COTTAGE CHEESE SOUP

Gluten-Free

The cottage cheese and milk in this soup are quick and easy sources of protein.

1 tablespoon oil (optional – use it only with fresh onion)
1 small onion, chopped, or 2 to 3 tablespoons dry chopped onion (optional)
3 to 4 cups of chopped fresh cauliflower or 1½ pounds frozen cauliflower
2 cups chicken broth or water
1 cup skim, low fat, or whole milk
1¼ cups low fat cottage cheese
Dash of salt and pepper, to taste (optional)

If you are using fresh onion, combine it with the oil in a saucepan. Cook it over medium heat until the onion is soft, about 3 minutes. When the onion is cooked, add the cauliflower and broth to the pan and bring it to a boil over medium-high heat. If you are not using fresh onion, combine the cauliflower and broth in the pan with or without the optional dry onion and bring it to a boil.

Reduce the heat and simmer the vegetables for ten minutes or until the cauliflower is tender. While the cauliflower is cooking, combine the cottage cheese and milk and puree them with a hand blender, blender or food processor until they are smooth.

When the cauliflower is cooked, remove about half of the cauliflower and a little of the broth from the pot and puree them with a hand blender, blender or food processor. Return the pureed cauliflower to the pot and add the cottage cheese puree. Reheat the soup gently over low heat, stirring frequently, until it steams and is just under the boiling point. Do not boil. Taste the soup and season with pepper and, if needed, salt to taste. Makes 4 servings each of which contains 2 protein units and 2 grams of fat.

Quick Stove-Top Lentil Soup

For a version of this soup that can cook unattended while you are away for the day, see "Crock Pot Lentil Soup" on page 132.

> 1 pound dry lentils
> Water
> 1 pound (about 5 large) carrots
> 3 to 5 stalks of celery
> ¼ teaspoon black pepper (optional)
> 1 15-ounce can diced tomatoes (optional)
> 1 to 1½ teaspoons salt, to taste

If you have time the night before you plan to serve this soup, rinse the lentils by running water over them in a strainer to remove any dirt. Put them in a 3-quart saucepan and cover them with cold water. Soak them overnight. In the morning, drain the water from the lentils, add fresh water to the pan, and drain the water again. Rinse the beans this way three times.* Drain off all the water after the last rinse.

If you do not have time to soak the lentils overnight, rinse them in a strainer as above. Put them in a 3-quart saucepan, cover them with three to four times their volume with cold water, bring them to a boil, and simmer them for two minutes. Remove the pan from the heat and let the lentils soak for an hour or longer. Then rinse them three times as in the paragraph above and drain the water completely.

Peel the carrots and cut them into ¼ inch slices. Slice the celery into ½ inch slices. Add the carrots, celery, and pepper to the lentils. Also add water – 6 cups if you are not using tomatoes or 5 cups if you do plan to use the tomatoes. Return the pan to a boil and simmer 40 minutes to 1 hour or until the lentils are tender. (The time required for the lentils to become tender may vary depending on the altitude, age of the lentils, their growing conditions, etc.) Add the salt and tomatoes if you are using them. Then bring the pan back to a boil, reduce the heat to a simmer, and cook for a few more minutes. Makes about 2½ quarts of soup or 9 servings which each contain 2 protein units and 1 gram of fat. The carbohydrates in cooked legumes are so high-fiber that Dr. Cheryle Hart does not count them. Leftover soup freezes well.

*__Note:__ Rinsing the lentils after soaking them removes indigestible carbohydrates that can cause intestinal gas.

CHANA DAL VEGETABLE SOUP

Gluten-Free

Chana dal is a "new" kind of legume that is extremely low on the glycemic index. Some diabetics swear by it for keeping their blood sugar on an even keel.

1 pound chana dal, such as Bob's Red Mill™ brand (See "Sources," page 277).
Water
1 pound carrots
4 stalks celery
½ cup chopped onion (optional or to taste)
½ teaspoon pepper (optional or to taste)
1½ teaspoons sweet basil (optional)
1 15-ounce can diced or crushed tomatoes (optional)
1½ teaspoons salt, or to taste

Pick over the chana dal beans and rinse them under running water in a strainer. Soak them overnight in at least four times their volume of water in a 3-quart saucepan or crock pot. If you are making this soup in the crock pot and will be pressed for time in the morning, prepare the vegetables as described below and refrigerate them in a plastic bag. The next morning, drain the soaking water from the beans. Replace it with cool water and drain it three times.

Stove-top preparation: Cover the drained beans in the saucepan with three times their volume of cold water. Bring them to a boil, reduce the heat to medium, and simmer for three minutes. Remove the pan from the heat and let it stand at room temperature for two hours. Drain and discard the soaking water. Add 7 cups of water to the drained beans in the soup pot. Peel and slice the carrots. Slice the celery and chop the onion. Add them to the pot with the pepper and basil. (Do not add the salt and tomatoes until near the end of the cooking time). Bring the pot back to a boil, reduce the heat, and simmer for 1½ to 2 hours or until the beans are beginning to soften. (Chana dal do not become as soft as most beans do when they are cooked). Check the soup occasionally. If it does not contain enough liquid to cover the beans during this time, add more water. Mash a few of the beans against the side of the pan to thicken the soup. (Do not cook the soup for an excessively long time after mashing the beans, just long enough to reheat it). Add the optional tomatoes and salt. If you are not using the tomatoes and the soup seems too thick for you, add water to bring it to the thickness you prefer. Return the soup to a boil and boil it for a just a minute or two. Makes about 2½ quarts of soup or 7 servings which each contain 2 protein units and 4 grams of fat. The carbohydrates in cooked legumes are so high-fiber that Dr. Cheryle Hart does not count them.

Crock pot preparation: Soak and rinse the beans as in the first paragraph above, Add 6 cups of water to the drained beans in the crock pot if you are not going to use the tomatoes or add 5 cups of water if you are planning to use the tomatoes. Peel and slice the carrots. Slice the celery and chop the onion. Add them to the pot with the pepper and basil. (Do not add the salt and tomatoes until near the end of the cooking time). Cook the soup for 6 to 8 hours on high or for 8 to 10 hours on the low setting. Mash a few of the beans against the side of the pot to thicken the soup. (Do not cook the soup for an excessively long time after mashing the beans, just long enough to reheat it). Add the optional tomatoes and salt. If you are not using the tomatoes and the soup seems too thick for you, add boiling water to bring it to the thickness you prefer. Cook on "high" for ½ hour or until it the soup is re-heated. (To speed the re-heating time, heat the tomatoes or water before adding them to the pot rather than adding them at room temperature). Makes about 2½ quarts of soup or 7 servings which each contain 2 protein units and 4 grams of fat. The carbohydrates in cooked legumes are so high-fiber that Dr. Cheryle Hart does not count them.

Multi-Bean Soup

Gluten-Free

Although it cooks in the crock pot all day, this soup takes only 20 minutes of your time to make – 5 minutes the evening before you want to eat it, 10 minutes the next morning, and 5 minutes near serving time. If you're pressed for time in the morning, the time required can be 10-5-5 minutes instead. This soup is delicious, nutritious and economical as well as quick.

> 1 pound mixed dry beans*
> Water
> ½ pound peeled mini-carrots or 3 to 5 whole carrots
> 3 stalks of celery
> ¼ teaspoon pepper (optional)
> 1 15-ounce can diced tomatoes OR 1 11-ounce can tomato puree (optional)
> 1½ to 2 teaspoons salt, to taste

The evening before you plan to serve this soup for dinner, put the beans in a strainer and run water over them thoroughly to remove any dirt. Put them in a 3-quart crock pot and fill the pot nearly full with water. Soak them overnight. If you will be pressed for time in the morning, prepare the carrots and celery the evening before as described below and refrigerate them in a plastic bag overnight.

In the morning, drain the water from the beans in the crock pot. Refill the pot with water and drain it two times more.* Add 5 to 6 cups of water to the pot and turn it to high. If you are using peeled mini-carrots, you may add them to the pot whole or cut them in half. (Using mini-carrots straight from the bag instead of whole carrots will save you about 5 minutes of time). If you are using whole carrots, peel them and slice them into ¼ inch slices. Wash the celery, lay the stalks together on a cutting board, and slice all three stalks into ½ inch pieces at the same time. Add the carrots and celery to the crock pot. Cook the soup on high for 5 to 6 hours or, if you are leaving for the day, turn it down and cook it on low for 8 to 10 hours.

When the beans are tender (after 5 to 6 hours if cooked on high), or slightly before serving time (if cooked on low), add the salt, pepper, and tomatoes. If you are not using the tomatoes and the soup seems too thick, add up to 1 cup of boiling water. If you are adding the tomatoes shortly before dinner time, warm them in the microwave before adding them to the pot to speed the reheating time. Cook the soup on high for ½ hour or until it is heated through.

This recipe makes about 2½ quarts of soup or 6 servings which each contain 2 protein units and 1 gram of fat. The carbohydrates in cooked legumes are so high-fiber that Dr. Cheryle Hart does not count them.

If you want to make a larger batch to freeze, use a 5-quart crock pot, double the amounts of all of the ingredients, and cook the soup on high for 8 to 10 hours. A double batch makes about 5 quarts of soup, or 12 servings. Leftovers freeze well.

*Notes about beans: Be sure that the bean mix does not contain barley or other gluten-containing grains or grains to which you are allergic. Bob's Red Mill™ 13-bean mix is all beans. Rinsing the beans after soaking them removes indigestible carbohydrates that can cause intestinal gas.

BLACK BEAN SOUP

Gluten-Free

This zesty soup will liven up any meal.

    1 pound dry black beans
    Water
    2 bell peppers, preferably one red and one green, seeded and diced
    1 small onion, diced (optional)
    1 teaspoon ground cumin (optional)
    ½ teaspoon black pepper or a 2-inch chili pepper or chile pequin, seeded and
        crumbled
    2 teaspoons oregano
    1 15-ounce can diced tomatoes or 1 pound tomatoes, chopped
    2 teaspoons salt

The night before you plan to serve this soup for dinner, rinse the beans by running water over them in a strainer to remove any dirt. Put them in a 3-quart crock pot and cover them with cold water. Soak them overnight. If you will be pressed for time in the morning, chop the peppers and onions the evening before as described below and refrigerate them in a plastic bag overnight.

In the morning, drain the water from the beans, add fresh water to the pot, and drain the water again. Rinse the beans this way three times.* Drain off all the water after the last rinse. Add 4 cups of water to the crock pot plus the peppers, onion, cumin, pepper, and oregano. Cover the crock pot with its lid and cook the soup on high for 6 hours or on low for 8 to 10 hours. Add the salt and diced or chopped tomatoes an hour before the end of the cooking time, or microwave the tomatoes to warm them and add them a few minutes before serving time. If the soup is thicker than you prefer, add a little boiling water to the pot near the end of the cooking time. Makes about 2½ quarts of soup or 8 servings which each contain 2 protein units and 1 gram of fat. The carbohydrates in cooked legumes are so high-fiber that Dr. Cheryle Hart does not count them. Leftover soup freezes well.

***Note:** Rinsing the beans after soaking them removes indigestible carbohydrates that can cause intestinal gas.

Navy Bean Soup

Gluten-Free

    1 pound dry navy beans
    Water
    2 carrots
    3 stalks celery
    2 teaspoons salt
    ¼ to ½ teaspoon pepper, to taste
    1 tablespoon parsley
    1 teaspoon sweet basil

The night before you plan to serve this soup for dinner, rinse the beans by running water over them in a strainer to remove any dirt. Put them in a 3-quart crock pot and cover them with cold water. Soak them overnight. If you will be pressed for time in the morning, prepare the carrots and celery the evening before as described below and refrigerate them in a plastic bag overnight.

In the morning, drain the water from the beans, add fresh water to the pot, and drain the water again. Rinse the beans this way three times.* Drain off all the water after the last rinse. Peel the carrots and cut them into ¼ inch slices. Slice the celery into ¼ inch slices.

Add 6 cups of water to the crock pot plus the carrots, celery, salt, pepper, parsley, and sweet basil. Cover the crock pot and cook the soup on high for 6 hours or on low for 8 to 10 hours. Check the soup near the end of the cooking time and add a little boiling water to the pot if the soup is thicker than you prefer. Makes about 2½ quarts of soup or 8 servings which each contain 2 protein units and 1 gram of fat. The carbohydrates in cooked legumes are so high-fiber that Dr. Cheryle Hart does not count them. Leftover soup freezes well.

***Note:** Rinsing the beans after soaking them removes indigestible carbohydrates that can cause intestinal gas.

SPLIT PEA SOUP

Gluten-Free

1 pound split peas
Water
3 to 4 carrots
3 stalks celery
1 to 2 teaspoons salt (Use less with the ham).
¼ teaspoon pepper
1 bay leaf
1 to 2 cups cubed cooked ham (optional)

The night before you plan to serve this soup for dinner, rinse the peas by running water over them in a strainer to remove any dirt. Put them in a 3-quart crock pot and cover them with cold water. Soak them overnight. If you will be pressed for time in the morning, prepare the carrots and celery the evening before as described below and refrigerate them in a plastic bag overnight.

In the morning, drain the water from the peas, add fresh water to the pot, and drain the water again. Rinse the beans this way three times.* Drain off all the water after the last rinse. Peel the carrots and cut them into ¼ inch slices. Slice the celery into ¼ inch slices.

Add 5 cups of water to the crock pot plus the carrots, celery, salt, pepper, ham, and bay leaf. Cover the crock pot with its lid and cook the soup on high for 6 hours or on low for 8 to 10 hours. Check the soup near the end of the cooking time and add a little boiling water to the pot if the soup is thicker than you prefer. Remove the bay leaf before serving. Makes about 2½ quarts of soup. If made without the ham, this is 8 servings which each contain 2 protein units and 1 gram of fat. If made with the ham, it is 10 servings which each contain 2 protein units and 2 gram of fat. The carbohydrates in cooked legumes are so high-fiber that Dr. Cheryle Hart does not count them. Leftover soup freezes well.

***Note:** Rinsing the peas after soaking them removes indigestible carbohydrates that can cause intestinal gas.

CROCK POT LENTIL SOUP

Because lentils may be the least allergenic legume, it you omit the optional tomatoes and pepper, this soup is likely to be tolerated by those with extensive food allergies.

> 1 pound dry lentils
> Water
> 3 to 5 carrots
> 3 stalks celery
> 2 teaspoons salt
> ¼ teaspoon pepper (optional)
> 1 15-ounce can diced tomatoes (optional)

The night before you plan to serve this soup for dinner, rinse the lentils by running water over them in a strainer to remove any dirt. Put them in a 3-quart crock pot and cover them with cold water. Soak them overnight. If you will be pressed for time in the morning, prepare the carrots and celery the evening before as described below and refrigerate them in a plastic bag overnight.

In the morning, drain the water from the lentils, add fresh water to the pot, and drain the water again. Rinse the beans this way three times.* Drain off all the water after the last rinse. Peel the carrots and cut them into ¼ inch slices. Slice the celery into ¼ inch slices. Add 5 cups of water to the crock pot plus the carrots, celery, salt, and pepper.

Cover the crock pot and cook the soup on high for 6 hours or on low for 8 to 10 hours. Add the optional tomatoes an hour before the end of the cooking time. Check the soup near the end of the cooking time and add a little boiling water to the pot if the soup is thicker than you prefer. Makes about 2½ quarts of soup or 9 servings which each contain 2 protein units and 1 gram of fat. The carbohydrates in cooked legumes are so high-fiber that Dr. Cheryle Hart does not count them. Leftover soup freezes well.

***Note:** Rinsing the lentils after soaking them removes indigestible carbohydrates that can cause intestinal gas.

Sandwiches

Although you must have bread to make a sandwich, those who avoid gluten, wheat, or yeast need not despair or forgo enjoying these lunch-time favorites. If your health food store sells good gluten-free or wheat-free bread that you tolerate and can afford, you will have a convenient, easy base for your sandwiches. To stay within the two carbohydrate units limit (30 grams net carbohydrate) per meal, read the nutrition label on purchased bread. Subtract the grams of fiber from the total grams of carbohydrate for one slice of bread. If the result is 15 grams net carbohydrates or less, you may use two slices for your sandwich. If the total net grams of carbohydrate for two slices of bread is more than 30 grams, reduce the size of the portion of bread to an amount that contains 30 grams or less. This may mean eating your sandwich open-faced. Try one piece of bread spread with your favorite natural nut butter or the garbanzo or lentil spreads on pages 116 to 117. For a sandwich with loose ingredients (meat, cheese, vegetables) use a leaf of lettuce or cabbage in place of the top slice of bread so you can pick up the sandwich to eat it easily

If you make bread using the recipes on pages 186 to 187 or pages 189 to 196, you can use lower GI flour[1] and vary the size of the pan in which you bake the bread, thus lowering number of grams of carbohydrate per slice. Norpro™ makes non-stick bread pans that yield slices of bread which are four inches wide. Their 4 by 10-inch or 4 by 12-inch bread pans are a good size for the amount of batter or dough made by the recipes in this book or in the books described on the last pages of this book. When using recipes from books that do not list carbohydrate unit information with the recipes, use this rule of thumb to calculate servings: Each slice of bread should be made with about ⅓ cup of flour in order to contain 15 grams of carbohydrate and to be one carbohydrate unit. Using a variety of pan sizes and a little math, you will be able to produce slices of bread that contain 15 grams of carbohydrate. Norpro™ bread pans can be purchased from Amazon.com or from Norpro.™ See "Sources," page 279.

Some types of bread made with alternative flours are crumbly. Crumbling is especially likely with non-yeast breads. To strengthen these breads for use in sandwiches, toast them thoroughly in a toaster oven. If you are on an allergy diet but do not need to avoid gluten, you may wish to try what I did about 30 years ago (back when I could eat grains) when I was first faced with taking a wheat-free sandwich to work in my lunch. I had discovered Wasa™ rye crispbreads in my health food store, but they were basically large crackers and would shatter into pieces when bitten into. I layered sliced turkey breast and cranberry sauce between two crispbreads in the evening, wrapped the sandwich in plastic wrap, and refrigerated it overnight. By lunchtime the next day I could

---

[1] Commercially made breads often contain mostly rice and tapioca flour. Rice is the only grain which has a high GI score eaten in its whole grain form, and tapioca flour is highly refined, so bread that you buy will have a much higher GI score than bread made from the recipes on pages 186 to 196.

bite into the sandwich without any mess. This sandwich is also good with sliced chicken or game meat. The recipe is below along with a few other sandwich recipes that my family enjoys.

TURKEY OR CHICKEN BLT

**Gluten-Free IF
made with GF bread**

With its generous amount of tasty protein, my husband has this sandwich almost every Saturday and finds that it very satisfying and blood sugar stabilizing.

- 2 slices of bread* which you tolerate, preferably whole grain
- 3 strips of cooked bacon
- 2 to 3 ounces of sliced cooked chicken or turkey breast
- 1 ounce of sliced cheddar or American cheese (optional)
- 1 small or ½ large tomato
- 1 leaf of lettuce
- 2 teaspoons of purchased diet mayonnaise, homemade mayonnaise, page 235, or "Super Smooth Sauce," page 234

Slice the tomato. Toast the bread, if desired, and spread it with the mayonnaise. Layer the turkey or chicken, cheese, bacon, tomato, and lettuce on one slice of bread or toast. Top with the second slice and serve. Makes one serving which contains 2 carbohydrate units, 3 to 4 protein units, and 15 grams of fat if made with diet mayonnaise.

***Note on the bread:** Each slice of bread should contain 15 grams or less of net carbohydrate (the grams of total carbohydrates minus the grams of fiber) to have this sandwich fit within 30 grams of carbohydrate per meal.

TURKEY AND CRANBERRIES SANDWICH

**Gluten-Free IF
made with GF bread**

Although turkey with cranberries is a tradition, cranberries give a tang and festive flair to any kind of meat in this sandwich.

- 2 slices of bread* which you tolerate, preferably whole grain
- 2 to 3 ounces of sliced cooked turkey breast, chicken, or roasted game meat
- 1 to 2 tablespoons of stevia sweetened "Cranberry Sauce,"** page 232

Toast the bread if desired. Spread one slice of it with the cranberry sauce. Layer the meat on top of the cranberries. Top with the second slice of bread or toast. Serve the sandwich. Makes one serving which contains 2 carbohydrate units, 2 to 3 protein units, and 5 grams of fat if made with turkey breast.

*Note on the bread: Each slice of bread should contain 15 grams or less of net carbohydrate (the grams of total carbohydrates minus the grams of fiber) to have this sandwich fit within 30 grams of carbohydrate per meal.

**Note on the cranberry sauce: If you want to use two slices of bread and keep your carbohydrate intake to 30 grams, you must make your cranberry sauce with stevia rather than using commercially made cranberry sauce. Serve this sandwich open-faced on one slice of bread if you must use commercially made cranberry sauce.

GRILLED CHEESE SANDWICH

**Gluten-Free IF
made with GF bread**

This sandwich is an old favorite. It is included here for the nutritional and serving size information.

> 2 slices of bread* which you tolerate, preferably whole grain
> 2 to 3 one-ounce slices of cheddar cheese of any type you tolerate (goat, soy, cow's milk, etc.), preferably low-fat
> 1 to 2 teaspoons of EFA-butter (recipe on page 236), softened butter or goat butter, or Earth Balance™ non-hydrogenated margarine

Spread one side of each piece of bread with EFA-butter, butter or margarine. Put one slice of the bread into a frying pan buttered side down. Lay the cheese on top of it. Top the sandwich with the second slice of bread buttered side up. Place the pan on the burner of your stove and turn the heat to low, medium-low, or medium. (You will have to find the setting on your stove and cooking time that produces the perfect grilled cheese sandwich by trial and error). Cover the pan with a lid; this helps the cheese melt. Cook the sandwich for 2 to 5 minutes, or until the bottom side is golden-brown. Turn the sandwich over and cook it until the other side is also golden-brown. Serve the sandwich immediately after it is cooked. Makes one serving which contains 2 carbohydrate units, 2 to 3 protein units, and 9 grams of fat.

*Note on the bread: Each slice of bread should contain 15 grams or less of net carbohydrate (the grams of total carbohydrates minus the grams of fiber) to have this sandwich fit within 30 grams of carbohydrate per meal.

Reuben Sandwich

With plenty of protein plus the fiber in the sauerkraut, this man-sized sandwich will keep you satisfied for hours.

    2 slices of bread* which you tolerate, preferably whole grain
    1 to 2 one-ounce slices of Swiss or Monterey Jack cheese of any type you
        tolerate (goat, soy, cow's milk, etc.), preferably low-fat
    1 slice (about 2 ounces) of cooked corned beef
    3 tablespoons (about 1½ ounces) of canned sauerkraut, drained
    1 to 2 teaspoons of EFA-butter (recipe on page 236), softened butter, or Earth
        Balance™ non-hydrogenated margarine

Spread one side of each piece of bread with EFA-butter, margarine, or softened butter. Press the sauerkraut between two pieces of paper towel to remove the moisture from it. If you want your sandwich heated through in record time, microwave the sauerkraut on the paper towel for about 15 to 30 seconds. Put one slice of the bread into a frying pan buttered side down. Put the corned beef on top of it. Put the sauerkraut on top of the corned beef. Lay the cheese on top of the sauerkraut. Top the sandwich with the second slice of bread buttered side up. Place the pan on the burner of your stove and turn the heat to low or medium-low. (You will have to find by trial and error the setting on your stove and cooking time will that produce a Reuben sandwich that contains melted cheese and is warm all the way through without being burned on the outside). Cover the pan with a lid; this helps the cheese melt. Cook the sandwich for 3 to 6 minutes, or until the bottom side is golden-brown. Turn the sandwich over and cook it for another 3 to 6 minutes until the other side is also golden-brown. Serve immediately. Makes one serving which contains 2 carbohydrate units, 3 to 4 protein units, and 17 grams of fat.

Note on the bread: Each slice of bread should contain 15 grams or less of net carbohydrate (the grams of total carbohydrates minus the grams of fiber) to have this sandwich fit within 30 grams of carbohydrate per meal.

DINNERS
MAIN DISHES

With the recipes in this chapter, you will discover that dinner doesn't have to be boring or just "plain meat" on a glycemic control diet. You will find dishes here that are not only tasty but are also exciting surprises such as the vegetarian stuffed peppers immediately below, enchiladas, lasagne, and pizza (the main dish that people I talk to most often miss on their special diets). Enjoy!

QUINOA STUFFED PEPPERS

Gluten-Free

Because quinoa contains high-quality protein, this is a very satisfying vegetarian main dish. You can substitute three cups of any other cooked grain for the quinoa and water if you wish. Round out a vegetarian meal with some legumes for additional protein to balance the carbohydrate in the quinoa.

 1½ cups quinoa
 3 cups water
 1 pound frozen chopped spinach
 2 tablespoons oil
 7 bell peppers of any color
 1½ teaspoons salt
 ¾ teaspoon pepper
 3 teaspoons sweet basil
 2 tablespoons paprika (optional - for color)
 Additional oil (optional)

Wash the quinoa thoroughly by putting it in a strainer and rinsing it under running water until the water is no longer foamy. Combine it with 3 cups of water in a saucepan. Bring it to a boil, reduce the heat, and simmer it for 15 to 20 minutes. Cook the spinach in the 2 tablespoons of oil, adding no water, for 5 to 10 minutes, or until it is barely tender. While the spinach and quinoa are cooking, use a paring knife to remove the stem, core, and seeds from the peppers. Mix the quinoa and spinach with the seasonings and stuff the mixture into the peppers.

To cook the peppers in the traditional way, put a little oil into a heavy frying pan, lay the peppers in the pan on their sides, cover the pan, and cook the peppers slowly, turning them to brown all sides, for 30 to 45 minutes. Or, if you would rather bake the peppers, parboil them for 5 minutes before stuffing them, stuff them, and bake them in an oiled casserole dish at 350°F for 45 minutes. Makes 7 servings, each of which contains 2 carbohydrate units, 1 protein unit, and 6 grams of fat.

TURKEY CURRY

Gluten-Free

This dish is loaded with anti-inflammatory foods including carrots, spinach, turmeric, and ginger.

> 1 to 1¼ pounds turkey breast meat, cut into strips about ¼ inch thick by 1 to 2 inches long
> 1 tablespoon oil plus additional oil if needed
> 3 large carrots to make about 1½ cups sliced carrots
> 2 slices of onion (optional)
> ½ to 1 teaspoon finely minced garlic (optional)
> 2 to 4 tablespoons grated ginger root, to taste*
> ¼ teaspoon cinnamon
> 1 teaspoon turmeric
> ½ teaspoon salt
> ¾ cup water
> Additional liquid ingredient of your choice such as ¾ cup canned tomatoes with juice or ½ cup yogurt or coconut milk
> 4 to 5 cups washed baby spinach leaves

Cut the turkey breast into strips ¼ inch thick, about ¾ inch wide, and 1½ to 2 inches long. Put the oil in a frying pan, heat it briefly, and then add the turkey and optional onion. Sauté for about 10 to 15 minutes, stirring and turning the turkey and onions, until the turkey is cooked through and most of the pieces have started to brown. While they are cooking, dice the garlic, peel and slice the carrots, and peel and grate the ginger. Measure out the spices so they can all be added to the pan quickly. Measure the water separately so it can be added quickly to halt the intense heating of the spices.

Push the turkey and vegetables to the side of the pan and add another teaspoon or two of oil to the empty side of the pan if all the oil originally added has been absorbed by the turkey and vegetables. Add the ginger, garlic and spices to the oil and sauté them for about 30 seconds or until the spices begin to emit their fragrance. Immediately stir in the water. Add the salt and tomatoes with juice if you are using them. If you are using whole tomatoes, cut them in pieces with a spoon as you are stirring them in the pan. Add the carrots, cover the pan with its lid, bring the mixture to a boil over medium heat, and reduce the heat and simmer for about 15 minutes. If the curry begins to dry out, add more water. After it has simmered for 15 minutes, add the yogurt or coconut milk if you are using either of them and return the pan to a low simmer. Stir in the spinach and put the lid back on the pan. Return it to a low simmer and cook it for a few minutes until the spinach is wilted. Makes 4 servings, each of which contains 3 to 4 protein units and 12 to 15 grams of fat.

***Note on amount of ginger:** If you're not used to eating hot ginger in food, the first time you make this recipe you may wish to use 2 tablespoons of grated ginger. Add more the next time if you like the heat and flavor.

TURKEY PICCATA

Gluten-Free

This recipe is a gourmet treat as well as being quick and easy to make.

> 1 to 1¼ pounds of sliced turkey breast
> 2 to 3 tablespoons tapioca starch, arrowroot, or cornstarch
> ¼ to ½ teaspoon salt
> Dash of pepper
> 2 tablespoons oil, preferably olive oil
> 2 tablespoons lemon juice
> ½ cup water or white wine*

Mix the starch, salt, and pepper together in a plate or on a piece of waxed paper. Dip the turkey slices into the mixture so both sides are coated. Heat the oil in a large frying pan (large enough to hold all the slices in a single layer) over medium to medium-high heat for a minute or so. Add the turkey breast slices to the pan and cook them for about 3 minutes on one side until they are beginning to brown. Turn them over and brown them on the other side for about 3 minutes. Add the lemon juice and wine to the pan. Reduce the heat and simmer uncovered for 3 to 5 minutes until the liquid begins to thicken. Turn the turkey slices. Cover the pan with a lid and simmer for another 5 minutes. Check the pan after 2 to 3 minutes and add more water or wine if the liquid is drying out. If necessary, at the end of the cooking time remove the lid and simmer until the liquid is very thick like a glaze covering the turkey. Serve immediately. Makes 4 servings, each of which contains 3 to 4 protein units, ¼ carbohydrate unit, and 13 grams of fat. If you are making this dinner for one or two people and do not have a large frying pan, halve the amounts of all the ingredients and cook it in a smaller pan.

***Note:** If you are allergic to yeast and wish to make this recipe, use the water instead of the wine.

QUICK STROGANOFF

1 8- to 13-ounce (dry weight) can mushrooms, drained, or ¾ pound fresh
 mushrooms, sliced* (optional)

1 small onion, chopped (optional)

1½ to 2½ tablespoons oil (Use the larger amount if more meat and vegetables
 are used).

1 to 1¼ pounds of boneless chicken breast, beef for stir-fry, or fairly tender
 beef or game meat steak

1 teaspoon salt, only if the beef broth is not used

2 tablespoons tapioca starch, arrowroot, or cornstarch

1 to 1¼ cups water, red wine*, or beef broth (Use the larger amount if
 more meat is used).

4 cups cooked noodles such as quinoa noodles or other noodles you tolerate
 cooked *al dente* as directed on page 163

If you are using the fresh mushrooms and/or onion, sauté them in the oil in a frying pan until they are tender. While the vegetables are cooking, prepare the meat by cutting it into thin strips about 2 inches long. Then bring the water for cooking the noodles to a boil while you wait. (Directions for cooking pasta are on page 163). When the vegetables are tender, remove them from the pan. If there is no oil left, add an additional tablespoon of oil to the pan and proceed as in the second paragraph below.

If you are not using the fresh vegetables, add 1½ tablespoons of oil to a frying pan. Prepare the meat as above. (Using pre-cut stir-fry meat will save you time on this step).

Cook the meat over medium-high heat in the oil for 5 to 7 minutes or until it is brown on all sides. Mix the starch with the wine, broth, or water and add the mixture to the meat. Add the cooked vegetables or canned mushrooms to the pan. Add the salt if you did not use the broth. Bring the pan to a boil over medium-high heat and cook for a few minutes until the sauce has thickened. Serve over hot cooked noodles. Makes 4 servings, each of which contains 3 to 4 protein units, ¼ carbohydrate unit, and 16 to 20 grams of fat. Also add the carbohydrate units from the noodles.

Game Stroganoff variation: Use any red game meat steak instead of beef or chicken. After browning the meat, add 1½ cups of water to the pan and simmer the meat for 45 minutes. Proceed with the recipe as above except use only ¾ cup of wine, broth or additional water to mix with the starch.

*Note: If you are allergic to yeast and wish to make this recipe, omit the mushrooms and use the broth or water instead of the wine.

CHICKEN MARSALA

Gluten-Free

2 whole skinless boned chicken breasts (about 2 pounds)
1½ to 2 tablespoon olive oil or other oil
Dash of salt
Dash of pepper
3 to 4 tablespoons tapioca starch, arrowroot, or cornstarch
1 4-ounce (dry weight) can of mushrooms, not drained*
½ to ¾ cup water, Marsala wine* or grape juice

Pound the chicken breasts with a meat tenderizer until they are thin. Mix the starch, salt and pepper together in a plate or on a piece of waxed paper. Dip the chicken into the mixture so both sides are coated. Heat the oil in a large frying pan (large enough to hold all the chicken in a single layer) over medium to medium-high heat for a minute or so. Add the chicken pieces to the pan and cook them for about 3 minutes on one side until they are beginning to brown. Turn them over and brown them on the other side for about 3 minutes. Add the mushrooms with their juice and the Marsala, juice or water to the pan. Cover the pan and bring the liquid to a boil. Reduce the heat and simmer for 15 minutes. Turn the pieces of chicken over half-way through the simmering time so both sides absorb the sauce. As the simmering time nears its end, check the pan and add more water or wine if the liquid is drying out. If the sauce does not thicken quickly enough, at the end of 15 minutes remove the lid from the pan and simmer another few minutes until the sauce is thick. Serve immediately. Makes 6 servings, each of which contains 4 to 5 protein units, ¼ carbohydrate unit, and 12 grams of fat. If you are making this dinner for one or two people and do not have a large frying pan, halve the amounts of all the ingredients and cook it in a smaller pan.

***Note:** If you are allergic to yeast and wish to make this recipe, omit the mushrooms and use juice or water instead of the wine.

Basil Roughy

This dish is delicious and tender, and it will be on the table in nearly no time. Bake "Nuke-n-Bake Carrots," page 172, in the oven with this for a quick meal.

> 1 pound orange roughy fillets
> 1½ to 2 tablespoons oil or melted butter
> 1 tablespoon lemon juice OR ¼ teaspoon unbuffered vitamin C powder plus
>   1 tablespoon water (optional)
> ⅛ teaspoon salt, or to taste
> Dash of paprika (optional)
> ½ teaspoon sweet basil

If you are using the vitamin C, mix it with the water in a corner of a 9-inch by 13-inch glass baking dish until it is dissolved. Combine the oil or melted butter with the vitamin C solution or lemon juice in the baking dish. Put the fillets into the dish and turn them over so they are coated with the oil mixture on both sides. Sprinkle them with the salt, paprika, and basil. Bake at 350°F for about 15 minutes, or until the fish flakes easily with a fork. Makes 2 servings, each of which contains 4½ protein units and 12 grams of fat.

Pepper Steak

This recipe cooks in the oven unattended while you are busy. The long cooking time makes less tender cuts of meat melt in your mouth. Serve with baked sweet potatoes (page 170) and an oven vegetable (pages 168 to 170) baked at the same time for an easy oven meal.

> 1 pound beef or game round steak, cut into serving-size pieces
> 1 to 2 bell peppers
> Dash of salt
> Dash of pepper
> Water

Remove the stems and seeds from the peppers and slice them into strips. Place the steak pieces into a glass baking dish. Add water almost to the top of the meat. Sprinkle the meat with salt and pepper and top it with the bell pepper strips. Cover the dish with its lid or with foil and bake it at 350°F for about 2 hours. As the baking time nears completion, check the steak as it is cooking and add more water if necessary to keep it from drying out completely. The water should have almost completely evaporated by serving time. If it seems to be evaporating too slowly, remove the lid during the last 15 minutes of baking and turn up the temperature if necessary so that the water evaporates and the meat browns. Makes 4 servings, each of which contains 3½ protein units and 11 grams of fat.

Buffalo Loaf

Gluten-Free

The fresh vegetables added to this meatloaf make it tender and give it excellent flavor.

1 pound ground buffalo
¼ small onion, finely chopped (optional)
½ small green pepper, finely chopped (about ⅓ cup chopped)
1 cup grated carrots
¾ teaspoon salt, or to taste
¼ teaspoon pepper (optional)
¼ teaspoon dry mustard (optional)
¼ cup water
¼ cup catsup, preferably unsweetened or fruit or agave sweetened (optional)

Mix together the buffalo, vegetables and seasonings. Shape the mixture into a loaf and put it into a 2- to 3-quart covered casserole dish with the water. Cover the casserole dish with its lid and bake the meatloaf at 350°F for 45 minutes. Then uncover it and bake it for another 30 minutes. Top it with the catsup during the last 15 minutes of baking, if desired. Makes 4 servings, each of which contains 3½ protein units and 2 grams of fat.

Oven Fried Chicken

Gluten-Free IF made with GF flour

3 pounds of skinless chicken breasts or chicken parts of any kind
½ to ¾ cup flour of any kind with a mild taste which you tolerate – sorghum flour (GF), brown rice flour (GF), cassava meal (GF), almond flour (GF), whole spelt flour, etc.
¼ teaspoon salt
⅛ teaspoon pepper (optional)

Skin the chicken and cut it into serving-sized pieces. Combine the flour, salt, and pepper in a plastic bag. Put the chicken pieces into the flour one or two at a time and shake the bag to coat the chicken thoroughly. Place the chicken pieces in a baking dish in a single layer. Turn your oven on to 375°F. Bake the chicken, uncovered, for one hour. Remove the pan from the oven and tilt it to allow the fat to run to one corner of the pan. Use a spoon or baster to pick up the fat and dribble it over the poultry. (If there is very little fat, you can baste the chicken with oil instead of pan drippings). Return the chicken to the oven and bake it for another hour, for a total cooking time of 2 hours. Remove it from the oven when it is browned and crisp. Makes 8 servings, each of which contains 4 protein units, ½ carbohydrate unit, and 13 grams of fat.

CROCK POT ROAST DINNER

Gluten-Free

This recipe makes economical cuts of meat taste like gourmet fare. It also makes great leftovers for tomorrow's dinner or roast beef sandwiches in your lunch.

> 1 2 to 2½-pound rump roast or pot roast of beef, buffalo, or other red game meat
> 10 to 12 small new red potatoes (about 1 pound), scrubbed or peeled and cut in half if desired (optional)
> 3 carrots, scrubbed or peeled and cut into 2-inch pieces
> 1 onion, peeled and sliced or cut into eighths (optional)
> ½ cup water, beef broth, or red wine*
> 1 tomato, chopped, 1 tablespoon tomato paste, or 2 to 3 tablespoons unsweetened or agave sweetened catsup (optional)
> Dash of salt
> Dash of pepper (optional)

Scrub or peel and cut up the vegetables and place them into the bottom of a three quart crock pot. Set the roast on top of the vegetables. Stir together the water, broth, or wine with the tomato, tomato paste or catsup. Pour the liquid over the roast. Sprinkle the roast with the salt and pepper. Cook on low for 10 to 12 hours or on high for 5 to 8 hours. This recipe is very tasty when made with red wine. The alcohol evaporates during cooking, leaving just its flavor. If you are allergic to yeast however, do not use the wine. If you prefer more juice with your roast, increase the amount of water, broth or wine to 1 cup and double the amount of tomato, tomato paste or catsup. Makes 7 servings, each of which contains 1 carbohydrate unit (only if the potatoes are used), 4 protein units, and 17 grams of fat.

***Note:** If you are allergic to yeast and wish to make this recipe, use the broth or water instead of the wine.

Superfood Beef or Game Meat Stew

This stew is easy to make in a crock pot and contains many anti-inflammatory ingredients including carrots, spinach or arugula, and black pepper. If you prefer a traditional-tasting stew, omit the arugula, but if you enjoy a change of pace, give it a try.

1½ to 2 pounds game meat or lean beef (such as round steak) cut into 1 or 2-inch pieces

1 pound new red potatoes or white sweet potatoes,* peeled and cut into 1-inch cubes

3 stalks celery, cut into 1-inch slices

3 large carrots, peeled and cut into 1-inch slices

¼ cup quick cooking (Minute™) tapioca (optional)

½ teaspoon ground black pepper

¾ to 1 teaspoon salt

1 to 1½ cups water

3 to 4 cups washed spinach or arugula (optional)

In a 3 quart crock pot, stir together the meat, potato cubes, carrots, celery, tapioca, pepper, and salt. Add the water: You will need only 1 cup of water if you omit the tapioca; if you are making this with tapioca for the first time, start with 1 cup of water. If you have made this stew before, are using the tapioca and like it juicier, add up to 1½ cups of water initially. Stir the stew again.

Cook on high for 4 to 5 hours or on low for 7 to 8 hours. At the end of that time, turn the crock pot temperature up to high if it has been on low. If you would like the stew juicier, add up to ½ cup boiling water. Add the spinach or arugula to the crock pot, put the lid back on, and cook on high for 15 to 30 minutes or until the spinach or arugula is wilted. Makes 6 servings, each of which contains 1 carbohydrate unit (only if the potatoes are used), 4 protein units, and 17 grams of fat.

*Note about the potatoes: White sweet potatoes have a mealy texture and neutral flavor. However, if white sweet potatoes are out of season, use orange sweet potatoes. Both new red potatoes and sweet potatoes are medium on the GI scale. In contrast, Russet potatoes have a high GI score.

CHICKEN AND BEAN ENCHILADAS

Gluten-Free IF
made with GF tortillas

3 cups shredded or cubed cooked chicken (about 16 ounces which can be
    prepared from about 1½ to 2 pounds of chicken breasts*)
½ medium onion
1 to 5 jalapeno peppers, to taste
2 to 3 teaspoons oil
1 15-ounce can black beans
1 15-ounce can kidney beans, canned without sugar (Salt-free beans often are
    sugar-free, or use a brand such as Westbrae™ from your health food store).
1 8-ounce can of tomato sauce, optional
8 ounces shredded low fat cheddar cheese (about 2 cups) of any kind you tolerate
16 to 20 6-inch thin corn tortillas or the number of other tortillas of any kind
    you tolerate which have an equivalent total net carbohydrate content
Oil or cooking oil spray

Prepare the chicken as directed on the next page or, for roasted chicken, as directed
in the recipe for "Italian Powerhouse Salad" on page 120. For convenience, prepare extra
chicken and freeze it for future use.

Slice the onion and cut the slices into ½ inch pieces. Combine the oil and onion
in a frying pan and sauté on medium heat for about 5 minutes. Quarter the jalapenos
lengthwise and slice the quarters crosswise. Add the peppers to the pan with the onion
and cook for another 5 minutes.

Rinse the beans under running water in a strainer. Using the pan you used to cook
the vegetables or a large bowl, combine the cooked vegetables, beans, chicken, tomato
sauce if you are using it, and about 1½ cups of the cheese. If you are allergic to tomatoes or prefer the flavor of these enchiladas without the tomato sauce, you may omit it.
However, it is easier to keep the filling together when you roll the enchiladas if you use
the tomato sauce.

Lightly oil two baking dishes, one large (9 by 13 inches) and one small (8 by 8
inches or a casserole dish will work). Preheat your oven to 350°F.

Spray or brush both sides of four tortillas with cooking oil spray or oil. Stack them
on a dish. Microwave them for 30 to 60 seconds or until they are warm and soft. Spoon
about ⅓ to ½ cup of the meat mixture onto each tortilla and roll them up. Lay them
seam side down in the baking dishes. Repeat with the remaining tortillas. Cover the
dishes with foil. Bake for 20 to 30 minutes or until the enchiladas are heated throughout. Remove the foil and sprinkle the remaining cheese over the enchiladas. Bake for
another 5 minutes or until the cheese is melted.

Makes 16 to 20 enchiladas. If you use 16 thin tortillas, a 4-enchilada serving contains 2 carbohydrate units, 5 protein units, and 11 grams of fat. If you use 20 thin tortillas, a 4-enchilada serving contains 2 carbohydrate units, 4 protein units, and 9 grams of fat.

If you use thick corn tortillas or other tortillas that contain 15 grams net carbohydrate each, eat only 2 enchiladas per serving. If you make 16 enchiladas with thick tortillas, each serving of 2 enchiladas will contain 2 carbohydrate units, 2½ protein units and 5½ grams of fat. If you make 20 enchiladas with thin tortillas, each serving of 4 enchiladas will contain 2 carbohydrate units, 4 protein units and 10 grams of fat. The carbohydrates in cooked legumes are so high-fiber that Dr. Cheryle Hart does not count them.

*Note on preparing chicken: To make enough cooked chicken for two to four batches of enchiladas, put 4 to 6 pounds of chicken breasts in a large pot with ½ teaspoon of salt. Cover the chicken with water and bring it to a boil over high heat. Then reduce the heat and simmer for 1 to 1½ hours. Cool the breasts. You may remove them from the broth to refrigerate them or refrigerate the whole pan at this point for several hours or overnight. The broth may gel if refrigerated overnight. When the breasts are cool, remove the skin and bones. Cut and/or break apart the meat with kitchen shears and your fingers, discarding any gristle or remaining bone. Use as much of the chicken as needed to make enchiladas and freeze the remainder in 3 cup portions for future use. Save and/or freeze the homemade chicken broth for use in recipes which call for chicken broth if desired. Six pounds of chicken yields about 10 to 12 cups of shredded chicken.

ENCHILADA CASSEROLE

**Gluten-Free IF
made with GF tortillas**

1 pound ground turkey, lean ground beef or other lean ground meat
1½ cups chopped bell pepper (about 1 large pepper total, any color or combination of colors)
½ cup chopped onion, optional
½ to 1 teaspoon chipotle powder or chili powder, to taste, optional (Use the smaller amount of chipotle powder with hot salsa).
1 6-ounce can tomato paste
3 to 3¼ cups bottled salsa, divided
2 to 3 cups (8 to 12 ounces) shredded cheese, preferably low fat cheddar, of any type you tolerate (goat, soy, cow's milk, etc.)
12 6-inch thin corn tortillas or the number of other tortillas you tolerate with an equivalent total net carbohydrate content*

Chop the onion and cut the peppers into about ½-inch pieces. For an eye-appealing dish, use half of an orange or red pepper and half of a green pepper. If you have no use for leftover halves of peppers, this dish is good made with one whole orange pepper. Cook the meat, onion and peppers in a skillet over medium heat, stirring and breaking the meat up, until the meat is brown throughout and the vegetables are soft.

Drain any fat. Add the chipotle powder, 1 to 1¼ cups of the salsa, and the tomato paste to the meat mixture and simmer about 5 to 10 minutes longer.

Set aside ½ cup of the cheese to sprinkle on the top of the casserole near the end of the baking time. Preheat your oven to 350°F.

Spread ½ cup of the salsa on the bottom of a 3-quart casserole dish. Top with a layer of slightly overlapping tortillas, using one third of the tortillas. (Depending on the size and shape of the dish, you may have to cut the tortillas to fit the dish). Top the tortillas with half of the meat mixture, half of the non-reserved cheese, and one third of the remaining salsa. Repeat with another layer of tortillas, meat, cheese, and salsa. Top with a final layer of tortillas and the remaining salsa.

Cover the dish with foil or its lid and bake for 30 to 45 minutes or until it is heated throughout. Remove the foil or lid, sprinkle with the reserved cheese, and bake for another 5 minutes or until the cheese is melted.

Makes 3 to 6 servings. If you use thick corn tortillas or other tortillas that contain 15 grams net carbohydrate each, this recipe makes 6 servings, each of which contains 2 carbohydrate units, 3½ protein units, and 10 grams of fat. If you use thin corn tortillas you can divide this batch into 3 servings with each serving containing 2 carbohydrate units, 7 protein units, and 20 grams of fat. Divide these numbers in half if you make 6 servings with thin corn tortillas. The carbohydrates in cooked legumes are so high-fiber that Dr. Cheryle Hart does not count them.

Rolled Enchiladas: If you have time, this recipe may be used to make rolled enchiladas. Make the meat and vegetable mixture as above using 2 to 2¼ cups of the salsa. Add all but ½ cup of the cheese to the mixture. Spread about ½ cup of the reserved salsa on the bottom of a 13 by 9 inch baking dish. Preheat your oven to 400°F.

Spray or brush both sides of four tortillas with oil. Stack them on a dish. Microwave them for 30 seconds or until they are warm and soft. Spoon about ⅓ cup of the meat mixture into each tortilla and lay them seam side down in the baking dish. Repeat with the remaining tortillas. Spread the tops of the enchiladas in the baking dish with enough of the remaining salsa to cover them. Cover the dish with foil. Bake for 20 to 30 minutes or until they are heated throughout. Remove the foil and sprinkle the reserved cheese over the enchiladas. Bake for another 5 minutes or until the cheese is melted. Makes 12 enchiladas or 3 to 6 servings. If you use thick corn tortillas or other tortillas that contain 15 grams net carbohydrate each, this recipe makes 6 2-enchilada servings, each of which contains 2 carbohydrate units, 3½ protein units, and 10 grams of fat. If you use thin corn tortillas you can have 3 4-enchilada servings, with each serving containing 2 carbohydrate units, 7 protein units, and 20 grams of fat. Divide these numbers in half if you make 6 servings with thin corn tortillas.

*Note on tortillas: If you are not allergic to corn, you may want to use corn tortillas in this recipe because they are traditional in and go very well with Mexican food as well as being gluten-free. If you purchase the thin "frying" variety rather than the thicker "bread" variety of tortillas you will get less carbohydrate. Read the nutrition label on the back of the tortilla package to determine how many (2 or 4) tortillas contain 30 grams of net carbohydrate (total carbohydrate grams minus grams of fiber). I use Mission™ Extra Thin Yellow Corn Tortillas which contain 28 grams of net carbohydrate in 4 tortillas. If you use other tortillas, adjust the serving size so the total net carbohydrate does not exceed 30.

ECONOMY CHILI

Gluten-Free

This recipe is very economical as well as great to have in your freezer for future meals. My original version is not very hot. My son Joel makes his chili more exciting by substituting salsa for the tomato sauce and adding jalapeno peppers and crumbled dry chili pequin peppers for heat and flavor; his variations on the recipe are included. See "Sources," page 282 if you cannot find chili pequin peppers locally.

  1 pound dry kidney beans
  Water
  1½ to 2 pounds of lean ground turkey, lean ground beef, buffalo, or game meat
  1 12-ounce can tomato paste
  1 16-ounce can tomato sauce (For Joel's hot chili, substitute 2 cups of salsa).
  1 small onion, chopped, or 3 tablespoons dry chopped onions (optional)
  1 teaspoon salt
  1 to 3 teaspoons of chili powder, to taste, or 2 to 5 crumbled 1-inch long dried
       chile pequin peppers, to taste (Use the chile pequin for Joel's hot chili).
  2 to 4 jalapeno peppers, chopped, or 1 to 2 4-ounce cans sliced jalapeno
       peppers, drained (optional – omit for mild chili and use with the seeds for
       the hottest chili).

The evening before you plan to serve the chili, rinse the beans by running water over them in a strainer to remove any dirt. Put them in a 3-quart crock pot and cover them with cold water. Allow the beans to soak overnight.

Preparation of the meat should be done the evening before if you will not be home at least an hour or two before dinner, or it can be done the afternoon of the day you serve this recipe if time allows. In a separate pan on the stove, brown the ground meat.

Add the optional fresh onion and fresh jalapeno peppers and cook for a few minutes more. Drain and discard the fat. If you are doing this the evening before, refrigerate the meat mixture. If you want to eat quickly when you get home the next day, warm it in the microwave oven before adding it to the crock pot. If you have more time to let the flavors meld, you can add it to the crock pot cold or freshly cooked and cook the chili with the meat for one to four hours before serving time.

In the morning, drain the water from the beans, add fresh water to the pot, and drain the water again. Rinse the beans this way three times. (This soaking and rinsing process removes difficult-to-digest carbohydrates which can cause intestinal gas). Add enough water to the beans in the pot to cover them. Cook on high for 4 to 6 hours or on low for 8 to 10 hours.

When the beans are tender, drain the water until it is about half the level of the beans in the pot. Stir the tomato paste into the pot thoroughly. Add the cooked meat or meat and vegetable mixture, dry onions (if you are using them), tomato sauce or salsa, canned jalapeno peppers (if you are using them), and seasonings. If you like your chili juicer, add some boiling water and drain less of the bean cooking liquid the next time you make this recipe. If you are adding these ingredients shortly before dinner, cook the chili on high for 20 minutes or until heated through. If you have more time, the flavor will be best if you can cook the chili for another 1 to 2 hours on high. Makes 8 to servings, each of which contains 4 protein units and 7 grams of fat. The carbohydrates in cooked legumes are so high-fiber that Dr. Cheryle Hart does not count them.

If you wish to make a larger batch of this chili in a 5-quart crock pot, multiply the ingredient amounts by 1½.

SPEEDY MICROWAVE CHILI

Gluten-Free

If you are in a real hurry and need dinner for only one or two people, see the note on how to make a small batch extra quickly at the end of this recipe. This recipe was originally developed for college students to make in dormitory microwave ovens.

   1 pound lean ground turkey or beef
   3 8-ounce cans tomato sauce
   3 15-ounce cans kidney beans canned without sugar, drained
   ¼ teaspoon salt
   ½ to 1 teaspoon chili powder, or to taste

Crumble the ground turkey or beef into a hard plastic colander set in a large casserole dish. Microwave on high for 5 to 8 minutes, stirring and breaking up the meat every 2 minutes, until the meat no longer has any pink spots. Drain the grease from the casserole and discard it. Add the cooked meat and tomato sauce to the casserole, cover it with the lid or plastic wrap, and microwave on high for 5 minutes, stirring half way through the cooking time.

Drain the bean liquid in the cans and add the beans to the casserole dish. Add the seasonings and microwave on high for another 5 to 7 minutes, stirring every 2 to 3 minutes. Makes 6 servings, each of which contains 4 protein units and 7 grams of fat. The carbohydrates in cooked legumes are so high-fiber that Dr. Cheryle Hart does not count them.

Note: To make a large serving for one person or medium-sized servings for two in less time, use ⅓ pound ground beef, 1 can of tomato sauce, 1 can of beans, and a dash of salt, and chili powder to taste. Microwave the meat for 3 to 5 minutes, the meat and tomato sauce for 5 minutes, and all of the ingredients together for another 5 minutes.

Mexican Mix

Gluten-Free

To save work on future meals, double this recipe and put three-fourths of it in the freezer to have three easy-to-finish meals.

> 1 Anaheim pepper, chopped (about ¾ cup chopped)
> ½ to 2 jalapeno peppers, finely chopped, to taste
> 1 small or ½ to ¾ of a medium or large bell pepper,* chopped (about 1 cup chopped)
> ¾ cup finely chopped onion (about 3 slices)
> 1 pound lean ground turkey, lean ground beef, buffalo, or other lean game meat
> 1 15-ounce can whole tomatoes, cut or crushed into large pieces
> 1 15-ounce can black beans, drained
> 1 4.5-ounce can chopped olives, drained
> 1 teaspoon salt, or to taste

Chop the onion and peppers. Retain and use the seeds from the jalapeno pepper if you like your Mexican food hot. Cook the meat, peppers, and onions in a frying pan over medium heat, stirring and breaking up the meat, until the meat is thoroughly cooked and the vegetables are tender. Drain and discard any fat that is in the pan. Cut or crush the tomatoes into large pieces, drain and rinse the beans, and drain the olives. Add the beans, tomatoes, olives and salt to the pan and simmer for five minutes. Makes about 7 cups of mix or enough for two batches of "Tamale Casserole," below. Freeze any mix you are not going to use within a day or two for future easy meals. A half-batch of this mix contains 7 protein units and 30 grams of fat. The carbohydrates in cooked legumes are so high-fiber that Dr. Cheryle Hart does not count them.

*Note on peppers: Green bell peppers contain the anti-nflammatory compound luteo-lin: orange peppers may also be anti-inflammatory and have a great flavor. For a single batch, I like to use ½ small pepper each of green and orange

Easy Fajitas: To make fajitas, roll ½ to ¾ cup of this mix in a tortilla with any desired additions (cheese, guacamole, etc.), use a toothpick to hold the tortilla closed, and microwave until hot. To have your serving provide the desired amount of protein, ½ cup of this mix is one protein unit; ⅞ to 1 cup is 2 protein units. Each ounce of cheese used will add 1 protein unit.

Tamale Casserole

Gluten-Free

3½ cups "Mexican Mix," above
1 cup water
½ cup cornmeal
½ to 1 cup (2 to 4 ounces) shredded cheese, preferably low-fat cheddar, of any
    type you tolerate (goat, soy, cow's milk, etc.), optional

If you are starting with frozen pre-made Mexican mix, put half a batch (about 3½ cups) of mix in a pan. If you just made the mix, remove all but 3½ cups from the frying pan you prepared it in. Add the water to the pan and bring it to a simmer. Stir in the cornmeal. Put the mixture in a 2½ to 3 quart casserole dish and cover it with a lid or foil. Bake at 350°F for 15 to 20 minutes or until the water is all absorbed, stirring it halfway through the baking time. Remove the casserole from the oven, stir it again, and sprinkle the cheese over the top. Bake it uncovered for another 5 to 10 minutes or until it is hot throughout and the cheese is melted. Makes 4 servings, each of which contains 1 carbohydrate unit, 2½ protein units, and 9 grams of fat. (You can increase the serving size up to double and stay within 30 grams of carbohydrate). The carbohydrates in cooked legumes are so high-fiber that Dr. Cheryle Hart does not count them.

PIZZA

**Gluten-Free IF
made with a GF crust**

Yes, you can have pizza on a glycemic control diet if you monitor your portion size. Because gluten-free dough is dense, it takes more of it – measured by the amount of flour used – to fill a pizza pan. To remain within two carbohydrate units (30 grams of carbohydrate) per meal, each person should have a portion of pizza containing about ⅖ cup of flour in the dough.

Pizza sauce for two 12-inch pizzas

> 1 6-ounce can tomato paste
> 1 8-ounce can tomato sauce
> ⅓ cup water
> 1 teaspoon oregano
> ½ teaspoon thyme
> ½ teaspoon sweet basil
> 1 tablespoon olive oil (optional)

Topping ingredients for a 12-inch pizza

(When making a 12-inch quinoa pizza which will serve 4, you may wish to increase the amount of these toppings if ¼ pizza is not enough to satisfy).

> 4 ounces (about 1 cup) grated part-skim mozzarella cheese of any type you tolerate (goat, soy, cow's milk, etc.)
> 2 tablespoons Romano cheese (optional – Try all-sheep Romano if you are allergic to cow's milk).
> 4 ounces cooked lean ground turkey, lean ground beef, or ground buffalo
> Vegetables toppings such as sliced bell peppers, olives, etc. (optional)

Pizza dough - choose one option below

Quinoa Pizza Dough, recipe on page 155
Yeast bread dough: amaranth, buckwheat, whole spelt, barley, etc.
> (Use a portion of the recipe which uses about ⅖ cup of flour for a 2-carbohydrate unit serving; recipes on pages 184 to 194 of *The Ultimate Food Allergy Cookbook and Survival Guide*)

Non-yeast bread dough: amaranth, buckwheat, teff, whole spelt, barley, etc.
> (Use a portion of the recipe which uses about ⅖ cup of flour for a 2-carbohydrate unit serving; recipes on pages 186 to 187 of this book or pages 151 to 153 of *The Ultimate Food Allergy Cookbook and Survival Guide*)

Stone Ground Whole Wheat Pizza dough, recipe on page 242, for your non-allergic eating plan companions

Combine the sauce ingredients in a saucepan. Cook the sauce on medium heat until it just begins to boil. Reduce the heat to low and simmer the sauce for 30 to 40 minutes, stirring every ten minutes to keep the sauce from sticking to the bottom of the pan. When it is thick, remove the sauce from the heat until you are ready to use it. This makes enough sauce for two 12-inch pizzas. Freeze the sauce you don't use immediately for future use

While the sauce is cooking, prepare the yeast dough of your choice and allow it to rise the first time. If you are using non-yeast dough, measure out the dry ingredients into a large bowl and stir them together. Measure and combine the liquid ingredients so they will be ready to add to the dry ingredients immediately before you assemble the pizza. Halve or otherwise reduce the amount of dough ingredients for the bread recipes listed above to yield portions that take about ⅔ cup of flour for each serving of pizza that you wish to make.

Prepare the toppings while the sauce is cooking. Brown the meat in a frying pan and thoroughly drain any fat. Chop or slice the vegetable toppings.

For a yeast dough pizza, lightly oil a 12-inch pizza pan. If you are making a smaller batch, oil half – or the appropriate fraction – of a pizza pan or a baking sheet. Stretch the dough thinly in a lightly oiled pizza pan or on the baking sheet. If you want a "thin crust" pizza, top it immediately as directed below. If you want a "thick crust" pizza, place the pizza in a warm spot in your kitchen and let the dough rise for 5 to 10 minutes. Pre-heat your oven to 400°F. While the oven is heating, spread the pizza dough with sauce and add the desired toppings. Bake for 20 to 25 minutes or until the edge is golden brown. The baking time may vary slightly with the type of dough used.

If you are using a non-yeast dough, preheat your oven to 400°F. Oil and flour a pizza pan or baking sheet. After the toppings are all prepared, stir the liquid ingredients into the dry ingredients for the dough. Do not over-mix. Immediately, flour your hand and pat the dough out to the edges of the pan or to the desired size on the baking sheet. Top with the sauce and toppings quickly and place the pizza into the oven without delay. Bake for 20 to 30 minutes or until the edge is golden brown. The baking time may vary slightly with the type of dough used.

Although making your own pizza dough gives you total control over what is in it and the balance between carbohydrates and protein as well as yielding the most tasty pizza, we don't always have time for making dough. You can use a pre-made gluten or wheat-free pizza crust, but watch portion sizes. Most of the crusts in the freezer at my health food store range from 24 to 32 grams of carbohydrates for a quarter of an 8-inch pizza crust and contain very little fiber (The fiber values range from "less than 1 gram" to 1 gram). Rustic Crust™ gluten-free pizza crust is an exception with only 12 grams of carbohydrate per quarter of an 8-inch pizza. With this brand, you could have half of an 8-inch pizza which is not an extremely small serving (in contrast with less than a quarter of the pizza for some of the other brands). Top a 2-carbohydrate-unit portion of crust from your health food store with pizza sauce and enough of the toppings above to yield at least two units of protein (2 ounces of meat plus cheese, or ¼ batch of the toppings), and bake as directed on the crust package.

The pizza toppings above (without the dough) yield 4 servings, each of which contains 2 protein units and 8 grams of fat. If made with quinoa dough and the topping amounts listed above, one pizza makes 4 servings, each of each of which contains 2 carbohydrate units, 2½ protein units, and 17 grams of fat

Quinoa Pizza Dough

Gluten-Free

This dough is my favorite example of gluten-free pizza dough but is not the only allergy or gluten-free dough you might use. See the bread recipes on pages 151 to 153 (yeast-free) or 184 to 194 of The Ultimate Food Allergy Cookbook and Survival Guide for more kinds of dough. For your non-allergic companions, make stone ground whole wheat pizza dough using the recipe on page 242.

> 1⅓ cups quinoa flour
> 1½ teaspoons active dry yeast
> 1½ teaspoons guar gum
> A scant ¼ teaspoon salt
> ⅔ cup water
> ⅓ cup apple juice concentrate, thawed
> 2 tablespoons oil

Put the flour, yeast, guar gum, and salt in a large mixer bowl. Mix on low speed for about 30 seconds. In a small saucepan, warm the water, apple juice and oil to 115 to 120°F. (Measure the temperature with a digital or a yeast thermometer). With the mixer running on low speed, add the liquids in a slow stream to the dry ingredients. Continue mixing until the dry and liquid ingredients are thoroughly mixed. Beat the dough on medium speed for 3 minutes. Scrape the dough from the beaters and the sides of the bowl into the bottom of the bowl. Cover the bowl, put it in a warm place (85°F to 90°F; see page 188 for more about this) and let the dough rise for one hour or until doubled. Beat the dough again for three minutes at medium speed.

If you have a bread machine, use the dough cycle to make the dough, adding the ingredients above to the machine in the order your instruction manual specifies. Mix the guar gum into the flour before adding it. Run the dough cycle to completion. Then restart the cycle and allow it to knead for 3 to 5 minutes after it begins kneading quickly (if your knead cycle has gentle start) to remove the gas from the dough.

Oil a 12-inch pizza pan or baking sheet. Scrape the dough out of the bowl or bread machine pan and onto the prepared pan. Then oil your hand and use it to spread the out to the edges of the pizza pan or to flatten it to the desired thickness on a baking sheet. Preheat your oven to 400°F. While the oven is heating, spread the pizza dough with ½ batch of pizza sauce and one batch of toppings or more toppings to provide satiety. Add at least two or more ounces of protein (meat plus cheese) per serving or 8 ounces for the whole pizza (at 4 servings per pizza) to make ¼ of a pizza enough to satisfy and to balance the carbohydrate in the crust. Top with vegetable toppings. Bake for 20 to 25 minutes or until the edge is golden brown. Makes 4 servings, each of which contains 2 carbohydrate units, 2½ protein units, and 17 grams of fat.

Lasagne

Gluten-Free IF made with GF pasta

When I make this most recent version of my lasagne recipe, the sauce cooks in a crock pot with minimal stirring and does not splash all over my kitchen the way it did when cooked on the stove.

Sauce ingredients

> 2 pounds lean ground turkey, beef, buffalo, or other meat
> 2 12-ounce cans tomato paste
> 1 28-ounce can tomato puree
> 1½ cups water
> 1 teaspoon salt
> ⅛ teaspoon pepper (optional)

Additional ingredients

> About 2 to 2½ boxes no-boil lasagne noodles, any type you tolerate
> 3 15-ounce containers of part-skim ricotta cheese, any type you tolerate (goat, soy, cow's milk etc.)
> ½ cup grated Romano or Parmesan cheese (optional – Use all sheep Romano if you are allergic to cow's milk).
> 32 ounces of part-skim mozzarella cheese, any type you tolerate (goat, soy, cow's milk etc.)
> 1½ tablespoons chopped dried parsley (optional)

Start making the sauce early in the morning on a day when you have adequate time to cook if you want to serve, refrigerate, or freeze the lasagne that evening. Or, if you want to spread the work out a little, make the sauce at least one day before you plan to serve, refrigerate, or freeze this lasagne.

Combine the tomato paste, tomato puree, water, salt and pepper in a 3-quart crock pot and turn it to "high." Cook the meat in a frying pan over medium heat, breaking it up and stirring it often, until it is well browned. Pour off and discard the fat. Add the meat to the crock pot and stir thoroughly. If you are having the lasagne the next day or later, you may turn the temperature control on the crock pot to low and allow the sauce to cook unattended for 8 to 10 hours total cooking time. However, if you will be at home and want to shorten the cooking time and/or have thicker sauce, you may cook it on high for four to six hours, stirring it every 1 to 1½ hours. Cooking the sauce on high will allow you to assemble the lasagne the same day that you make the sauce.

When the sauce is almost cooked, I do not stir it within about the last hour of the cooking time. This allows the meat to settle so the sauce at the top of the crock pot is lower in meat content than the sauce at the bottom. I use a large spoon to remove some of the low-meat sauce from the top of the pot to use both under the first layer of pasta and on top of the last layer of pasta when I assemble the lasagne. After I've taken off enough of the lower-meat sauce, I stir the remaining sauce before removing it from the pot. However, if you like meaty sauce at the top and the bottom of your lasagne, stir it thoroughly before taking any from the pot.

This size batch of lasagne sauce plus the cheese filling contains 75 protein units and 320 grams of fat. If you use it to make 18 servings of lasagne, each serving contains 4 protein units and 18 grams of fat. See the last paragraph of this recipe to determine how many servings you should make with the type of pasta you use.

The sauce may be refrigerated overnight or frozen. Makes about 2½ quarts of sauce. If you wish to make lasagne often, make a double batch of sauce in a 5-quart crock pot and freeze some of the sauce. Then when you want to make more lasagne, the sauce will be ready to go.

Lasagne assembly instructions:

In a bowl, combine the ricotta cheese, Romano or Parmesan cheese, and parsley. Mash them together with a potato masher. Slice the mozzarella cheese thinly.

Spread about 1½ to 2 cups of the sauce (total amount for all pans) over the bottoms of a deep 13 inch by 9 inch cake pan or a similar-sized deep casserole dish PLUS a 2½ to 3-quart casserole dish. If you have a large stainless steel lasagne pan/roaster which will hold the whole batch, spread the 1½ to 2 cups of the sauce in the bottom of it. Lay dry lasagne pasta in a single layer over the sauce. (The amount of pasta you need may vary with the type of baking dishes you are using). Spread the pasta with about 3 to 3½ cups of the sauce. Layer about half of the mozzarella cheese over the sauce. Spread half of the ricotta mixture over the mozzarella. Add another layer of pasta to the dish, followed by another 3 to 3½ cups of sauce, the rest of the mozzarella, and the rest of the ricotta mixture. Add a third layer of pasta to the dish(es) and top it with about 2 cups of sauce. Serve any remaining sauce on the side with the lasagne. If you wish to, you may refrigerate or freeze the lasagne at this point. Cover the dish(es) with plastic wrap to refrigerate or freeze the lasagne. The lasagne also may be baked before being frozen. If you are sending one portion-sized pieces to college with a special student, bake the lasagne before cutting and freezing it, thus allowing the student to warm it in a microwave oven.

When you are ready to bake the lasagne, thaw it completely in the refrigerator if it has been frozen. Cover it with aluminum foil or with the lid of the casserole dish. Bake the lasagne at 350°F for about 1½ hours or until it is hot throughout and bubbly at the edges. If you refrigerated or froze the lasagne before baking it, allow about an extra ½ hour or more of baking time. If it was frozen and is not completely thawed before baking it, you will have to add more baking time.

To calculate the size of 2-carbohydrate unit serving for this recipe, keep track of how many pieces of pasta you use to assemble the lasagne. Calculate the total net carbohydrates in the casserole using the carbohydrate units minus fiber units from the pasta package. Then divide the casserole so each serving contains 30 grams of net carbohydrate. Because this dish contains a generous amount of meat and cheese, there will be enough protein for balance in each serving. The full batch of lasagne sauce and the cheese fillings contains 75 protein units and 320 grams of fat. These numbers can be divided by the number of servings dictated by the pasta to determine how much protein and fat there is in a serving.

SIDE DISHES, VEGETABLES AND SALADS

A husband once told me that if he said that he really enjoyed a side dish at dinner-time but did not mention the main dish, his wife didn't consider it a complement for her cooking. Although the main dish is the part of a meal that usually takes the most time to prepare and may be the most expensive, side dishes are often the stars of the meal for nutrition since they contribute fiber , vitamins, minerals, and anti-inflammatory phyto-nutrients such as bioflavonoids and carotenoids. This chapter will introduce you to some new ways of making side dishes exciting enough to draw rave reviews.

Several of the side dishes in the chapter can be baked in the oven with a main dish. This simplifies meal preparation when you are going to be working at home in the afternoon. Just put all the components of the meal into the oven and let things cook while you work. For oven vegetable and side dish recipes, see pages 160 to 162 and 168 to 171. Put a roast, pepper steak (page 142), or oven-fried chicken (page 143) into the oven with these dishes, and you will have a complete meal that will tend itself while you get something else done. This chapter also contains some recipes for vegetables which are first microwaved for a few minutes and then baked or broiled. Serve these microwave-plus-conventional veggies with entrées such as poached fish or broiled meat that cook more quickly than the dishes mentioned above.

Another way to save yourself work is to make good use of your crock pot. The "Crock Pot Baked Beans" recipe on page 164 does not contain the sugar of canned beans and can be made tomato-free for those who are allergic to tomatoes without requiring the tending that oven-baked beans require. For basic recipes and techniques for cooking vegetables conventionally or with a microwave oven, read the packages of frozen vegetables or refer to a general cookbook such as *Easy Cooking for Special Diets* as described on the last pages of this book.

Finally, this chapter contains recipes for simple but nutrient-packed salads and basic salad dressing recipes that avoid problem allergens such as the vinegar and corn found in commercially prepared dressings. Making your own dressing also allows you to incorporate the healthiest of oils which are high in essential fatty acids. Additionally, the use of an oil-containing dressing increases the absorption of nutrients from the salad as well as adding to your satisfaction and enjoyment. Thus, for best nutrition, economize on grams of fat in another part of your meal rather than the salad dressing.

Quinoa Pilaf or Poultry Stuffing

Quinoa boasts a generous level of high quality protein and a low GI score of 53. Thus it is a great substitute for rice. This tasty grain-free side dish is also delicious as poultry stuffing. Be sure to rinse the soap-like coating off of the quinoa before cooking it.

> 2 cups sliced celery
> ¼ small onion, chopped (optional)
> 3 to 4 tablespoons oil
> 1 cup quinoa, thoroughly washed
> 2 cups water
> ½ to 1 teaspoon salt, or to taste
> ¼ teaspoon pepper
> 1 tablespoon dried parsley
> 1 teaspoon sweet basil
> ¼ teaspoon ground rosemary (optional)

Rinse the quinoa in a strainer under running water until the water is no longer sudsy in order to remove its natural soapy coating. Sauté the celery and onion in oil in a saucepan until they just begin to brown. Add the quinoa and water, bring the mixture to a boil, and simmer it for 15 to 20 minutes, or until the quinoa is translucent. Stir in the seasonings thoroughly and allow the quinoa to stand for a few minutes so that the flavors can blend. Serve it as a side dish or stuff it into a large chicken and then roast the chicken. If you use this stuffing for a turkey, double the recipe for a 12-pound turkey or triple it for a 24-pound turkey. Makes 4 to 8 servings. If you divide this into 4 servings, each contains 2 carbohydrate units, ¾ protein unit, and 12 grams of fat. For 8 servings, halve these unit amounts.

Oven Grains

These grains are easy to prepare in the oven while the main dish is cooking yet are so delicious that they make an oven meal special.

Quinoa
> 1 cup quinoa
> 2½ cups water
> ½ teaspoon salt, or to taste
> 1 tablespoon oil
Cooking time: 1 hour

Buckwheat

>1 cup white or roasted buckwheat groats
>3½ cups water
>½ teaspoon salt, or to taste
>1 tablespoon oil
Cooking time: 1 to 1½ hours

Teff

>1 cup teff
>3 cups water
>½ teaspoon salt, or to taste
>1 tablespoon oil
Cooking time: 1 to 1½ hours

Brown rice

>1 cup brown rice
>2½ cups water
>1 tablespoon oil
>½ teaspoon salt
Cooking time: 1 to 1½ hours

Wild rice

>1 cup wild rice
>4 cups water
>1 tablespoon oil
>½ teaspoon salt
Cooking time: 1½ to 2 hours

Choose one set of ingredients from the list above. If you are cooking quinoa, be sure to rinse it in a strainer under running water until the water is no longer sudsy in order to remove its natural soapy coating. Stir together the grain, water, oil and salt in a 2 to 3-quart glass casserole dish with a lid. Cover the dish and bake at about 350°F until the grain is tender and all the water is absorbed. The baking time is flexible so these grains can usually be baked the same amount of time as the entrée of an oven meal. Approximate baking times for each type of grain are given at the end of each ingredient list above. If you will be baking the grain for much longer than these times or at a high temperature, you may need to add a little more water. Check it near the end of the cooking time the first time you make it and note how much extra water you added, if it was indeed needed. Record how much extra water you used for the next time you cook it at a high temperature or for a longer time.

Makes about 2 cups of cooked grain or 4 to 10 servings. If you make 4 servings of quinoa, each contains 2 carbohydrate units, ¾ protein unit, and 6 grams of fat. If you make 4 servings of buckwheat, each contains 2 carbohydrate units, ⅔ protein unit, and 5 grams of fat. If you make 4 servings of teff, each contains 2 carbohydrate units, ½ protein unit, and 4 grams of fat. If you make brown rice, you will need to divide the recipe into 5 servings; each contains 2 carbohydrate units, ½ protein unit, and 5 grams of fat. If you make 4 servings of wild rice, each contains 2 carbohydrate units, ⅔ protein unit, and 4 grams of fat. For 8 servings of each grain except brown rice or 10 servings of brown rice, halve these unit amounts for each grain.

Stove-Top Grains

Gluten-Free

Amaranth
1 cup amaranth
2½ cups water
¼ teaspoon salt
Cooking time: 30 to 35 minutes

Quinoa
1 cup quinoa
2 cups water
¼ teaspoon salt
Cooking time: 20 minutes; Quinoa should be thoroughly rinsed under running water in a strainer before cooking.

Buckwheat
1 cup buckwheat
2½ cups water
½ teaspoon salt
Cooking time: 20 to 30 minutes

Teff
1 cup teff
3 cups water
¼ teaspoon salt
Cooking time: 15 to 20 minutes

Brown rice
1 cup brown rice
2½ cups water
¼ teaspoon salt
Cooking time: 45 to 50 minutes

Wild rice

    1 cup wild rice
    4 cups water
    ¼ teaspoon salt
  Cooking time: 60 minutes

Choose one set of ingredients above. Bring the water to a boil in a saucepan. Add the grain and salt. Put the lid on the pan. Allow the water to return to a boil, then lower the heat and simmer for the time specified at the end of the ingredient list above. Remove the pan from the heat. Allow the grain to stand for a few minutes, fluff and serve. Makes about 2 cups of cooked grain or 4 to 10 servings. If you make 4 servings of amaranth, each contains 2 carbohydrate units and 1 protein unit. If you make 4 servings of quinoa, each contains 2 carbohydrate units and ¾ protein unit. If you make 4 servings of buckwheat, each contains 2 carbohydrate units and ⅔ protein unit. If you make 4 servings of teff, each contains 2 carbohydrate units and ½ protein unit. If you make brown rice, you will need to divide the recipe into 5 servings; each contains 2 carbohydrate units and ½ protein unit. If you make 4 servings of wild rice, each contains 2 carbohydrate units and ⅔ protein unit. If you divide the recipe into 8 servings of any grain except brown rice or 10 servings for brown rice, halve the unit amounts per serving.

PASTA COOKED AL DENTE

**Gluten-Free IF
GF pasta is used**

Pasta is an enjoyable and versatile addition to your meals, but it must be cooked properly – al dente rather than overdone – to have a moderate glycemic index score. If you are gluten-intolerant or allergic to wheat, there are many varieties of gluten and wheat-free pasta on the market. Although rice pasta is very common, try other types, such as quinoa pasta, which has a lower glycemic impact than rice.

    10 ounces to 1 pound of pasta - quinoa pasta, bean pasta, Purity Foods™ spelt
        pasta, or other wheat-free or gluten-free pasta you tolerate
    3 to 6 quarts of water
    ½ to 1 teaspoon salt

Put the water and salt in a large pot. (The purpose of the salt is to increase the boiling temperature of the water slightly). Bring the water to a rolling boil over high heat. Add the pasta and stir to keep it from sticking together. If you are cooking spaghetti and it is too long for the pan, don't break it. Just hold one end in the pan, let it soften a little, and then stir it all in. Return the water to a boil and then reduce the heat slightly to keep the pasta from boiling over while still maintaining a good boil. Begin timing the cooking of the pasta from the time the water returns to a boil. Set a large colander in your kitchen sink so you will be ready to drain the pasta when the right time comes.

The best estimate of how long to cook the pasta will be what the package says for cooking time. This varies with the size and shape of the pasta, the type of flour it is made from, and the altitude at which you are cooking. At the minimum cooking time given on the package, take a piece of pasta from the pan and taste it. It should be *al dente* when you bite into it, or offer some resistance "to the tooth," without being hard. If it is not done, continue to boil it, retesting it at one to two minutes intervals until it is done. Then immediately pour it though the colander to drain. Do not run cold water on it unless it is to be used in a cold salad recipe. After draining the pasta, put it back into the pan or a serving bowl and toss it with a little oil or pasta sauce to keep it from sticking together. Serve immediately with grated cheese and pasta sauce if desired. Makes about 6 to 8 servings. Use the nutrition facts on the box to calculate how much pasta is a 2 carbohydrate unit (30 grams net carbohydrate) serving and be sure to balance each serving with two units of protein in your meal.

CROCK POT BAKED BEANS

Gluten-Free

1 pound small white or small navy beans
Water
¾ cup apple juice concentrate, thawed (optional) or ⅛ to ¼ teaspoon pure white
      stevia powder such as Protocol for Life Balance™ brand (optional, to taste)
1-6 ounce can tomato paste or 1½ teaspoons paprika (optional)
1 tablespoon finely chopped onion or 1 teaspoon dried onion flakes (optional)
1 teaspoon dry mustard powder (optional)
1 teaspoon sweet basil
1½ teaspoons salt
¼ teaspoon pepper

The night before you plan to serve this dish, wash the beans by putting them in a strainer and running cold water over them. Remove and discard any shriveled beans. Put the beans in a 3 quart crock pot and fill the pot almost to the top with water. The volume of the water should be two to three times the volume of the beans. The next morning, drain the soaking water from the beans, replace it with fresh water and drain it again two or three times. (This soaking and rinsing process removes indigestible carbohydrates that can cause gas). Pour off all the water after the last rinse. Add 4 cups of water to the crock pot and put the lid on the pot. Cook the beans 4 to 6 hours on high or until they are very tender. Check them during cooking and add more water if necessary. It is all right if the level of the water goes a little lower than the level of the beans in the pot.

If you are using the tomato paste, stir it into the apple juice or into ¾ cup water until the mixture is smooth. Add this mixture (or just the apple juice if you're not using the tomato paste) and the seasonings and stevia (if you are using it) to the crock pot. Stir these ingredients into the beans thoroughly. Cover the pot and cook the beans on high another 3 to 5 hours. Check them during cooking and add more water if necessary. If you like a thick sauce, smash a few beans against the side of the pot an hour or so before the end of the cooking time. If the sauce still isn't thick enough, set the lid ajar so some of the liquid can evaporate. For very thick, oven-style baked beans, start cooking the beans in the middle of the day. Add the seasonings and apple juice in the evening and then cook the beans on low overnight. Refrigerate or freeze the beans until you want to use them or you can even eat them for breakfast! Makes 7 servings which are contain 2 protein units each; if made with the apple juice, each serving also contains 1½ carbohydrate units. The carbohydrates in cooked legumes are so high-fiber that Dr. Cheryle Hart does not count them. Leftovers freeze well.

PARSLEY POTATOES

Gluten-Free

6½ ounces of new red potatoes
1 to 2 teaspoons butter, Earth Balance™ non-hydrogenated margarine, or oil
Dash of salt, to taste
Dash of pepper (optional)
¼ teaspoon dry or 1 teaspoon fresh chopped parsley

Scrub the potatoes. If they are small (about 1 inch in diameter) leave them whole. Cut larger potatoes in half or in quarters. Put them in a saucepan with enough water to cover and heat on high until they come to a boil. Boil for 20 to 30 minutes or until they are tender when pierced with a fork. Drain the water from the pan. Add the butter, margarine, or oil and cover the pan with its lid again. Let the potatoes stand for a minute or two to allow the butter or margarine to melt. Stir the potatoes gently to coat them with the butter, margarine, or oil. Put the potatoes in a serving dish if desired, sprinkle them with the seasonings, and serve. Makes one serving which contains 2 carbohydrate units and 4 to 8 grams of fat. The quantities in this recipe may be multiplied by the number of 2 carbohydrate unit servings you wish to have or halved for a 1 carbohydrate unit serving.

OVEN FRIES

My husband likes these made with turnips because they do not add any carbohydrates to his meal. This means he can have a hamburger in a bun with his fries.

1 pound of sweet potatoes (preferably white sweet potato), new red potatoes, or turnips
1 tablespoon oil
¼ teaspoon salt

Preheat your oven to 400°F for the potatoes or to 425°F for the turnips. Peel the vegetables and cut them into ⅜ to ½ inch sticks or "fries." Put them in a bowl and toss them with the oil. Spread them out in a single layer on a baking sheet, preferably a non-stick baking sheet. Bake them for about 20 minutes. Remove the baking sheet from the oven and turn the fries over with a spatula. Bake them for another 15 to 20 minutes, or until they are nicely browned. If you use red potatoes, this recipe makes 5 servings which each contain 1 carbohydrate unit and 3 grams of fat. If you use sweet potatoes, this recipe makes 7 servings which each contain 1 carbohydrate unit and 2 grams of fat. If made with turnips, the whole batch contains 14 grams of fat and 0 carbohydrate units since turnips do not contained concentrated carbohydrate.

MASHED NEW RED POTATOES

Leaving the skin on potatoes gives you more fiber and nutrients. Since red potatoes have thin skins, the skins mash nicely into the potatoes.

6½ ounces of new red potatoes
2 tablespoons milk, preferably nonfat or low fat, of any kind you tolerate (optional)
1 teaspoon butter, Earth Balance™ non-hydrogenated margarine, or oil
¹⁄₁₆ to ⅛ teaspoon salt, to taste
Dash of pepper (optional)

Scrub the potatoes and peel them if desired. If they are peeled and small (about 1 to 1½ inches in diameter) leave them whole. Cut larger potatoes in half or in quarters. If you leave the peel on, cut the potatoes into ½ to ¾ inch cubes so the pieces of peel in the potatoes will be small.

Put the potatoes in a saucepan with enough water to cover and heat on high until they come to a boil. Boil for 20 to 30 minutes or until the potatoes are tender when pierced with a fork. Drain most of the water from the pan, but reserve some of the water you drained. Add the milk, butter and seasonings and mash the potatoes. Add some of the reserved water if the potatoes seem dry. Makes one serving which contains 2 carbohydrate units and 4 grams of fat. The quantities in this recipe may be multiplied by the number of 2 carbohydrate unit servings you wish to have or halved for a 1 carbohydrate unit serving.

Dairy-free mashed potatoes: When the potatoes are cooked, drain less of the water than above, and do reserve some water. Mash the potatoes with Earth Balance™ non-hydrogenated margarine or oil and salt, adding some of the reserved water to bring them to the right consistency. Makes one serving which contains 2 carbohydrate units and 4 grams of fat.

Onion Scented Peas

Gluten-Free

My mother cooked peas this way when I was a child, with just enough onion to give them an enticing flavor.

> 1 slice of onion about ½ inch thick, chopped (about ⅓ to ½ cup)
> 2 teaspoons oil
> 1 pound frozen peas
> 4 teaspoons to 2 tablespoons water
> Salt to taste

In a saucepan, sauté the onion in the oil over low to medium heat until the onion begins to brown. Add the peas and 4 teaspoons of water and cook over medium heat until the peas are heated through and the water is evaporated. Watch the pan closely and if you hear it sizzling, add some of the additional water. Makes 4 servings of peas which each contain 2 grams of fat. The carbohydrates in non-starchy vegetables do not count so this recipe contains zero carbohydrate units.

Quick version of oven scented peas: Substitute 1½ teaspoons minced dry onion for the raw onion. Add all of the ingredients to the saucepan using 2 tablespoons of water and heat until peas are heated through and the water is evaporated. Watch the pan closely and if you hear it sizzling, add additional water.

OVEN CARROTS

This dish will make you a cooked carrot lover, especially if made with whole organic carrots.

    2 to 2½ pounds whole carrots or pre-peeled mini carrots
    ⅓ cup water
    ½ teaspoon salt
    2 to 3 tablespoons oil

If you are using pre-peeled mini carrots, bake them without any water or salt in a covered casserole dish at 350°F for an hour. Drain off the water at this point in the recipe. If you are using whole carrots, peel or scrub them and cut them lengthwise into quarters or into eighths if they are very large. Lay the carrot sticks parallel to each other in a 2 to 3 quart glass casserole dish with a lid. To the partially cooked mini carrots or the raw whole carrot sticks, add the salt and water and drizzle the oil over the top of the carrots. Cover the dish with its lid and bake the carrot sticks at 350°F for about 1 to 1½ hours or the mini-carrots for an additional hour, or until they begin to brown and become caramelized. Makes 8 servings which each contain 3 grams of fat. The carbohydrates in non-starchy vegetables do not count so this recipe contains zero carbohydrate units.

OVEN CABBAGE

This method of cooking cabbage brings out its delicious sweet flavor.

    1 head of cabbage weighing about 1½ to 1¾ pounds
    ½ teaspoon salt
    ¼ teaspoon pepper (optional)
    ⅓ cup water
    3 tablespoons oil

Coarsely chop the cabbage and put it into a 3-quart glass casserole dish with a lid. Add the salt, pepper, and water. Drizzle the oil over the top of the cabbage. Cover the dish with its lid and bake at 350°F for 1 to 2 hours, stirring once or twice during the cooking time if possible. Makes 8 servings which each contain 5 grams of fat. The carbohydrates in non-starchy vegetables do not count so this recipe contains zero carbohydrate units.

OVEN PEAS OR BEANS

Gluten-Free

Because you start with frozen vegetables, this is very quick and easy to prepare.

1 10-ounce package frozen peas, cut green beans, or lima beans
⅓ cup water
⅛ teaspoon salt
1 tablespoon oil

Combine all of the ingredients in a 1 to 1½ quart glass casserole dish. Cover the dish with its lid and bake at 350°F for 1 to 1½ hours for the beans or 20 minutes to 1 hour for the peas. Makes 4 servings which each contain 3 grams of fat. The carbohydrates in non-starchy vegetables do not count so this recipe contains zero carbohydrate units.

BRAISED CAULIFLOWER

Gluten-Free

Here is another family recipe – Italian, of course. Vegetables were never boring at our house when I was a child and often were fresh from the garden in the summertime.

1 head of cauliflower, about 2½ pounds, or 2 pounds of cauliflower florets
2 tablespoons oil, preferably olive oil for its flavor and heat stability
¼ teaspoon salt
Generous sprinkling of pepper, or to taste
Water
1 to 2 tablespoons grated Romano cheese, optional

Rinse the head of cauliflower. Cut the leaves and core from the cauliflower and cut it into florets. In a 12-inch or larger frying pan, sauté the cauliflower in the oil over medium heat for 10 to 15 minutes or until most of the florets have at least one side that is browned. Add 3 tablespoons of water and the salt and pepper to the pan. Cover the pan and cook over low heat until the cauliflower is tender, about 10 to 20 minutes. While it is cooking, stir it occasionally and add more water as needed. (You will probably need another 2 to 4 tablespoons of water). Allow the pan to dry out and the florets to brown a little more in the oil at the end of the cooking time. Sprinkle the cauliflower with Romano cheese if desired. Makes 6 servings which each contain 5 grams of fat. The carbohydrates in non-starchy vegetables do not count so this recipe contains zero carbohydrate units.

If you do not have a large 12 inch frying pan with a lid, cut the amounts of all of the ingredients in half and cook the cauliflower in an 8 to 10 inch frying pan.

SPECIAL OVEN SQUASH

Gluten-Free

The easiest way to prepare winter squash in the oven is to cut it in half, remove the seeds, and bake it cut side down. (See the recipe below). However, if you have a little time and would like a change from plain squash, this is very tasty.

  2½ pounds butternut squash
  ¼ teaspoon salt
  2 tablespoons oil

Peel the squash. Cut it in half lengthwise and remove the seeds. Slice it into ¼-inch slices. Put the slices into an 11 inch by 7 inch baking dish, sprinkle them with the salt, and drizzle them with the oil. Stir to coat all of the slices. Bake at 350°F for 1½ to 2 hours, turning the slices after the first hour. Makes 8 servings which each contain 3 grams of fat. The carbohydrates in non-starchy vegetables do not count so this recipe contains zero carbohydrate units.

EASY BAKED STARCHY VEGETABLES

Gluten-Free

These are the easiest side dishes to have with your oven entrée. Try baking a mealy squash such as kabocha or hokkaido for an extra-satisfying treat. Serve squash with a generous sprinkle of Penzey's Vietnamese cinnamon for extra help with blood sugar stability.

Small new red potatoes, white or orange sweet potatoes, or winter squash

Scrub and pierce the potatoes. Cut the squash in half and remove the seeds. Place the squash cut side down on a baking dish or a baking sheet with an edge. You may place white potatoes directly on the oven rack. Orange sweet potatoes sometimes ooze sticky liquid so use a baking dish or baking sheet with an edge for them. Bake these with the rest of your oven meal for 1 to 2½ hours at 350°F to 450°F or until they are tender when squeezed and your main dish is done. (Use a longer cooking time with the lower temperatures). One 6½ ounce serving of new red potatoes or a 8 ounce sweet potato is two carbohydrate units. Although an average serving size for squash is ⅓ to ½ pound per person, enjoy as much of this nutritious and filling food as it takes to satisfy your hunger. Winter squash does not contain concentrated carbohydrate so this recipe contains zero carbohydrate units if made with squash.

CRISPY OVEN RED POTATOES OR SWEET POTATOES

Gluten-Free

It is quickest to bake potatoes as in the previous recipe, but if you want to make a special dish and have time for slicing, these potatoes are delicious.

> 2 pounds new red potatoes or sweet potatoes (preferably white, but orange are
>   also good)
> 2 tablespoons oil
> ½ teaspoon salt
> Pepper or herbs to taste (optional)

Peel or scrub the potatoes and slice them into ¼-inch slices. Put the slices into an 11 inch by 7 inch baking dish, sprinkle them with the salt and optional pepper or herbs, and drizzle them with the oil. Stir to coat all of the slices. Bake at 350°F for 1½ to 2 hours, turning the slices after the first hour. If you use sweet potatoes, this recipe makes 8 servings which each contain 1 carbohydrate unit and 3 grams of fat. If you use red potatoes, this recipe makes 10 servings which each contain 1 carbohydrate unit and 3 grams of fat.

NUKE-N-BAKE WINTER SQUASH

Gluten-Free

The hardest part of cooking many winter squashes is cutting them in half before you bake them. This recipe makes that easy.

> 1 large winter squash weighing about 3 pounds

Pierce the squash with a knife in at least two places making sure that you go all the way into the center cavity. This keeps it from exploding in the microwave. Cook it in the microwave on full power for 8 minutes. Cut the squash in half and remove the strings and seeds. Place the halves cut side down in a glass baking dish and microwave for another 4 minutes. Preheat your oven to 450°F while the squash is microwaving. Transfer the squash to the oven and cook it for another 15 minutes. Drier types of winter squash, such as kabocha and hokkaido, will be more mealy when cooked this way than if just microwaved. Makes about 6 to 8 servings. An average serving size for squash is ⅓ to ½ pound per person, but enjoy as much of this nutritious and filling food as it takes to satisfy your hunger. Winter squash does not contain concentrated carbohydrate so this recipe contains zero carbohydrate units.

NUKE-N-BROIL CARROTS

This is a great way to cook carrots if you have your broiler already heated to cook steaks or broil fish.

    1 pound peeled mini-carrots
    ¼ cup water
    ¼ teaspoon plus a dash of salt
    1 to 2 tablespoons oil

Put the carrots in a glass baking dish with ¼ cup of water and ¼ teaspoon of salt. Cover and microwave on high for 8 minutes. If possible stir the carrots after the first 4 minutes of microwaving. (The microwave time may vary with the power of your microwave and how well done you like your vegetables). Drain the carrots and put them into an 8 or 9 inch square metal cake pan, drizzle them with the oil and sprinkle them with salt to taste. Stir and arrange the carrots so they are mostly in one layer. Broil at the temperature required by the entrée for 10 minutes. They will have begun to brown and can be eaten at this point if desired. However, if you have time to cook them longer, stir and re-arrange them and then broil them another 5 to 10 minutes or until they are well-browned. Makes 4 servings which each contain 4 grams of fat. The carbohydrates in non-starchy vegetables do not count so this recipe contains zero carbohydrate units.

NUKE-N-BAKE CARROTS OR GLAZED CARROTS

Carrots prepared by long baking in the oven are so delicious that once you have eaten them, you will not want steamed or boiled carrots ever again. However, there will be days when you do not have enough time to prepare "Oven Carrots" (recipe on page 168). This recipe and the recipe above provide two microwave-plus-conventional recipes that approximate the taste of oven carrots in much less time.

    1 pound peeled mini-carrots
    ¼ cup water
    ¼ teaspoon plus a dash of salt
    1 to 2 tablespoons oil
    1 tablespoon agave, Fruit Sweet™ or honey (optional)

Put the carrots in a flat glass baking dish or 1-quart casserole dish with ¼ cup of water and ¼ teaspoon of salt. Cover and microwave on high for 8 minutes. Preheat your oven to 500°F (or whatever temperature your entrée requires) while they are microwaving. If possible, stir them after the first 4 minutes of microwaving. (The microwave time may vary with the power of your microwave and how well done you like your vegetables). Drain the carrots. Drizzle them with the oil and sprinkle them with salt to taste. For glazed carrots, also drizzle them with the agave, Fruit Sweet™ or honey. Stir and arrange the carrots so they are mostly in one layer. Bake uncovered at 350°F to 500°F for ½ to 1½ hours, using higher temperatures with shorter baking times. If you wish you may stir them mid-way through the baking time if you will be around to do so; if you are baking them hot and fast, stirring is recommended. The longer you bake them, the more they will caramelize. Makes 4 servings which each contain 4 grams of fat. If the agave, Fruit Sweet™ or honey is used, each serving also contains ¼ carbohydrate unit. The carbohydrates in non-starchy vegetables do not count.

TOSSED SALAD

Gluten-Free

This salad is a powerhouse of nutrition when made with greens or lettuce other than iceberg lettuce. The more darkly colored the lettuce or greens, the more nutritious. Try pre-washed blends that contain red leaf lettuce, endive, spinach or arugula in this salad.

4 cups of leaf lettuce or other greens, any variety or combination, torn into bite-sized pieces
¼ to ½ cup sliced carrots, cucumbers, and/or radishes
1 medium or large tomato, if tolerated, cut into eight to twelve pieces (optional)
½ to 1 avocado, peeled and cut into cubes (optional)
Optional additions to make the salad more substantial on protein:
2 tablespoons sunflower seeds
2 tablespoons crumbled or grated cheese of any kind tolerated
¼ to ⅓ cup cooked beans, such as garbanzo beans, drained
¼ to ⅓ cup of any salad dressing – commercially made allergen – or gluten-free diet Italian dressing or dressing made using the recipes on pages 177 to 178

Tear the lettuce or greens into bite sized pieces and put them in a large salad bowl. Slice the cucumbers, carrots, or radishes and cut up the tomato; add them to the salad bowl and toss. Add the dressing and toss. Sprinkle the top of the salad with the optional additions such as avocado, seeds, nuts, beans, or cheese. Serve immediately. Makes 3 to 4 servings which each contain 2 grams of fat if made with diet Italian dressing, or read the nutritional information for the salad dressing you are using and add any fat or carbohydrate units it contains. If you use ½ avocado, this adds only 4 to 5 grams of fat per serving. The carbohydrates in non-starchy vegetables do not count so this recipe contains zero carbohydrate units if made with sugar-free salad dressing.

THREE BEAN SALAD

The salt-free varieties of canned beans often do not contain sugar or additives. If you have canned beans you can eat, the preparation of this salad is a breeze.

1¼ cups cooked cut green beans or 1 15-ounce can green beans, drained
1 15-ounce can kidney beans, drained
1 15-ounce can garbanzo beans, drained
2 tablespoons chopped onion or 1 to 2 teaspoons dry chopped onion
    (optional)
½ cup chopped green pepper (optional)
2 tablespoons apple juice concentrate, thawed
¼ teaspoon salt
⅛ to ¼ teaspoon pepper (optional)
⅓ cup lemon juice or vinegar OR 2 teaspoons tart-tasting unbuffered vitamin
    C powder, as tolerated (See the comment on bowel tolerance below).
¼ cup oil

Combine the beans, onion, and green pepper in a large bowl. In a separate small bowl, stir together the apple juice, lemon juice or vinegar (if you are using either of them), salt, and pepper until the salt is dissolved. Pour this mixture and the oil over the beans, toss them thoroughly, and refrigerate until serving time. (This salad tastes best if the flavors soak into the beans for an hour to overnight).

If you are using the vitamin C powder, stir it into 2 tablespoons of water until it dissolves and add it to the salad just before serving. Vitamin C loses its tang in this salad if added too long before serving time. In addition, if a large serving is eaten, some individuals lack bowel tolerance for so much vitamin C. Makes 7 servings which each contain 1 protein unit and 9 grams of fat. The carbohydrates in cooked legumes are so high-fiber that Dr. Cheryle Hart does not count them.

MAKE-AHEAD TOSSED SALAD

Gluten-Free

This is an easy salad that you can make ahead of time when you have a large crowd of guests. For a small party, cut the recipe in half.

½ cup oil, preferably olive oil for monounsaturated fatty acids or walnut or canola oil for omega-3 fatty acids

1 clove of garlic, crushed (optional)

½ teaspoon oregano, sweet basil or parsley, or ¾ teaspoon Penzey's Italian herb blend (optional)

½ teaspoon salt

Dash of pepper

¼ to ⅓ cup vinegar or lemon juice

½ to 1 cup sliced carrots, cucumbers, and/or radishes

2 to 3 medium tomatoes, each cut into eight pieces

12 cups of leaf lettuce or other greens, any variety or combination, torn into bite-sized pieces

Optional additions to make the salad more substantial on protein:
    ⅓ cup sunflower seeds or chopped nuts
    ⅓ cup crumbled or grated cheese of any kind tolerated
    ¾ to 1 cup cooked beans such as garbanzo beans, drained

If you wish to use the garlic, crush it and put it and the oil in a glass jar. Refrigerate at least overnight. Remove the garlic from the oil and discard the garlic. Combine the oil with the seasonings and vinegar or lemon juice in a large salad bowl or 4- quart mixing bowl. Stir the dressing thoroughly. Add the carrots, cucumbers, radishes, and tomatoes to the dressing in the bowl. (They will prevent the lettuce from being immersed in the dressing before serving time). Put the lettuce and/or other greens on top of the cut vegetables. Cover the bowl with plastic wrap and refrigerate it until serving time.

At serving time, toss the salad. Sprinkle the top of the salad with your choice(s) of the seeds, nuts, cheese, and/or beans if desired. Makes 10 servings which each contain 10 grams of fat. The carbohydrates in non-starchy vegetables do not count so this recipe contains zero carbohydrate units. For a small party, cut the ingredient amounts in half.

COLESLAW

If you use packaged shredded cabbage or coleslaw mix instead of the cabbage and carrot, this salad will be ready in a jiffy.

¾ to 1 pound of cabbage,* about half of a large head
1 small carrot,* shredded
1 to 2 teaspoons grated onion, or to taste (optional)
3 to 5 tablespoons minced bell pepper, preferably orange for its sweetness
        (optional)
⅛ to ¼ teaspoon salt (optional)
¾ to 1 cup light mayonnaise, mayonnaise, or "Super Smooth Sauce," page 234
1 to 2 tablespoons lemon juice** or ⅛ to ¼ teaspoon unbuffered vitamin C
        powder
1 to 4 tablespoons water (less with light mayonnaise)

Wash and core the cabbage. Cut it into wedges and slice each wedge crosswise as thinly as possible or shred it with a food processor. Put the cabbage strips into a large salad bowl. Grate the carrot or shred it with a food processor. Grate the onion and finely chop the pepper. Combine all of the vegetables in the bowl. Stir together the salt, mayonnaise, lemon juice or vitamin C, and enough water to make a creamy dressing in a separate bowl or cup. Add them to the cabbage mixture and toss thoroughly until the cabbage is completely coated with the dressing. Store in the refrigerator. Makes 6 servings which each contain 10 grams of fat if made with light mayonnaise. The carbohydrates in non-starchy vegetables do not count so this recipe contains zero carbohydrate units.

*Note on vegetables: To save time, you can use a 1-pound bag of pre-shredded cabbage or coleslaw mix for the cabbage or cabbage and carrot.

**Note on lemon juice: To prevent your coleslaw from being too tangy, you may want to use the smaller amount of lemon juice if you are using bottled juice. Start with 1 tablespoon and then add more to taste if needed.

SPINACH SALAD

Gluten-Free

Pre-washed spinach makes this salad a snap.

> 4 cups of spinach leaves, washed and torn into bite-sized pieces
> 1 cup diced or sliced cooked beets (optional)
> 1 avocado, peeled, seeded, and cut into bite-sized pieces (optional)
> 2 slices of cooked bacon, crumbled (optional)
> ¼ cup of "Basic Vinaigrette Salad Dressing," below, gluten- and allergen-free
>   diet Italian dressing, or similar bottled gluten- and allergen-free dressing

Put the spinach in a large salad bowl. Slice or cut up the beets or avocado and add the pieces to the salad bowl. Add the dressing and toss. Crumble the optional bacon and sprinkle it on top of the salad if desired. Serve immediately. Makes 4 servings which each contain 7 grams of fat if made with the vinaigrette or 2 grams of fat made with diet Italian dressing. The bacon adds 2 grams of fat per serving. The carbohydrates in non-starchy vegetables do not count so this recipe contains zero carbohydrate units.

BASIC VINAIGRETTE SALAD DRESSING

Gluten-Free

Because they are not heated, salad dressings are a great place to add fragile oils which are high in essential fatty acids to your diet. Canola and walnut oils are good sources of omega-3 fatty acids which most of our diets lack in sufficient quantities. Olive oil is great for traditional flavor and also good for heart-healthy monounsaturated fatty acids.

> ½ cup olive oil for traditional flavor or walnut or canola oil for omega-3 fatty
>   acids
> ¾ teaspoons Penzey's Italian blend herbs or ½ teaspoon oregano, sweet basil or
>   parsley (optional)
> ½ teaspoon salt
> Dash of pepper
> ¼ to ⅓ cup wine vinegar or lemon juice OR 1 to 1½ teaspoons unbuffered
>   vitamin C powder plus 1 tablespoons water

Combine all of the ingredients in a jar and shake. Shake the dressing again to thoroughly mix it right before pouring it on your salad. Refrigerate leftover dressing if you make it with lemon juice or vitamin C. Makes about ¾ to 1 cup of dressing or 12 servings which each contain 9 grams of fat.

SWEET YOGURT DRESSING

1 cup plain yogurt, preferably nonfat or low fat (cow, goat, sheep, soy, or any
  other kind you tolerate)
2 tablespoons lemon juice or ¼ teaspoon unbuffered vitamin C powder
¼ cup apple or pineapple juice concentrate, thawed, OR 2 tablespoons of
  agave, Fruit Sweet™ or honey OR $\frac{1}{16}$ to ⅛ teaspoon of pure white
  stevia powder such as Protocol for Life Balance™ brand, to taste
¼ teaspoon salt
1 teaspoon poppy seeds (optional)

If you are using the vitamin C and/or stevia, thoroughly stir them into a few tablespoons of the yogurt. Add the rest of the ingredients and thoroughly stir them together.
Serve the dressing immediately or refrigerate it until meal time. Refrigerate any leftover
dressing. Makes about 1⅓ cups of dressing or 12 servings which each contain ¼ carbohydrate units (only if made with a sweetener other than stevia) and no fat if made with
nonfat yogurt.

HERBED YOGURT DRESSING

1 cup plain yogurt, preferably nonfat or low fat (cow, goat, sheep, soy, or any
  other kind you tolerate)
2 tablespoons of lemon juice or ¼ teaspoon unbuffered vitamin C powder
⅛ to ¼ teaspoon pepper, or to taste
¼ teaspoon salt
1 teaspoon oregano, sweet basil, or Penzey's Italian herb blend

If you are using the vitamin C, thoroughly stir it into a few tablespoons of the
yogurt. Add the rest of the ingredients and thoroughly stir them together. Serve the
dressing immediately or refrigerate it until meal time. Refrigerate any leftover dressing.
Makes about 1 cup of dressing or 8 servings which each contain no carbohydrate and
no fat if made with nonfat yogurt.

Muffins, Crackers and Bread

I chuckle when I see a free magazine at a health food store with "Gluten-free Recipes" blazoned on the cover and find that the recipes inside are for salmon with a special sauce, vegetables prepared in a unique way, a fennel and fruit salad, and rice pudding. Nearby are advertisements for sugar and fat-laden gluten-free cookie mixes and frozen rice bread. There is a problem with this scenario. It assumes that we only want to cook what we could have cooked (less creatively, however) without their recipes, and that gluten-free baking is too challenging to attempt without a mix, if at all.

Allergy and gluten- free baking is different, but it is not difficult. Our health problems don't need to make us captive to the health food industry, abdicating our decisions about which grains and sweeteners to use. Truly healthy baked goods are not mostly made from rice, do not contain sugar, and are not expensive because you can make them yourself. Furthermore, by using lower GI flours (amaranth, quinoa, buckwheat, etc. rather than rice), you can escape or reverse the weight gain that many experience when they are diagnosed with gluten intolerance or wheat allergy and switch from eating wheat products to commercially made rice bread, crackers, snacks, and cookies.

The information here is the key to success in wheat-free baking: The difference between ordinary and wheat-free baking is that the flour you are using usually contains less or even no gluten. The function of gluten in baked goods is to form layers and sheets of protein which trap the gas that makes the baked goods rise. Thus, gluten-free or low gluten baked goods must be handled more carefully in mixing and baking so that they do not deflate. Additionally, ordinary baking powder usually contains corn, a potent allergen, so the leavening systems used in allergy baking also need special care.

To succeed with the recipes in this chapter, be sure to use reliable ingredients, measure accurately (see pages 97 to 98 for more about this), and follow this procedure when you bake: Before you begin baking, preheat your oven. Prepare the baking pans ahead of time; oil and flour them with the same oil and flour used in the recipe. Mix the dry ingredients together in a large bowl and the liquid ingredients together in a measuring cup or another bowl. Tolerating no interruptions from this point on and working quickly, stir the liquid ingredients into the dry ingredients until they are **just mixed.** It is critical that you do not mix for too long or the leavening will produce most of its gas in the mixing bowl rather than in the baking pan in the oven. Only stir until the dry ingredients are barely moistened; a few floury spots in your batter or dough are all right. As soon as you have mixed just enough, quickly put the batter or dough into the prepared baking pans and pop them into the preheated oven. Bake and test your baked goods for doneness and cool them as directed in the recipe.

This chapter gives you a collection of wheat and gluten-free baking recipes. Because this book is written for those with food allergies as well as for the gluten-intolerant, pay attention to the ingredients in the recipe and the gluten-free comments (or lack thereof under the recipe title) with each recipe. Where options are given for ingredient choices, choose the options that fit YOUR intolerances. Not every recipe in this book fits every reader, but the ones that do fit you will help you restore your health and also lose weight.

This book is planned as the first in a series of cookbooks for glycemic control to be used by people with gluten intolerance and food allergies. Since this is the introductory book, it does not contain the full complement of recipes. (I did not want to delay the publication of this book for a few years in order to include all the recipes that should eventually be included). For more baking recipes, including both yeast-free and yeast-containing recipes made with sorghum, amaranth, teff, buckwheat, millet, quinoa, rice, chestnut flour, or the gluten-containing grains barley, oat, spelt, kamut, and rye, see *The Ultimate Food Allergy Cookbook and Survival Guide* as described on the last pages of this book. Unlike many gluten-free recipes, these recipes are suitable for those who are allergic to eggs.

BARLEY MUFFINS

These are delicious for breakfast and can be made with high-fiber Sustagrain™ barley flour for less impact on blood sugar levels.

> 2 cups Sustagrain™ barley flour or ordinary barley flour (See "Sources," page 278)
> ¼ teaspoon salt
> 1 teaspoon baking soda
> ¼ teaspoon unbuffered vitamin C powder
> ¼ cup oil
> 1¼ cups water or apple juice

Preheat your oven to 400°F. Line 12 wells of a muffin pan with paper liners or oil and flour them with barley flour. Mix the flour, salt, baking soda, and vitamin C powder in a large bowl. Stir optional variety* ingredients (see below) into the flour mixture. Mix the juice or water with the oil, pour them into the dry ingredients, and stir until they are just mixed in. Fill the muffin cups about ⅔ full. Bake for 30 to 35 minutes or until the muffins begin to brown and a toothpick inserted into the center comes out dry. Makes 12 muffins which each contain 1⅓ carbohydrate units and 5 grams of fat if made with water or 2 carbohydrate units and 5 grams of fat if made with apple juice concentrate.

*Note: For variety, add 1 teaspoon of cinnamon and/or ⅓ cup raisins plus ⅓ cup nuts or ⅔ cup of raisins or other diced dry fruit or ⅔ cup nuts to the muffins.

AMARANTH BLUEBERRY MUFFINS

Gluten-Free

If you can't finish eating a whole batch of these muffins within a day or so, freeze them to maintain their moistness.

1¾ cups amaranth flour

½ cup arrowroot

2 teaspoons baking soda

½ teaspoon unbuffered vitamin C powder

¼ teaspoon cinnamon or cloves (optional)

¾ cup apple or pineapple juice concentrate, thawed, OR ¾ cup water plus
    a scant ¼ teaspoon to ¼ teaspoon pure white stevia powder such as
    Protocol for Life Balance™ brand, to taste

¼ cup oil

1 cup fresh or frozen blueberries or ¾ cup dried blueberries

Preheat your oven to 375°F. Line 12 wells of a muffin pan with paper muffin cup liners. If you are using frozen blueberries, rinse them with cold water in a strainer and set them aside. Combine the amaranth flour, arrowroot, stevia (if you are using it), baking soda, and vitamin C powder in a large bowl. Stir in the dried blueberries if you are using them. Stir together the water or juice and oil. Pour the liquid ingredients into the dry ingredients and stir until they are just mixed. The batter will be stiffer than for most muffins. If you are using the frozen blueberries, quickly stir them into the batter. Put the batter into the prepared muffin tin filling the cups about ⅞ full. Bake for 20 to 22 minutes or until the muffins brown and a toothpick inserted in the center comes out dry. (Stevia-sweetened muffins will not brown much). Makes 12 muffins. If made with the juice, they each contain 1⅔ carbohydrate units and 6 grams of fat. If made with stevia, they each contain 1 carbohydrate unit and 6 grams of fat. If you can "afford" the extra ⅔ carbohydrate unit with your meal, this is a recipe in which juice produces a superior texture and taste.

AMARANTH CRACKERS

Gluten-Free

These crackers are so good that I would like to eat them every day.

    3 cups amaranth flour
    1 cup arrowroot
    2 teaspoons baking soda
    ½ teaspoon unbuffered vitamin C powder
    1 teaspoon salt
    ¾ cup water
    ½ cup oil

Preheat your oven to 375°F. Combine the amaranth flour, arrowroot, baking soda, vitamin C powder, and salt in a large bowl. Mix together the water and oil and pour them into the flour mixture. Stir until the dough sticks together, adding another few tablespoons of water if necessary to form a stiff but not crumbly dough. Divide the dough into thirds. Roll each third to about ⅛ inch thickness on an ungreased baking sheet and cut the dough into 2 inch squares. Sprinkle the tops of the crackers lightly with additional salt if desired. Bake for 15 to 20 minutes or until the crackers are crisp and lightly browned. If the crackers around the edges of the baking sheet brown before those in the center, remove them from the baking sheet and allow the crackers in the center to bake longer. Cool the crackers on paper towels. Makes about 9 dozen crackers or 21 5-cracker servings. A serving of 5 crackers contains 1 carbohydrate unit and 6 grams of fat.

QUINOA "GRAHAM" CRACKERS

Gluten-Free

    3 cups quinoa flour
    1 cup tapioca starch
    2 teaspoons baking soda
    ½ teaspoon unbuffered vitamin C powder
    ½ teaspoon cinnamon (optional)
    1¼ cups apple juice concentrate
    ½ cup oil

Preheat your oven to 350°F. Oil two large or three smaller baking sheets. (If your baking sheets are 14 by 18 inches or larger, you can bake these crackers using two sheets). Mix together the quinoa flour, tapioca starch, baking soda, vitamin C powder, and cinnamon in a large bowl. Combine the apple juice concentrate and oil and stir them into the dry ingredients until the dough sticks together. Divide the dough into halves or thirds depending on the size of your baking sheets. Put each portion on one of the prepared baking sheets. Flour a rolling pin and the top of the dough. Roll each portion of dough to just under ¼ inch thickness. Flour a knife and cut the dough into 1 inch by 3 inch bars. You may have to re-flour the knife between cuts. Prick each bar three times with a fork to resemble graham crackers. Bake for 10 to 15 minutes or until the crackers are lightly browned. Re-cut the crackers on the same lines if necessary. Remove the crackers from the baking sheet using a spatula, and allow them to cool on paper towels. Makes about 4 dozen rectangular crackers. A serving of 3 crackers contains 2 carbohydrate units and 9 grams of fat.

QUINOA SESAME SEED CRACKERS

Gluten-Free

If you are new to quinoa and are not accustomed to its flavor, this is the recipe to try. The sesame seeds made these satisfying crackers taste great!

    3 cups quinoa flour
    1 cup tapioca starch*, arrowroot, or Hi-Maize™ cornstarch
    ⅜ cup sesame seeds
    2 teaspoons baking soda
    ½ teaspoon unbuffered vitamin C powder
    1 teaspoon salt
    1¼ cups water
    ½ cup oil

Preheat your oven to 350°F. Mix together the quinoa flour, tapioca starch, sesame seeds, baking soda, vitamin C powder and salt in a large bowl. Combine the water and oil and stir them into the dry ingredients until the dough roughly comes together. Divide the dough into halves or thirds. (If your baking sheets are 14 by 18 inches or larger, you can bake these crackers using two sheets; otherwise divide the dough into thirds). Press each portion of the dough together on the baking sheet and sprinkle the top with quinoa flour. Roll each part to a little over ⅛ inch thickness on an ungreased baking sheet using an oiled rolling pin. If the dough sticks to the rolling pin, lightly flour the top of the dough again. After rolling, cut the dough into 1½ inch squares and sprinkle the tops of the crackers with salt if desired. Bake for 15 to 25 minutes, or until the crackers are crisp and lightly browned. The crackers around the edges of the baking sheet will probably brown before those in the center. Remove them from the baking sheet and allow the crackers in the center to bake 5 minutes longer. Then remove any others that are brown and allow the remaining crackers to bake 5 minutes longer again. Makes about 9 dozen crackers or 21 5-cracker servings. A serving of 5 crackers contains 1 carbohydrate unit and 7 grams of fat.

Note on tapioca starch: I usually use tapioca starch in this recipe but you can substitute arrowroot in the same amount if you tolerate it better. I made these crackers with Hi-Maize™ cornstarch because it is higher in fiber and should therefore lower the glycemic impact of the crackers. My admittedly fussy husband preferred the original tapioca flour containing recipe, but if you tolerate corn and want to lower the absorption rate of the carbohydrate in these crackers by adding more fiber, you may substitute Hi-Maize™ in the same amount as the other starches.

ALMOND SESAME SEED CRACKERS

Gluten-Free

These tasty crackers made with almond flour are a protein snack eaten alone and do not need to be balanced with a protein food unlike most other crackers.

> 3 cups finely ground blanched almond flour such as Honeyville™ brand (See "Sources," page 281).
> 1 cup sesame seeds
> 1 teaspoon salt
> 2 large eggs OR ½ cup "Flaxseed Egg Substitute," page 237, at room temperature or cooler
> 2 tablespoons oil

Preheat your oven to 350°F. Prepare two large baking sheets by cutting parchment paper to fit them. Then cut a third piece of parchment paper the same size.

In a large bowl stir together the almond flour, sesame seeds and salt. If you are using the flaxseed egg substitute, measure it out and vigorously stir in the oil or use a hand blender to mix the oil into it thoroughly. If you are using the eggs, beat them until the yolk and white are well combined with a fork and stir the oil into the eggs thoroughly. Add the liquid ingredients to the dry ingredients and stir and mash until they are mixed together well. Divide the dough into two parts and put each half on one of the baking sheets. Top one of the dough halves with the extra piece of parchment paper. Roll the dough about ¹⁄₁₆ to ⅛ inch thick. Remove the parchment paper and cut the dough into 1½ to 2 inch squares with a sharp knife. Re-use the spare piece of parchment paper to roll the second half of the dough. Bake the crackers until they are golden brown – for 12 to 16 minutes if the crackers were made with the flaxseed egg substitute or for 14 to 17 minutes if the crackers were made with egg. Remove them from the oven and re-cut them on the lines from the previous cutting if needed. Slide the parchment paper off the baking sheet onto a cooling rack to cool. Makes about 5 to 5½ dozen crackers or 25 3-cracker servings. A serving of 3 crackers contains 1 protein unit and 7 grams of fat.

CHOOSE-YOUR-COUNTRY CRACKERS

Gluten-Free

The caraway version of these crackers is delicious and reminds me of the way caraway Rye Krisp™ tasted. Like the crackers in the previous recipe, they are a protein snack eaten alone.

3½ cups finely ground blanched almond flour such as Honeyville™ brand (See "Sources," page 281).

¾ teaspoon salt

Seasoning of your choice:

    1½ tablespoons dry sweet basil for Italian crackers

    2 tablespoons caraway seed for German crackers

    1 to 2 teaspoons chili powder, to taste, for Mexican crackers

2 large eggs OR ½ cup "Flaxseed Egg Substitute," page 237, at room temperature or cooler

2 tablespoons oil

Preheat your oven to 350°F. Prepare two large baking sheets by cutting parchment paper to fit them. Then cut a third piece of parchment paper the same size.

In a large bowl, stir together the almond flour, one seasoning of your choice, and salt. If you are using the flaxseed egg substitute, measure it out and vigorously stir in the oil or use a hand blender to mix the oil into it thoroughly. If you are using the eggs, beat them until the yolk and white are well combined with a fork and stir the oil into the eggs thoroughly. Add the liquid ingredients to the dry ingredients and stir and mash until they are mixed together well. Divide the dough into two parts and put each half on one of the baking sheets. Top one of the dough halves with the extra piece of parchment paper. Roll the dough about ⅟₁₆ to ⅛ inch thick. Remove the parchment paper and cut the dough into 1½ to 2 inch squares with a sharp knife. Re-use the spare piece of parchment paper to roll the second half of the dough. Bake the crackers until they are golden brown – for 12 to 16 minutes if the crackers were made with the flaxseed egg substitute or for 14 to 17 minutes if the crackers were made with egg. Remove them from the oven and re-cut them on the lines from the previous cutting if needed. Slide the parchment paper off the baking sheet onto a cooling rack to cool. Makes about 5 dozen crackers or 24 3-cracker servings. A serving of 3 crackers contains 1 protein unit and 5 grams of fat.

NON-YEAST BREAD

Gluten-Free IF made with GF flour

Teff (GF)
3 cups teff flour
¾ teaspoon salt
3 teaspoons baking soda
¾ teaspoon unbuffered vitamin C powder
⅜ cup oil
2¼ cups water

Quinoa (GF)
2¼ cups quinoa flour
¾ cup tapioca flour
1 teaspoon salt
2 teaspoons baking soda
½ teaspoon unbuffered vitamin C powder
¼ cup oil
1½ cups water

Rice (GF)
3 cups brown rice flour
¾ cup tapioca starch or arrowroot
1 teaspoon salt
1 tablespoon guar gum or xanthan gum
2 teaspoons baking soda
½ teaspoon unbuffered vitamin C powder
¼ cup oil
2½ cups water

Rye
3 cups rye flour
1 teaspoon salt
1½ teaspoons baking soda
½ teaspoon unbuffered vitamin C powder
2 to 3 teaspoons caraway seed (optional, to taste)
⅓ cup oil
1½ cups water

Spelt

> 3½ cups whole spelt flour
> 1 teaspoon salt
> 2 teaspoons baking soda
> ½ teaspoon unbuffered vitamin C powder
> ½ cup oil
> 1¼ cups water

Choose one set of the above ingredients from the previous page or above. Preheat your oven to 350°F. Rub oil all around the inside of an 8 by 4 inch or 9 by 5 inch loaf pan. Put 1 to 2 tablespoons of flour of the same kind you are using in the recipe in the pan and shake it around until the bottom and all the sides are coated with flour.

Stir together the flour(s), salt, baking soda, vitamin C powder, guar or xanthan gum (if used) and caraway seed (if used) in a large bowl. Thoroughly mix the oil and water in another bowl or measuring cup. Before the liquid ingredients have time to separate, pour them into the bowl with the dry ingredients. Stir together the liquid and dry ingredients until they are just mixed. DO NOT OVER-MIX. Quickly scrape the batter into the prepared pan. Put the bread into the oven and bake it for 45 to 55 minutes, or until it is beginning to brown. Insert a toothpick into the center of the loaf. If it comes out dry, remove the loaf from the oven. Turn the bread out onto a cooling rack and cool it completely before slicing it. If you wish, you can freeze leftover sliced bread. When you want to eat it, toast the slices in a toaster oven while still frozen. If you want to make sandwiches with the more fragile varieties of this bread, toast the bread thoroughly using a toaster oven in which you can lay the slices of bread flat. Makes one loaf of bread.

The teff, quinoa, and rye bread loaves can be sliced into 13 to 15 slices for one-carbohydrate unit slices. The rice bread and spelt bread contains more carbohydrates so the rice bread "costs" 2 carbohydrate units per thin slice; spelt bread is 1½ units for a thicker slice. For these breads, you may want to use a narrow bread pan, such as the Norpro™ pans described on page 133, to be able to produce 1-carbohydrate unit slices. If you use the Norpro™ pan for the other breads, you may find it easier to use the bread sliced less thinly. See "Sources," page 279, for information about purchasing Norpro™ pans.

One slice of teff bread (at 14 slices per loaf) contains 1 carbohydrate unit and 7 grams of fat. One slice of quinoa bread (at 15 slices per loaf) contains 1 carbohydrate unit and 6 grams of fat. One slice of rice bread (at 14 slices per loaf) contains 2 carbohydrate units and 7 grams of fat. One slice of spelt bread (at 12 slices per loaf) contains 1½ carbohydrate units and 10 grams of fat. One slice of rye bread (at 13 slices per loaf) contains 1 carbohydrate unit and 6 grams of fat.

About Yeast Breads

Although I grew up baking bread the old-fashioned way, now I prefer to make yeast bread more easily using an appliance such as a mixer or a bread machine. However, if you makr yeast bread by hand and prefer not to use a machine, you can make the spelt bread recipe on page 192 the traditional way by using the ingredient list and the by-hand method to which you are accustomed. (The hand method can be used only for gluten-containing bread). The two gluten-free recipes below must be made by the mixer method or with a bread machine to develop the structure of the guar or xanthan gum.

If you already have a bread machine, you may not be able to make bread in it start-to-finish unless you can program a shorter last rising time. However, you will probably be able to use it to simplify making special diet breads. Add the ingredients to the machine in the order listed in your machine's instruction booklet (usually liquids first, salt and other seasonings, flour, and finally yeast). Use the machine's dough cycle to per-form the initial mixing and kneading and the first rise for your bread. Then restart the cycle and allow the dough to knead for another 3 to 5 minutes. (If your machine mixes slowly at first, begin timing this after it switches to kneading more quickly). Remove the dough from the machine and put it in a prepared loaf pan. Proceed with the second rise and bake the bread in your oven as directed in the following recipes.

The recipes here direct that the bread should rise in a warm (85 to 90°F) place. Unless you have a very cozy corner in your kitchen, while the dough is mixing in your mixer or completing the first rise in your bread machine, begin preparing your oven to be a rising spot for the dough. If you have a gas oven, the pilot light will probably keep the oven at just about the right temperature, 85 to 90°F. If you have an electric oven, turn it to 350°F and let it preheat. Turn it off, open the oven door, and let it cool for 8 to 10 minutes until the temperature inside the oven is about 85 to 90°F. Then close the oven door. Use a thermometer to verify that the oven is at the correct temperature the first few times you do this. After you gain experience, you will be able to tell the right temperature by the feel of the oven when you place your dough in it to rise.

Most gluten-free bread recipes call for a combination of several flours plus multiple stabilizers. This seems to produce bread with a more conventional texture. However, as you have read previously, this book takes a different approach to combining several grains in each recipe both to save time on measuring and, more importantly, to prevent the development of allergies to foods that are eaten every day. Therefore, the recipes in this book are made with a single grain or grain alternative or a single grain or grain alternative plus a starch which acts as a binder.

For more information about making bread by hand, see *Allergy Cooking With Ease* or *The Ultimate Food Allergy Cookbook and Survival Guide* which are described at the end of this book. For more information on how to make yeast bread by hand, mixer, or bread machine and how to choose the bread machine that will work best for your special diet, see *Easy Breadmaking for Special Diets* as described on the last pages of this book.

My two favorite gluten-free yeast bread recipes are included in this chapter as well as a recipe for spelt yeast bread. For more bread recipes made with a wide variety of grains and grain alternatives using the hand method, a mixer, or a bread machine, see the books mentioned above.

The final recipe in this chapter is for wheat and gluten-free buckwheat sourdough bread which is made possible by the new freeze-dried sourdough bacteria that you can get from King Arthur Flour. (See "Sources," page 280. Unlike traditional sourdough starters, these new starters do not contain wheat flour). Sourdough bread has a lower GI score than bread made from the same grain that has not undergone the sourdough fermentation. Therefore, a wheat and gluten-free sourdough bread recipe is very exciting to be able to include in this chapter. At the time of this writing, Zojurushi has just come out with a programmable bread machine with a sourdough cycle. Although I have not been able to acquire the new machine yet, I hope it will simplify sourdough bread making and that future books in this series will have many more sourdough recipes. I also have ideas for oven-baked English muffins and other favorite foods you may miss. Stay tuned for the next episode!

QUINOA RAISIN YEAST BREAD

Gluten-Free

This tasty bread has an amazingly whole wheat-like texture for a gluten-free loaf. Try it toasted for breakfast.

> ¼ cup water
> ⅓ cup apple juice concentrate
> About 4 large or 3 extra large eggs* (enough to measure ¾ cup in volume) at
>   room temperature
> 2 tablespoons oil
> ¾ teaspoon salt
> 1 teaspoon cinnamon
> 4 teaspoons guar or xanthan gum**
> 2½ cups quinoa flour
> ¾ cup tapioca starch
> 2¼ teaspoons (1 package) active dry yeast
> ½ cup raisins

If you wish to use a bread machine to mix the dough for this bread, prepare the dough using the dough cycle as described in the second paragraph on the previous page.

After the first rise, start the cycle again and re-mix the dough for 3 to 5 minutes. (If your machine mixes slowly at first, begin timing this after it switches to kneading more quickly). Add the raisins and mix for a minute or two more until they are evenly distributed in the dough. Proceed with this recipe as in the third paragraph of these directions below.

To make this bread with a mixer, heat the water and apple juice concentrate to about 115°F. Beat the eggs slightly and measure ¾ cup. Stir together the dry ingredients in a large electric mixer bowl. With the mixer running at low speed, gradually add the juice mixture, eggs and oil. Beat the dough for three minutes at medium speed. Scrape the dough from the beaters and the sides of the bowl into the bottom of the bowl. Oil the top of the dough and the sides of the bowl, and cover the bowl with plastic wrap and then with a towel. Put the bowl in a warm (85°F to 90°F) place*** and let the dough rise for about 1 hour or until it doubles in volume. Beat the dough again for three minutes at medium speed. Stir in the raisins by hand.

Oil and flour an 8 by 4 inch loaf pan. Put the dough in the pan and allow it to rise in a warm place*** for about 20 to 30 minutes or until it barely doubles. Preheat the oven to 375°F. Bake the loaf for about 50 to 70 minutes, loosely covering it with foil after the first 15 minutes to prevent excessive browning. Remove the loaf from the pan and cool it completely on a cooling rack. Makes one loaf or 15 slices of bread each of which contains 1½ units of carbohydrate and 4 grams of fat. If you want thicker 2-carbohydrate unit slices (great toasted for breakfast), divide the loaf into 11 slices.

This bread can also be made from start to finish in a programmable machine using the following cycle: Knead – 20 minutes; Rise 1 and 2 – Off; Rise 3 (or the last rise) – 30 minutes; Bake – 60 minutes. Be prepared to tweak this cycle to fit your machine and baking conditions. If the loaf over-rises and falls, decrease the time of the last rise.

*Note on eggs: If you are allergic to eggs, use ¾ cup warm water in their place. If you do not take the eggs out of the refrigerator early enough for them to come to room temperature before you are ready to bake, put them in a bowl of warm water for 5 or 10 minutes before cracking them to use in this recipe.

**Note on guar or xanthan gum: When making the dough for this bread in a bread machine, mix the guar or xanthan gum into the flour before adding them to the machine. If you just add the ingredients to the machine in the order listed, during the warm-up time before mixing begins, the water and gum can form lumps that routine mixing may not completely eliminate.

***Note on a warm rising place: To use your oven as a cozy place for bread to rise, see the third paragraph on page 188.

BUCKWHEAT "RYE" BREAD

The caraway seeds and rye flavor powder give this bread a delicious rye-like taste. If you have rye fans at your house, watch out! I have to freeze part of the loaf to keep the whole loaf from vanishing in a day or two. If you do not like rye or are allergic to the corn the flavor contains, this bread is also delicious without the rye flavor.

½ cup water

¼ cup apple juice concentrate

About 4 large or 3 extra large eggs*, or enough to measure ¾ cup in volume, at room temperature

3 tablespoons oil

1¼ teaspoon salt

1 tablespoon caraway seed (optional)

¾ teaspoon rye flavor powder, to taste (optional – This is gluten free but contains corn. See "Sources," page 281).

1 tablespoon guar or xanthan gum**

2 cups buckwheat flour

1⅜ cup tapioca starch or arrowroot

2¼ teaspoons (1 package) GF active dry yeast

If you wish to use a bread machine to mix the dough for this bread, use the method described in the second paragraph on page 188. After the first rise, re-start the cycle and remix the dough for 3 to 5 minutes. (If your machine mixes slowly at first, begin timing this after it switches to kneading more quickly). Then proceed with this recipe as in the third paragraph of these directions below.

To make this bread using a mixer, heat the water and apple juice concentrate to about 115°F. Beat the eggs slightly and measure ¾ cup. Stir together the dry ingredients in a large electric mixer bowl. With the mixer running at low speed, gradually add the juice mixture, eggs and oil. Beat the dough for three minutes at medium speed. Scrape the dough from the beaters and the sides of the bowl into the bottom of the bowl. It will be very sticky. Oil the top of the dough and the sides of the bowl. Then cover the bowl with plastic wrap and finally with a towel. Put the bowl in a warm (85°F to 90°F) place*** and let the dough rise for 1 to 1½ hours. Beat the dough again for three minutes at medium speed.

Oil and flour an 8 by 4 inch loaf pan. Put the dough in the pan and allow it to rise in a warm place*** for about 20 to 35 minutes, or until it barely doubles. Preheat the oven to 375°F. Bake the loaf for about 50 to 65 minutes, loosely covering it with foil after the first 30 to 45 minutes if it is getting excessively brown. Remove the loaf from the pan and cool it completely on a cooling rack. Makes one loaf or 15 slices of bread each of which contains 1½ units of carbohydrate and 5 grams of fat. If you want thicker 2-carbohydrate unit slices, divide the loaf into 11 slices.

This bread can also be made from start to finish in a programmable machine using the following cycle: Knead – 20 minutes; Rise 1 and 2 – Off; Rise 3 (or the last rise) – 25 minutes; Bake – 57 minutes. Be prepared to tweak this cycle to fit your machine and baking conditions. If the loaf over-rises and falls, decrease the time of the last rise.

*Note on eggs: If you are allergic to eggs, use ¾ cup warm water in their place. If you do not take the eggs out of the refrigerator early enough for them to come to room temperature before you are ready to bake, put them in a bowl of warm water for 5 or 10 minutes before cracking them to use in this recipe.

**Note on guar or xanthan gum: When making the dough for this bread in a bread machine, mix the guar or xanthan gum into the flour before adding them to the machine. If you just add the ingredients to the machine in the order listed, during the warm-up time before mixing begins, the water and gum can form lumps that routine mixing may not completely eliminate.

***Note on a warm rising place: To use your oven as a cozy place for bread to rise, see the third paragraph on page 188.

Spelt Yeast Bread

This bread is so normal in taste and texture that guests may be surprised that they are not eating wheat. It can be made on the basic bread cycle of almost* any bread machine. Always use Purity Foods™ flour to make spelt yeast bread. (See page 97 for the reasons why).

> 1 cup water
> ¼ cup apple juice concentrate, thawed
> 1½ tablespoons oil
> 1 teaspoon salt
> About 3¼ to 3¾ cups whole spelt flour**
> 2¼ teaspoons (1 package) active dry yeast

To make this recipe with a bread machine, add the ingredients to the pan in the order listed by your bread machine's instruction manual using the smaller amount of the flour. (For most machines this will be the order given above). Chose the basic cycle and a loaf size of 1½ pounds. Start the machine. After a few minutes of mixing, look in the machine. If the dough is very soft, begin adding more flour about 2 tablespoons at a time until it reaches a consistency that is not sticky. After about 10 minutes of mixing, re-check the consistency of the dough and add flour if needed. It should not be too soft or sticky and be starting to become elastic. Re-check the dough near the end of the kneading time, such as when the "add raisins" timer sounds, because spelt dough can soften during kneading and may need more flour. Then allow the rest of the cycle to run.

To make this recipe with a mixer, put one-half to two-thirds of the flour, the yeast, and the salt in the mixer bowl. Mix on low speed for about 30 seconds. Warm the liquid ingredients to 115 to 120°F. With the mixer running on low speed, add the liquids to the dry ingredients in a slow stream. Continue mixing until the dry and liquid ingredients are thoroughly mixed. If your mixer is not a heavy-duty mixer, at this point beat the dough for 5 to 10 minutes. You will be able to tell that the gluten is developing because the dough will begin to climb up the beaters. Then knead the rest of the flour in by hand, kneading for about 10 minutes, or until the dough is very smooth and elastic. If your mixer is a heavy-duty mixer, after the liquids are thoroughly mixed in, with the mixer still running, begin adding the rest of the flour around the edges of the bowl ½ cup at a time, mixing well after each addition before adding more flour, until the dough forms a ball and cleans the sides of the bowl. Knead the dough on the speed directed in your mixer manual for 5 to 10 minutes or until the dough is very elastic and smooth. If it softens during kneading, add more flour. Turn the dough out onto a floured board and knead it briefly to check the consistency of the dough, kneading in a little more flour if necessary. Put the dough into an oiled bowl and turn it once so that the top of the ball is also oiled. Cover it with plastic wrap and then with a towel and let it rise in a warm (85°F to 90°F) place*** until it has doubled in volume, about 45 minutes to 1 hour.

While the dough is rising, prepare your baking pan. Spelt is different from other types of bread in that it can be very difficult to get the bread out of the pan. Rub the inside of an 8-inch by 4-inch or 9-inch by 5-inch loaf pan with oil. Cut a piece of parchment or waxed paper the length of the pan and put it in the pan so the bottom and sides are covered with the paper. Oil the paper also. When the dough has doubled in volume, punch it down and shape it into a loaf. Put the loaf into the prepared loaf pan. Allow it to rise until double again. Bake bread at 375°F for 45 minutes to an hour or until it is nicely browned. Check it midway through the baking time, and if it is already getting brown, cover it with a piece of foil to prevent over-browning. At the end of the baking time, remove the loaf from the pan. You may need to run a knife along the ends of the pan which are not lined with paper to loosen the loaf. If it is done, the loaf should sound hollow when tapped on the bottom. Cool it completely on a cooling rack before slicing it. If you can't wait to eat it, slice it carefully with a serrated knife.

Makes one loaf or 13 slices of bread each of which contains 1½ units of carbohydrate and 1 gram of fat. If you want 1-carbohydrate unit slices for sandwiches, use a long, narrow Norpro™ bread pan (see page 183) and divide the loaf into 16 slices.

Note on bread machines: An exception to this working well in almost any bread machine is that it will not work in machines that over-knead the dough. This bread will not come out well in the programmable Breadman Ultimate™ bread machine, which kneads so vigorously and almost violently that it over-kneads spelt flour. I have another Breadman machine which makes a 1-pound loaf and which also kneads exceptionally vigorously and doesn't work well with spelt. The gentle knead of Zojirushi machines is ideal for spelt.

Note on flour: Even if you use Purity Foods™ flour, spelt flour is variable from batch to batch on how much flour it takes to make dough of the right consistency. Most bread machine recipes do not require much adjustment, and gluten-free recipes should be made "as written" the first time, because their dough may be the consistency of a stiff batter. However, in this recipe, you may have to check the dough several times throughout the kneading time and add more flour because spelt bread softens as it kneads.

***Note on a warm rising place:** To use your oven as a cozy place for bread to rise, see the third paragraph on page 188.

Buckwheat Sourdough Bread

Gluten-Free

Sourdough bread has a lower GI value than regular bread made with the same grain. Now, with new freeze-dried starters, we can make sourdough bread gluten- and wheat-free and without keeping a starter. You will love this bread!

Sponge
¼ teaspoon LA-4 French sourdough starter (See "Sources," page 280).
¾ cup bottled (non-chlorinated) water
1½ cups buckwheat flour

Dough
2 extra-large eggs* at room temperature, or 2 large* eggs at room temperature
    plus enough warm non-chlorinated water to bring the volume up to ½ cup
¼ cup apple juice concentrate, lukewarm
3 tablespoons oil
1¼ teaspoon salt
1 tablespoon caraway seed (optional)
1 tablespoon guar or xanthan gum
½ cup buckwheat flour
1⅜ cup tapioca starch
2 teaspoons active dry yeast

To make this bread with a programmable bread machine, program one of the home-made menu cycles on your machine for these times: Knead 1: 10 minutes, Rise 1: 20 hours. All the other parts of the cycle should be set to zero minutes. To make it without using a bread machine, plan to be home for most of two days and use your mixer on medium speed to do the mixing. Do not keep the sponge or dough in a metal mixing bowl; rather use plastic or glass. Allow the sponge and starter to rise in a warm place. (If you are using your oven for the warm place, this will probably tie up your oven for most of two days!)

About noon of the day before you want to serve this bread, measure the ingredients for the sponge. Mix them with your mixer for 5 minutes or put the ingredients for the sponge into the pan of your bread machine. Let it mix for three minutes at slow speed, using a spatula to make sure that all of the ingredients are well combined. Then it will mix for 7 minutes at a faster speed. (These are the two components of the knead part of the cycle on the Zojirushi BBCC-X-20). Cover the pan of your machine loosely with plastic wrap and leave it in the machine for 18 to 20 hours, or cover the glass or plastic dough bowl with plastic wrap and then with a towel and let it rise in a warm (85 to 90°F) place** for 18 to 20 hours. After this time the sponge should have expanded in volume by ⅓ or more and should smell sour.

The morning of the day you plan to serve this bread, mix the guar or xanthan gum with the ½ cup buckwheat flour and tapioca starch. If you are using a bread machine, add the flour mixture and the rest of the dough ingredients to the sponge and restart the sourdough cycle you programmed. Allow it to mix for 10 minutes and then rise for 30 to 40 minutes. Then cancel the cycle and re-start it. Stop it after 10 minutes at the end of the mixing time. If you are using your mixer, add the flour mixture and the rest of the ingredients to the sponge and beat it for 5 minutes. Allow it to rise in your warm place for 30 to 40 minutes and then beat it again for 5 minutes.

While the dough is mixing for the final time, oil and flour a 9 by 5 inch loaf pan. When the dough is finished mixing, put it in the pan and allow it to rise in a warm** (85 to 90°F) place for about 20 to 30 minutes, or until it barely doubles in volume. Preheat your oven to 375°F. Bake the loaf for about 50 to 65 minutes, loosely covering it with foil after the first 30 to 45 minutes if it is getting excessively brown. Remove the loaf from the pan and cool it completely on a cooling rack. The final loaf should sound hollow when tapped on the bottom. It will be about 3 inches high. Makes one loaf or 15 slices of bread each of which contains 1½ units of carbohydrate and 4 grams of fat. If you want thicker 2-carbohydrate unit slices, divide the loaf into 11 slices.

Note on eggs: If you are allergic to eggs, use ½ cup warm water in their place. If you do not take the eggs out of the refrigerator early enough for them to come to room temperature before you are ready to bake, put them in a bowl of warm water for 5 or 10 minutes before cracking them to use in this recipe.

**Note on a warm rising place: To use your oven as a cozy place for bread to rise, see the third paragraph on page 188. Since your oven will not retain the heat for the 18 to 20 hours needed to ferment the sponge, you will have to adjust the temperature by either reheating and cooling the oven or monitoring the oven temperature with a thermometer and turning the oven on for about 15 seconds occasionally to raise the temperature as needed.

DESSERTS AND TREATS

It is difficult to modify our eating habits on the long-term basis needed for permanent weight loss if we feel deprived of pleasure. The recipes in this chapter will give you an escape from this feeling and thus help you succeed with your healthy eating plan.

In her bariatric (weight loss) medical practice, Dr. Cheryle Hart allows her patients to have controlled splurges with pleasurable foods to enable them to stay on the diets she prescribes long-term. Because chocolate contains substances that raise the level of feel-good neurotransmitters in the brain, many of her patients enjoy one ounce of dark chocolate several times a week. If you are not allergic to chocolate, this chapter contains several chocolate recipes that you will enjoy. By making these chocolate recipes sugar-free, you may be able to have dessert after a carbohydrate-containing meal without exceeding 30 total grams of carbohydrate. If you are allergic to chocolate, try "Carob Brownies," page 200, or the other recipes in this chapter. Keep an allergen or gluten-free treat on hand in your freezer at all times so you can have a controlled splurge when you need it before the feeling of deprivation gets too strong.

The recipes in this chapter were developed to yield portion sizes that are not extremely small. Somehow, a recipe that says, "You can eat this cake on your healthy eating plan as long as you limit the serving size to a 2-inch cube of cake" seems to fall short of the goal of this chapter, which is to satisfy a craving before it gets out of hand. I know a 2-inch cube of cake would not satisfy me! The problem with most sweet treats is that they contain both flour and a sweetener. When these are the main ingredients of a food, it is easy to exceed the 30 gram carbohydrate limit. With the advent of the new stevia (see page 96 for more about this), we have a healthy and tasty solution to this problem since stevia contains no carbohydrate. Many of the recipes in this chapter can be made with your choice of either stevia or a non-sugar nutritive sweetener. This gives the option of having a larger portion of the dessert if you make it with stevia. Although allergic individuals often have problems with it, Equal™ is included as a non-nutritive sweetening option for your non-allergic eating plan companion(s) in a few recipes in this book that do not need to be baked.

The other sweeteners used in this chapter are lower on the glycemic index scale than sugar. These include agave (with a GI score of between 11 and 32 depending on the source), single source honey, Fruit Sweet™, other fruit sweeteners, and coconut sugar (with a GI score of 35). Listen to your body if you decide to use coconut sugar, however. It contains mostly sucrose, the same type of sugar as white table sugar, but is less refined. Several people I have talked to, myself included, report that it increases their hunger. It is used in the buckwheat chocolate brownie recipe here because a dry sweetener is required for traditional brownie texture.

As you enjoy the recipes in this chapter, remember to control the portion size and link and balance these treats with protein. Then they will be a sanity-saving part of your healthy eating plan without destabilizing your blood sugar.

STEVIA-SWEETENED CHOCOLATE CANDY OR CHOCOLATE CHIPS

Gluten-Free

This candy does not add any carbohydrates to a snack or meal because it is sweetened with stevia. It is easy to make using a microwave oven.

> 4 ounces unsweetened baking chocolate
> ¼ cup cocoa butter
> 2 to 2¼ teaspoons pure white stevia powder such as Protocol for Life Balance™ brand
> 1 tablespoon vegetable oil

Remove the lid from the jar of cocoa butter and put the jar in the microwave oven. Microwave it on high power, checking it with a fork at 30 second intervals, until the cocoa butter can be broken into pieces when pierced with the fork. Put enough of the broken pieces into a glass measuring cup to reach the ¼ cup line. Microwave the cocoa butter in the cup on reduced power, stirring it every minute. After it liquefies, add and submerge more chunks of cocoa butter to bring the level up to the ¼ cup line. Microwave and stir the cocoa butter at 30 second intervals until it is all melted. The glass measuring cup will feel hot.

Break the chocolate into ½ ounce pieces or, if you are short on time for melting and cooling the chocolate, into smaller pieces. Add the pieces to the melted cocoa butter. Allow the mixture to stand for 5 or 10 minutes if time allows. Then stir it with a rubber spatula until the chocolate is melted. If you have time, allow the chocolate to stand until it is just warm.

While the chocolate is cooling, generously grease a 12 by 8 inch* metal pan (if you are making chocolate chips) or an 8 or 9-inch square metal pan (if you are making chocolate candy squares) with butter, cocoa butter which has been softened in the microwave, or goat butter. In a small bowl, thoroughly stir together the stevia powder and vegetable oil.

When the chocolate is cooled (or you can do this when it is hot if you're in a rush), use a spatula to scrape all the stevia-oil mixture out of the bowl and into the chocolate. Stir it thoroughly; then scrape down the sides into the middle of the chocolate and stir it more so all of the chocolate gets combined with the stevia mixture.

Pour the chocolate into the prepared pan. The thickness should be between ⅛ and ¼ inch. Set it in the refrigerator and let it harden for about 5 minutes or up to 15 minutes if the chocolate was hot. The middle should be set but not firm.

For chocolate candies, use a large knife to cut the chocolate into four strips in each direction, making 16 chocolate squares which are about 2 inches square. Then run your knife around the edges of the pan. Put the pan back in the refrigerator and let the chocolate harden thoroughly. Remove it from the refrigerator, turn the pan upside down and flex the bottom. The chocolate should fall out. If not, use a spatula to remove the chocolate and grease the pan more generously the next time you make this. Wrap the squares in plastic wrap if desired and store them in the refrigerator.

To make chocolate chips, use a large knife to cut the solidifying chocolate into strips about ¼ inch wide. Then cut the chocolate strips in a direction perpendicular to the first cuts to form ¼ inch squares. Run your knife around the edges of the pan. Put the pan back into the refrigerator and let the chocolate harden thoroughly. Remove it from the refrigerator, turn the pan upside down and flex the bottom. The chocolate should fall out. If not, use a spatula to remove the chocolate and grease the pan more generously the next time you make this. Break any sections of chips that are stuck together into individual chips (or do this at serving time) and store the chocolate chips in the refrigerator. Serve the chips as a candy or sprinkled on ice cream (recipes on pages 220 to 221). These chips are not suitable for baking in cookies because they melt completely in the oven and the chocolate runs out of the cookies and onto the baking sheet.

If you wish to make special occasion candy, use candy molds. Most of them do not need to be greased. If they came with instructions saying that you should grease them, use a very light coating of softened butter or goat butter. Make the chocolate as above, adding nuts (see below) if desired. Cool the chocolate to near its hardening point and pour it into the molds. Put the molds in the refrigerator. Unmold when the chocolate is completely hard and wrap the candies in plastic wrap or colored foil if desired.

Makes about 1¼ cup chocolate chips or 6 ounces of chocolate candy. Although this chocolate does not contain carbohydrates, it does contain saturated fat, so eat it slowly for maximum enjoyment and use it to satisfy your pleasure needs in moderation. Each 2-inch square of chocolate candy contains 8 grams of fat and weighs about ⅜ of an ounce. A half-ounce serving of chocolate chips contains 11 grams of fat.

Chocolate almond bar variation: After mixing the stevia into the chocolate, stir about ¾ cup (4 ounces) of whole almonds into the chocolate. Pour it into the prepared 8 or 9 inch square pan and distribute the almonds evenly in the pan. Put the pan in the refrigerator for 5 to 15 minutes. Check it every few minutes after the first 5 minutes. When it begins to set up, cut the chocolate into 16 squares with a knife as directed above, cutting through the nuts. Then refrigerate until it is thoroughly chilled and hardened. Remove the candy from the pan as directed above. Break the candy into squares along the cut lines and wrap each piece in foil, colored foil, or plastic wrap. Makes 16 candy squares which are very satisfying due to the protein and crunch added by the almonds. Each square contains 11 grams of fat and ⅓ of a protein unit.

*Note on pans: A 12 by 8 inch foil pan is especially good to use for chocolate chips because the flexibility of the pan makes the chips easy to remove.

Cookies

Cookies have always been small morsels of delight. Because of their traditional size, you can have a small serving and it will feel just right. A cookie is a perfect treat that will not cause you to exceed the carbohydrate limit for a meal or snack. Some of the cookies in this section contain only half a carbohydrate unit each.

CAROB BROWNIES

Gluten-Free

These gluten- and grain-free fruit-sweetened brownies are a delicious and satisfying treat for those who must avoid chocolate.

> 1 cup amaranth flour
> ¼ cup arrowroot
> ⅓ cup carob powder
> ½ teaspoon baking soda
> ¾ cup apple juice concentrate, thawed
> ¼ cup oil

Preheat your oven to 350°F. Oil and flour a 9 inch by 5 inch metal loaf pan. If your carob powder contains lumps, press it through a strainer with the back of a spoon to remove the lumps before measuring it. Combine the amaranth flour, arrowroot, carob powder and baking soda in a bowl. In another bowl or measuring cup stir together the apple juice concentrate and oil. Stir the liquid ingredients into the dry ingredients until just mixed and immediately put the batter into the prepared pan. Bake for 20 minutes. The batter will puff up during baking and then collapse either near the end of the baking time or after you remove the brownies from the oven. Do not over-bake. The toothpick test on page 99 does not apply to these brownies; if you test them with a toothpick, the toothpick will come out with wet dough on it. These brownies have a moist, chewy texture. At the end of the baking time, remove the pan from the oven and cool the brownies completely before cutting. Makes 10 brownies each of which contains 1⅔ carbohydrate units and 6 grams of fat.

Stevia-sweetened carob brownies: Stir ⅛ teaspoon of unbuffered vitamin C powder and ⅛ to ¼ teaspoon of pure white stevia powder such as Protocol for Life™ brand into the dry ingredients. Omit the apple juice concentrate and instead use ¾ cup of water with the oil. Makes 11 brownies each of which contains 1 carbohydrate unit and 6 grams of fat. To cut 11 brownies, mentally or using a ruler, divide the length of pan into 11 equal segments. Cut one of these segments across the end of the pan. Then cut the rest of the pan down the center of the long direction and then crosswise into five segments.

CHOCOLATE BROWNIES

Gluten-Free

These rich brownies are favorites with the most discriminating of my recipe tasters.

> 2 1-ounce squares unsweetened chocolate
> ⅜ cup oil
> 1 cup coconut sugar
> 2 large eggs
> ½ teaspoon salt
> ¾ cup buckwheat flour
> ½ teaspoon baking powder such as Featherweight™ brand*

Preheat your oven to 350°F. Oil an 8-inch square metal baking pan. Line the bottom and two opposite sides of the pan with an 8-inch wide strip of parchment or waxed paper. Then oil the paper. Melt the chocolate in a double boiler over boiling water or carefully microwave it in a glass bowl, stirring often, until it is just melted. Stir the oil into the melted chocolate thoroughly. Add the coconut sugar, eggs, and salt and stir thoroughly. In a separate bowl, stir together the flour and baking powder. Add the dry ingredients to the chocolate mixture and stir until just mixed. Spread the batter in the prepared pan. Bake for 25 to 30 minutes or until a toothpick inserted into the brownies comes out dry or with just a few moist crumbs on it. Cool in the pan. Then cut into squares. Makes 16 brownies each of which contains 1 carbohydrate unit and 8 grams of fat.

*Note on baking powder: If you are allergic to corn, use Featherweight™ brand baking powder which contains potato starch instead of corn starch.

QUINOA ALMOND COOKIES

This cookie has several different personalities depending on which sweetener and how much liquid you use. Try all the varieties – they're delicious in different ways.

1½ cups quinoa flour
½ cup almond meal or flour (Bob's Red Mill™ almond meal is fine in this recipe).
¾ teaspoon baking soda
¼ teaspoon unbuffered vitamin C powder
¼ cup sliced almonds
½ cup oil
½ teaspoon almond flavoring (optional)
½ cup agave or honey (for crisp cookies, with honey being more crisp)
   OR ½ cup agave or honey plus ½ cup water (for soft cookies)
   OR 1 cup apple juice concentrate, thawed (for fruit-sweetened soft cookies)

Preheat your oven to 375°F. Oil your baking sheets or, if you are using the agave, line your baking sheets with parchment paper for easiest cookie removal. Combine the flour, almond meal, baking soda, vitamin C and almonds in a large bowl. Thoroughly mix the oil and almond flavoring with the agave, honey, agave or honey plus water, or juice in a measuring cup or small bowl. Immediately pour the liquid ingredients into the dry ingredients and stir the dough until it is just mixed. Drop it by teaspoonfuls onto the prepared baking sheets. For the crisp cookies, flatten the cookies with an oiled glass bottom or your fingers held together. Bake the cookies for 7 to 10 minutes or until golden brown. Remove them from the cookie sheets and place them on paper towels to cool. Makes about 2 dozen crisp or 3 dozen soft cookies. The soft cookies each contain ½ carbohydrate unit and 4 grams of fat. The crisp cookies each contain ¾ carbohydrate unit and 6 grams of fat.

Very crisp cookie variation: Make the crisp cookie variation of this recipe using ½ cup agave or honey for the sweetener and no water, but also decrease the flour to 1 cup. If you are using the agave, be sure to line your baking sheets with parchment paper to avoid the struggle to remove cookies. There is no need to flatten the cookies with your fingers or a glass because the batter will be much thinner and will spread readily. Place the cookies at least 3 to 4 inches apart on the baking sheet. Bake at 375°F for 6 to 9 minutes. Slide the parchment paper and cookies off onto a cooling rack or, if you did not use parchment paper, let the cookies cool on the cookie sheet for about 2 minutes before removing them with a spatula and placing them on paper towels to cool. Makes about 1½ dozen cookies which each contain ¾ carbohydrate unit and 8 grams of fat.

CASHEW BUTTER COOKIES

Gluten-Free

This delicious and satisfying alternative to peanut butter cookies is gluten-free — made with amaranth flour. People who doesn't like peanut butter cookies love these!

1½ cups amaranth flour
½ cup arrowroot or tapioca starch
½ teaspoon baking soda
⅛ teaspoon unbuffered vitamin C powder
⅔ cup cashew butter
¼ cup oil
¾ cup agave or Fruit Sweet™
1 teaspoon vanilla (optional)

Preheat your oven to 400°F. If you are using the agave, line your baking sheets with parchment paper for easiest cookie removal or lightly oil the baking sheets. Combine the flour, starch, baking soda, and vitamin C powder in a large bowl. In a small bowl thoroughly mix together the cashew butter, oil, agave or Fruit Sweet™ and vanilla. (A hand blender is helpful for thorough mixing especially if the cashew butter is fairly solid from having been refrigerated). Stir and mash the cashew butter mixture into the dry ingredients. Drop the dough by heaping teaspoonfuls onto an ungreased baking sheet. Use an oiled fork to flatten the balls of dough, making an "X" on the top of them with the fork tines. Bake the cookies for 8 to 10 minutes or until they are golden brown. Remove them from the cookie sheets and place them on paper towels to cool. Makes about 3 dozen cookies which each contains ⅘ carbohydrate unit and 4 grams of fat.

CHOCOLATE ALMOND FLOUR COOKIES

Gluten-Free

Here's a chewy "chocolate fix" in a high protein package.

3½ cups finely ground blanched almond flour such as Honeyville™ brand
¼ cup cocoa
¼ teaspoon salt
½ teaspoon baking soda
¾ cup agave, Fruit Sweet™ or single source honey
⅛ cup (2 tablespoons) water
⅓ cup oil
2 teaspoons gluten- and alcohol-free vanilla extract such as Frontier Naturals™
    brand (optional)

Line two large baking sheets with parchment paper. Preheat your oven to 350°F. Mix together the flour, cocoa, salt, and baking soda in a large bowl. Combine the sweetener, oil, water and vanilla and stir them into the flour mixture until they are mixed in. Drop the batter by level tablespoonfuls onto the prepared cookie sheets, leaving at least 2 inches between the cookies. Flatten the dough with your fingers held together. Bake for 18 to 24 minutes or until the cookies are set to the touch in the center. Allow them to stand on the baking sheets for at least 20 minutes after removing them from the oven. Then slide the parchment paper and cookies onto a table or countertop to finish cooling. Makes three dozen cookies each of which contains ⅔ carbohydrate unit, ⅔ protein unit, and 4 grams of fat.

CHOCOLATE OR CAROB CHIP ALMOND FLOUR COOKIES

Gluten-Free

Here is everybody's favorite cookie made high-protein and grain and gluten-free by using almond flour.

3¼ cups finely ground blanched almond flour such as Honeyville™ brand
¼ teaspoon salt
½ teaspoon baking soda
½ cup agave, Fruit Sweet™ or single source honey
½ cup oil
1 teaspoon gluten- and alcohol-free vanilla extract such as Frontier Naturals™ brand (optional)
½ cup chocolate or carob chips, optional

Line two large baking sheets with parchment paper. Preheat your oven to 350°F. Mix together the flour, salt and baking soda in a large bowl. Combine the sweetener, oil, and vanilla and stir them into the flour mixture until they are mixed in. Stir in the chips. Drop the batter by level tablespoonfuls onto the prepared cookie sheets, leaving at least 2 inches between the cookies. Flatten the dough with your fingers held together. Bake for 7 to 10 minutes or until the cookies are brown on the edges. They will continue to brown after being removed from the oven. Allow them to stand on the baking sheets for at least 20 minutes after removing them from the oven. Then slide the parchment paper and cookies onto a table or countertop to finish cooling. Makes 30 to 32 cookies each of which contains ⅝ carbohydrate unit, ¾ protein unit, and 6 grams of fat if made without the chips. If made with chocolate chips, each cookie contains ⅔ carbohydrate unit, ¾ protein unit, and 7 grams of fat.

Cinnamon Raisin Almond Flour Cookies

Gluten-Free

These simple cookies are chewy and delicious. I enjoy them without the raisins or dried fruit as a basic lightly spiced cookie.

3¼ cups finely ground blanched almond flour such as Honeyville™ brand
¼ teaspoon salt
½ teaspoon baking soda
1 to 1½ teaspoons cinnamon
½ cup agave, Fruit Sweet™ or single source honey
½ cup oil
1 teaspoon gluten- and alcohol-free vanilla extract such as Frontier Naturals™ brand (optional)
⅓ cup raisins or other dried fruit cut into small pieces, optional

Line two large baking sheets with parchment paper. Preheat your oven to 350°F. Mix together the flour, salt, baking soda, and cinnamon in a large bowl. Combine the sweetener, oil and vanilla and stir them into the flour mixture until they are mixed in. Stir in the raisins or dried fruit if you are using them. Drop the batter by level tablespoonfuls onto the prepared cookie sheets leaving at least 2 inches between the cookies. Flatten the dough with your fingers held together. Bake for 7 to 10 minutes or until the cookies are brown on the edges. They will continue to brown after being removed from the oven. Allow them to stand on the baking sheets for at least 20 minutes after removing them from the oven. Then slide the parchment paper and cookies onto a table or countertop to finish cooling. Makes 30 to 32 cookies each of which contains ⅝ carbohydrate unit, ¾ protein unit, and 6 grams of fat if made without the raisins. If made with raisins, each cookie contains ⅔ carbohydrate unit, ¾ protein unit, and 6 grams of fat.

CARROT COOKIES

These cookies are packed with nutrition and can be sweetened with either fruit juice or stevia.

> 3 cups quinoa or spelt flour
> 1 cup tapioca starch or arrowroot
> 1½ teaspoons baking soda
> ⅜ teaspoon unbuffered vitamin C crystals if you are using the apple juice OR
> ⅛ teaspoon unbuffered vitamin C crystals if you are using the stevia and
> water
> 1½ teaspoons cinnamon
> 2¼ cups grated carrots
> 1 cup raisins or chopped dates or other dried fruit (optional)
> 1⅜ cups apple juice concentrate, thawed, OR 1⅜ cups water plus ¾ to 1
> teaspoon pure white stevia powder such as Protocol for Life Balance™
> brand, to taste
> ½ cup oil

Preheat your oven to 350°F. Mix together the flour, starch, baking soda, vitamin C crystals, cinnamon and stevia (if you are using it) in a large bowl. Stir in the carrots and raisins or chopped dried fruit. Combine the juice or water and oil and stir them into the flour mixture until they are just mixed in. Drop the batter by heaping teaspoonfuls onto an ungreased cookie sheet and bake for 12 to 15 minutes. The stevia-sweetened cookies will not brown very much, but they will feel dry when they are touched. Remove them from the cookie sheets and place them on paper towels to cool. Makes 4 to 5 dozen cookies each of which contains ⅔ carbohydrate unit and 2 grams of fat if made with apple juice or ½ carbohydrate unit and 2 grams of fat if made with stevia. The raisins add about 1 gram of carbohydrate per cookie, a negligible amount if the serving size is not extremely large.

Cobblers and Pies

Desserts such as pies or cobblers are a traditional part of holiday dinners. With the recipes here, you will not feel deprived nor have to spend hours in the kitchen preparing dessert. The cobbler recipes below are especially easy.

To make a pie for your non-allergic eating plan companion(s), you may use a regular pie crust rolled thinly and with the thick or extra pasty edge trimmed off to produce servings of crust which will be under one carbohydrate unit each. When combined with the filling, their piece of pie will be within 30 grams of carbohydrate, making this a dessert to have two or more hours after the meal, balanced with protein, of course. Keep in mind, however, that the white flour in mix (or from-scratch) pie crust is high on the GI scale, so pie in a regular crust should be a rare treat rather than a commonly eaten food.

If you prefer to have dessert immediately after your holiday meal, make pumpkin pudding (pumpkin pie filling made using a non-nutritive sweetener as pumpkin pudding without the crust). A few of the recipes here also give Nutrasweet™ (Equal™) as a non-nutritive sweetener option for your companion(s) who may not be accustomed to stevia.

APPLE COBBLER

Gluten-Free

Here's an alternative to apple pie that's quick and easy to make especially if you use the canned apples.

> 4 to 5 apples, peeled, cored, and sliced to make 3½ to 4 cups of slices OR
>   1 20-ounce can of sliced apples canned in water such as Mussleman's™
>   brand, drained
> ½ cup apple juice concentrate OR ½ cup water plus ¼ teaspoon pure white
>   stevia powder such as Protocol for Life™ brand
> 4 teaspoons tapioca starch or arrowroot
> 1 teaspoon cinnamon
> "Nutty Topping," page 209

Drain the canned apples or peel, core and slice the fresh apples. If you are using fresh apples, put them in a saucepan with the all but 2 tablespoons of the liquid, bring to a boil, and then reduce the heat and simmer for 15 to 20 minutes until the apples are tender. If you are using the canned apples, add all but 2 tablespoons of the liquid to the pan and bring to a boil. Stir the starch into the reserved 2 tablespoons of liquid. Add this starch mixture, the cinnamon and the stevia (if you are using it) to the pan. Bring the mixture back to a boil over medium heat, stirring it constantly. When it comes to a boil, boil it for one minute. Put the fruit into a 2½ to 3 quart casserole dish. Top with nutty toping just before serving time and serve warm or cool. Divide this cobbler filling into 7 servings which contain 1½ carbohydrate unit each if made with apple juice or into 6 servings which contain 1 carbohydrate unit each if made with stevia. Remember to add the number of nutritional units for the correct serving size of the nutty topping which you serve with this cobbler.

BLUEBERRY COBBLER

Gluten-Free

This is very easy to make using frozen blueberries. If you keep some nutty topping and blueberries in your freezer at all times, you can whip up this dessert at a moment's notice.

4 cups fresh blueberries OR a 1 pound bag of unsweetened frozen blueberries
½ cup apple or pineapple juice concentrate, thawed, OR ½ cup water plus
       ¼ teaspoon pure white stevia powder such as Protocol for Life™ brand
5 teaspoons arrowroot or tapioca starch
"Nutty Topping," page 209

In a saucepan combine the blueberries, juice concentrate (if you are using it) or water, stevia (if you are using it), and starch. Bring the mixture to a boil over medium heat, stirring it constantly. When it comes to a boil, boil it for one minute. Put the fruit into a 2½ to 3 quart casserole dish. Top with nutty toping just before serving time and serve warm or cool. Makes 6 servings of filling which each contain 1⅓ carbohydrate units if made with apple juice and ¾ carbohydrate unit if made with stevia. Remember to add the number of nutritional units for the correct serving size of the nutty topping which you serve with this cobbler.

NUTTY TOPPING

This is delightful on top of ice cream. If you keep a jar of this topping on hand, you will be able whip up a cobbler very quickly. Just make any cobbler filling* and sprinkle it with this topping for a dessert you and your guests will really enjoy.

⅔ cup unsweetened coconut (shredded to a medium coarseness)

⅓ cup chopped almonds or pecans or ½ cup sliced almonds

¼ cup almond or pecan meal or flour (See "Sources," page 281)

¼ teaspoon cinnamon (optional)

2 tablespoons oil

2 tablespoons agave, Fruit Sweet™ or apple juice concentrate, thawed

Preheat your oven to 400°F. Stir together the coconut, nuts, nut meal and cinnamon in a bowl. Add the oil and sweetener and stir until the nut mixture is well moistened throughout. If there are still dry particles after thorough mixing, the coconut used may have been more finely shredded than what was used to develop this recipe. Add a little more oil until all the particles are moistened. If the mixture is quite wet, the coconut may have been coarsely shredded. Add more coconut until the topping is no longer excessively wet.

Oil an 8 or 9 inch square metal cake pan. Spread the nut mixture evenly in the pan. Bake it for 5 to 10 minutes or until the coconut is just beginning to brown. Remove the pan from the oven and stir the nut mixture. Watching it carefully, bake it for an additional 2 to 10 minutes until it is all lightly browned. Stir the mixture again when you remove it from the oven. Cool it completely in the pan. Store it in a jar with an airtight lid at room temperature or in the freezer. Serve it on warm or cooled cobbler filling (pages 207 to 208) for an instant cobbler. Makes enough topping for 1 to 1⅓ batches of fruit cobbler filling. It is also delicious served on ice cream. Makes 6 servings of nutty topping which each contain ⅔ carbohydrate unit, ⅓ protein unit and 14 grams of fat, or divide the batch into 8 servings of nutty topping which each contain ½ carbohydrate unit, ¼ protein unit and 11 grams of fat.

*Note on other fruit fillings to use with this cobbler topping: For more cobbler filling options to use with this topping, see pages 224 to 227 of *The Ultimate Food Allergy Cookbook and Survival Guide,* pages 187 to 190 of *Allergy Cooking With Ease,* or pages 51 5o 54 of *I Love Dessert* as described on the last pages of this book.

No-Bake Pumpkin or Sweet Potato Pie or Pudding

You can make your traditional Thanksgiving pie with or without the crust to fit your healthy eating plan and your schedule. If you have dessert in the mid-afternoon, make it with the crust. To have dessert with the meal, make pumpkin pudding. Either way the spices are good for you — ginger is anti-inflammatory and cinnamon aids blood sugar control.

> 1 envelope unflavored gelatin OR 1 tablespoon agar flakes
>
> 1 cup water or milk of any kind you tolerate (soy, goat, cow's, etc.)
>
> 1 15-ounce can pumpkin or 1¾ cups mashed baked sweet potatoes (from about 1¼ to 1½ pounds of sweet potatoes)
>
> ¾ teaspoon pure stevia powder such as Protocol for Life™ brand, to taste, OR 18 to 24 packages of Equal™ for your non-allergic companions
>
> 1 teaspoon cinnamon
>
> 1 teaspoon nutmeg
>
> ¼ teaspoon ground cloves
>
> ¼ teaspoon allspice
>
> ¼ teaspoon ginger
>
> 1 baked pie crust,* recipes on pages 215 and 218 (optional – omit for pudding)

If you are making sweet potato pie, bake the sweet potatoes at 400°F for an hour (longer for very large potatoes) or until they feel soft when you squeeze them. Allow them to cool enough to handle or refrigerate them overnight. Scoop the potato out of the skin and measure 1¾ cups of potato.

Prepare and bake the pie crust as directed in the recipes on the following pages. If you are using a nut meal crust, bake it until it is fairly brown before filling it. Cool the crust thoroughly.

Put the water or milk in a saucepan and sprinkle the gelatin or agar over the surface of the liquid. Heat the water over medium heat, stirring occasionally, until it comes to a boil and the gelatin or agar dissolves. If you are using the milk, heat it slowly over low heat to a bare simmer, stirring to dissolve the gelatin or agar flakes. Thoroughly stir in the rest of the ingredients. If the sweet potatoes are lumpy, blend the mixture with a hand blender, blender or food processor. For pudding, put the mixture into a serving bowl and refrigerate it at this point.

For pie, cool the filling to at least room temperature or cooler before putting the mixture into the pie shell to keep the shell from becoming soft. If you are making the nut meal crust, this is especially important. For the best results, put the pan containing the filling into a sink full of cool water and stir it every few minutes until it is quite cool and beginning to seem thicker (i.e. it is on the verge of gelling) before putting the filling into the crust. Refrigerate the pie for several hours until it is thoroughly chilled before serving. Serve with whipped cream (recipe on the next page) if desired.

This recipe makes 8 servings of pie filling or pudding. If made with sweet potato, each serving contains 1 carbohydrate unit. Pumpkin is a squash rather than a source of concentrated carbohydrate and thus pumpkin pie filling or pudding does not contribute to the carbohydrate units of a meal or snack.

Flavoring option for sweet potato pie: If you like a milder sweet potato pie, use 1 teaspoon vanilla and ½ teaspoon cinnamon in place of all of the spices listed above.

Less assertive flavoring option for pumpkin pie: Use 1 teaspoon Ceylon cinnamon (instead of Vietnamese or "grocery store" cinnamon), ¼ teaspoon nutmeg, ⅛ teaspoon allspice, ⅛ teaspoon cloves, and omit the ginger.

*Note on crust: If you are making this pie for your non-allergic companions, see the second paragraph of the "Cobblers and Pies" introduction on page 207 about using a regular pie crust.

STABILIZED WHIPPED CREAM

Gluten-Free

This is delicious on the pies and cobblers here. It's just as good made without the thickener if you are allergic to corn or if you will be making it shortly before serving time.

> ½ pint (1 cup) whipping cream
> 2 teaspoons to 1 tablespoon agave, 1 to 2 stevia spoons* of pure white stevia
>   powder such as Protocol for Life™ brand, to taste, or 2 packages of Equal™
> 2 teaspoons Signature Secrets Culinary Thickener,™ optional (Omit if you are
>   allergic to corn. See "Sources," page 280, to order).

Beat the cream at high speed until soft peaks form. Add the sweetener and beat it in thoroughly. Add the thickener and blend it on low speed until it seems well mixed into the cream. Then beat on high speed for one to two more minutes until the cream forms stiff shapes. The surface of the cream will look chunky. Refrigerate the whipped cream. It will stay whipped for at least several days. If you are allergic to corn, omit the thickener and whip the cream up to an hour or two before you plan to serve it. The cream will look smooth on the surface but have stiff peaks when it has been whipped enough. Makes about 2 cups of whipped cream or 16 2-tablespoon servings which contain 6 grams of fat each.

*Note on the stevia spoon measurement: Protocol for Life Balance™ and several other brands of pure white stevia powder come with a small plastic spoon that holds an amount of stevia equivalent to about 2 teaspoons of sugar in sweetening power. Use this plastic spoon to measure the stevia in this recipe.

APPLE PIE

6 to 7 apples, peeled, cored and sliced to make about 5 cups of slices or 1½
    20-ounce cans water-packed apple slices, such as Mussleman's™ brand, drained
¾ cup water, divided
¼ to ½ teaspoon pure white stevia powder such as Protocol for Life Balance™
    brand, to taste, OR 6 packages of Equal™ or to taste
1 teaspoon cinnamon
2 tablespoons arrowroot or tapioca starch OR 3 tablespoons of quick-cooking
    (Minute™) tapioca
1 baked pie crust,* recipes on pages 215 to 218

If you are using the canned apples, drain the liquid from the cans. In a saucepan combine the fresh or canned apple slices, ½ cup water, ¼ teaspoon stevia and cinnamon. Bring them to a boil and reduce the heat to a simmer. For fresh apples, simmer for about 15 to 20 minutes or until they are tender. If you are using canned apples, simmer for just a few minutes to heat them. While they are cooking, in a separate cup stir together the additional ¼ cup water with the starch or tapioca. If you are using quick-cooking tapioca, let it stand for 5 minutes in the cup before adding it to the apples. Stir the starch or tapioca mixture into the saucepan at the end of the simmering time for the apples. Continue to simmer until the fruit mixture returns to a boil. Cook and stir it for one minute if you are using the quick-cooking tapioca or until it thickens if you are using the starch. Remove the pan from the heat.

If this is the first time you have made this pie, taste the filling after 3 minutes of cooling. If it is not sweet enough for you, sprinkle an additional ⅛ teaspoon of stevia powder over the surface and then stir it in very thoroughly. Taste the filling again. If it is still not sweet enough, add another ⅛ teaspoon of stevia. Record how much you use for next time. If you are using the Equal,™ stir it into the apples thoroughly after about 5 minutes of cooling. Allow the filling to cool, stirring it occasionally, for 15 to 30 minutes or until it is lukewarm or cooler and thickening but not set. Put the filling in the pie crust. Chill the pie in the refrigerator for a few hours before serving. Makes 8 servings of pie filing which contain one carbohydrate unit each. Add the carbohydrate units and grams of fat for the crust you use to these numbers to get the total units for a piece of pie.

*Note on crust: If you are making this pie for your non-allergic companions, see the second paragraph of the "Cobblers and Pies" introduction on page 207 about using a regular pie crust.

BLUEBERRY PIE

Gluten-Free

There are some people who cannot become accustomed to stevia (especially if they can't get Protocol for Life™ brand). These pie fillings are among the rare cooked recipes where you can use Nutrasweet™ (Equal™) without it breaking down due to the heat because you stir it into the filling after cooking it.

> 16 to 20 ounces fresh or frozen blueberries (about 5 to 6 cups fresh or 1 to 1¼ 1-pound bags frozen blueberries)
>
> 1 cup water
>
> 2 to 3 tablespoons quick-cooking (Minute™) tapioca or 2½ tablespoons tapioca starch or arrowroot
>
> ⅜ to ⅝ teaspoon pure white stevia powder such as Protocol for Life™ brand or 6 packages of Equal™
>
> 1 baked pie crust,* recipes on pages 215 to 218

Combine the blueberries, water, thickener, and ⅜ teaspoon of the stevia (if you are using it) in a saucepan. If you are using the Minute™ tapioca, allow the mixture to stand for 5 minutes. Then cook it over medium heat, stirring occasionally, until it comes to a boil. Cook and stir it for one minute if you are using the quick-cooking tapioca or until it thickens if you are using the starch. Remove the pan from the heat.

If you are using the stevia and this is the first time you have made this pie, taste the filling after 3 minutes of cooling. If it is not sweet enough for you, sprinkle an additional ⅛ teaspoon of stevia powder over the surface and then stir it in very thoroughly. Taste the filling again. If it is still not sweet enough, add another ⅛ teaspoon of stevia. Record how much stevia you use for the next time you make this.

If you are using the Equal™, stir it into the blueberries thoroughly after about 5 minutes of cooling. Allow the filling to cool, stirring it occasionally, for 15 to 30 minutes or until it is lukewarm or cooler and thickening but not set. Put the filling in the pie crust. Chill the pie in the refrigerator for a few hours before serving. Makes 8 servings of pie filing which are one carbohydrate unit each. Add the carbohydrate units and grams of fat for the crust you use to these numbers to get the total units for a piece of pie.

*Note on crust:** If you are making this pie for your non-allergic companions, see the second paragraph of the "Cobblers and Pies" introduction on page 207 about using a regular pie crust.

CHERRY PIE

Because pie cherries are fairly tart, this recipe may require more stevia than some to taste sweet enough. I prefer my pie a little on the tart side to minimize the stevia taste and so use ¾ teaspoon of stevia powder, but you may prefer it sweeter.

> 2 16 ounce cans water-packed tart pie cherries, drained
> ¾ cup reserved cherry juice
> ¾ teaspoon pure white stevia powder such as Protocol for Life™ brand, or a
>   little more to taste OR 15 to 18 packages of Equal™
> 3 tablespoons arrowroot or tapioca starch OR ¼ cup quick-cooking (Minute™)
>   tapioca
> 1 baked pie crust,* recipes on pages 215 and 218

Thoroughly drain the liquid from the canned cherries and reserve ¾ cup of the liquid. Combine the stevia and thickener with the cherry juice in a saucepan. If you are using quick-cooking tapioca, let it stand in the liquid for at least five minutes before you begin cooking the filling. Add the cherries and stir. Heat the fruit mixture over low to medium heat, stirring frequently, until it comes to a boil and thickens. Boil it for one minute if you are using the quick-cooking tapioca.

If this is the first time you have made this pie and you are using the stevia, taste the filling after 3 minutes of cooling. If it is not sweet enough for you, sprinkle an additional ⅛ teaspoon of stevia powder over the surface and then stir it in very thoroughly. Taste the filling again and adjust the sweetness to your liking. Record how much stevia you use for the next time you make this. If you are using the Equal™, stir it into the filling after about 5 minutes of cooling.

Allow the filling to cool in the pan, stirring occasionally, for 15 to 30 minutes or until it is lukewarm or cooler and thickening but not set. Put it in the baked cooled pie crust and refrigerate until it is cool. Makes eight servings of pie filing which contain 1 carbohydrate unit each. Add the carbohydrate units and grams of fat for the crust you use to these numbers to get the total units for a piece of pie.

*Note on crust: If you are making this pie for your non-allergic companions, see the second paragraph of the "Cobblers and Pies" introduction on page 207 about using a regular pie crust.

Nut Meal Pie Crust

Gluten-Free

This recipe gives those who are allergic to almonds the option of making a nut-based low carbohydrate pie crust with other kinds of nuts.

1¼ cups pecan, hazelnut, or almond meal* (See "Sources," page 281)
¼ cup tapioca starch or arrowroot
Dash of salt
½ teaspoon baking soda
⅛ teaspoon unbuffered vitamin C powder
2 tablespoons oil
1½ to 2½ tablespoons water

Oil a 9-inch pie plate. Preheat your oven to 375°F. Combine the nut meal, tapioca starch or arrowroot, salt, baking soda and vitamin C in a large bowl and stir them together thoroughly. Add the oil and cut it in with a pastry cutter. Stir the nut meal mixture with a fork while gradually adding enough of the water to make the dough come together. It does not have to come together all in one ball. You may not need all of the water or may need slightly more depending on how finely or coarsely ground the nut meal is. If you are using the almond meal, this will probably be 1½ to 2 tablespoons; for the pecan or hazelnut meal you will probably need 2 to 2½ tablespoons of water.

Since this is a baking soda and vitamin C leavened crust, finish the rest of this recipe without too much delay. Transfer the crust to the prepared pie plate. Oil your fingers and press the ball of dough out to cover the bottom and sides of the pie plate, pushing the dough from the bottom up the sides until the plate is evenly covered. Bake for 15 to 25 minutes or until it is light brown. Make sure it is thoroughly baked if you are going to fill it with pumpkin filling. Cool it thoroughly before filling it. If you fill this crust with a high-liquid filling (such as pumpkin), try to eat the pie within a few days to keep the crust from becoming soft. Makes 1 crust or 8 servings which each contain ½ carbohydrate unit, 1 protein unit and 7 grams of fat.

*Note on nut meal: Bob's Red Mill™ almond flour/meal, which is available in many health food stores, works well in this recipe. You can purchase hazelnut or pecan meal online from King Arthur Flour. See "Sources," page 281.

Quick-Mix No-Roll Pie Crust

Gluten-Free IF
made with a GF grain

This amaranth crust has a delicious nutty taste. If you are allergic to wheat but not gluten-intolerant, you might enjoy the spelt crust.

Amaranth (GF)

> 1½ cups amaranth flour
> ¾ cup arrowroot
> ½ teaspoon salt
> ½ teaspoon baking powder such as Featherweight™ brand
> ⅝ cup oil
> ¼ cup cold water

Rice (GF)

> 3 cups brown rice flour
> ½ teaspoon salt
> ½ teaspoon baking powder such as Featherweight™ brand
> ¼ teaspoon cinnamon (optional)
> ⅔ cup oil
> ⅓ cup cold water or apple juice

Spelt

> 2¾ cups spelt flour
> ½ teaspoon salt
> ½ teaspoon baking powder such as Featherweight™ brand
> ⅜ cup oil
> ¼ cup cold water

Chose one set of ingredients above. In a large bowl, stir together the flour(s), salt, baking powder, and optional cinnamon. Measure the water or juice and oil into the same measuring cup and stir them together thoroughly. Before they have a chance to separate, pour them into the bowl with the flour. Stir the ingredients together quickly; if the flour does not all come together into the dough readily, cut the mixture with the side of the spoon to help it become a crumbly mixture. Do not stir or cut the dough for very long; you should not over-work the dough.

For two one-crust pies, press half of the dough on to the bottom and sides of each of two pie plates. Preheat your oven to 400°F. Bake for 10 to 15 minutes or until the pie crust is lightly browned. If you have a leftover crust, it will freeze well. You may also cut the amounts of the ingredients in half to make a single crust. This recipe also may be used to make a double crust pie by crumbling half of the dough over the filling before you bake the pie.

Makes two single pie crusts, each of which contains 8 servings. Each serving of amaranth crust contains ¾ carbohydrate unit and 8 grams of fat, a serving of rice crust contains 1½ carbohydrate units and 10 grams of fat, and a serving of spelt crust contains 1 carbohydrate unit and 6 grams of fat.

ALMOND FLOUR PIE CRUST

Gluten-Free

You can enjoy a pie made with this crust and the pumpkin pie filling on page 210 any time without adding carbohydrate units to your meal. This pie also makes a great stand-alone snack because the crust supplies one protein unit per serving.

> 1½ cups finely ground blanched almond flour, such as Honeyville™ brand (See "Sources," page 281).
> Dash of salt
> ¼ teaspoon baking soda
> 3 tablespoons oil
> Water – 2 tablespoons if you are using stevia or no sweetener OR 1 tablespoon if you are using agave or Fruit Sweet™
> 1 tablespoon agave or Fruit Sweet™ OR 1 stevia spoon* of pure stevia powder such as Protocol for Life Balance™ brand (optional)

Oil a 9-inch pie plate. Preheat your oven to 375°F. Combine the almond flour, salt, baking soda, and optional stevia in a large bowl and stir them together thoroughly. In a separate bowl or cup stir together the oil, water, and optional agave or Fruit Sweet.™ Stir the liquid ingredients into the flour mixture until thoroughly mixed. Press the mixture into the pie plate. Bake for 12 to 18 minutes or until it is nicely browned. Cool the crust thoroughly before filling it. If you fill this crust with a high-liquid filling (such as pumpkin), try to eat the pie within a few days to keep the crust from becoming soft. Makes 1 crust or 8 servings which each contain 1 protein unit and 9 grams of fat.

*Note on the stevia spoon measurement: Protocol for Life Balance™ and several other brands of pure white stevia powder come with a small plastic spoon that holds an amount of stevia equivalent to about 2 teaspoons of sugar in sweetening power. Use this plastic spoon to measure the stevia in this recipe.

COCONUT PIE CRUST

2 cups unsweetened shredded or very finely shredded coconut (See "Sources,"
    page 281 for finely shredded coconut).
Coconut oil – ¼ cup with shredded coconut OR ⅜ cup with finely shredded
    coconut

Preheat your oven to 300°F. Melt about ½ cup coconut oil in a small saucepan over
low heat or in the microwave. Measure the amount of coconut oil you expect to need.
Measure the coconut into a glass pie dish. Pour the coconut oil onto the coconut. Mix
the oil and coconut thoroughly using a spoon and your hands. Press the mixture evenly
onto the bottom and sides of the dish. Bake the crust for 12 to 15 minutes or until it
begins to brown. Cool the crust completely on a wire cooling rack. Fill the crust with
cooled fruit or pumpkin filling, pages 210 to 214. Makes 1 crust or 8 servings which
each contain ⅕ protein unit and 19 grams of fat.

Ice Cream

Ice cream is my husband's favorite dessert on his healthy eating plan because milk
products do not add to the carbohydrate count of his dinner. Thus he can have ice
cream sweetened with stevia or Equal™ with a meal without exceeding 30 grams of
carbohydrate.

Ice cream is easy to make even without an ice cream maker, thus allowing you to use
lower GI sweeteners and avoid cow's milk. (Coconut milk makes wonderful ice cream!)
You need no special equipment for the still-freezing method below. However, if you have
a food processor, you can use it to make ice cream.

Homemade ice cream is best eaten shortly after you make it rather than after it has
been stored in the freezer for days or weeks because it does not contain the stabilizers
that commercial ice cream usually contains. However, if you do have leftovers you need
to store, take them out of the freezer about 20 minutes before serving. The ice cream
will soften up and be delicious and easy to scoop by serving time. If you plan to make
homemade ice cream for guests, one or two hours in the freezer will firm your ice cream
but not produce a hard texture. Make it an hour or two before you expect to serve it, put
it in the freezer, and the consistency will be fine.

STILL FREEZING METHOD FOR FREEZING ICE CREAM

The still freezing method is best suited to high-fat ice creams such as those made with cream, half-and-half, or full-fat coconut milk or to ice cream that contains a good quantity of fiber from fruit. The fat or fiber helps promote a creamy texture.

To still freeze ice cream, mix the ingredients and put them in a shallow metal cake pan, loaf pan(s) or old-fashioned ice cube tray(s) without the dividers. Put the pan(s) or tray(s) in the freezer and allow to freeze until the mixture is firm around the edges and slushy in the middle, about 20 to 45 minutes. Remove the pan from the freezer and stir it until the consistency is uniform throughout. Put the pan back in the freezer and freeze it for another 10 to 25 minutes until the mixture becomes firm around the edges again. Remove it from the freezer and stir it again. Repeat this one or two more times until the stirred mixture is the consistency you prefer. Serve the frozen dessert immediately or scoop it into a container and freeze it. If it has been frozen for more than a few hours before serving time, allow it to stand at room temperature for about 20 minutes to soften before serving.

FOOD PROCESSOR OR BLENDER METHOD FOR FREEZING ICE CREAM

To make ice cream using a food processor or blender, start the day before you wish to serve the frozen dessert. Mix the ingredients, put them into ice cube trays, and freeze overnight.

The next day, at least a half hour to forty five minutes or more before you wish to serve the ice cream, remove the frozen cubes from the freezer. Allow them to stand at room temperature for 10 to 20 minutes or until they are just barely beginning to soften. Add about three cubes to the blender or food processor and process until the mixture is smooth. Add cubes two at a time and process until all of the dessert mixture has been processed. (If you are using a blender, you may have to do this in several small batches rather than processing it all together). Serve immediately or transfer it to a container and freeze the ice cream a few hours until serving time. If it has been frozen for more than a few hours, allow it to stand at room temperature for about 20 minutes to soften before serving.

Vanilla Ice Cream

Gluten-Free

2½ cups cream, half-and-half, milk of any kind (cow, goat, soy, etc.), or
    coconut milk (about 1½ 14-ounce cans)
⅜ cup agave, Fruit Sweet™ or honey OR ½ to 1 teaspoon pure stevia* powder
    such as Protocol for Life Balance™ brand stevia OR 9 to 12 packets of Equal™
1 tablespoon vanilla extract OR a 2-inch piece of vanilla bean, cut open

Combine the milk, sweetener, and vanilla. If you are using a vanilla bean rather than
vanilla extract for flavoring, add it to the milk mixture and let the mixture sit overnight
in the refrigerator. In the morning scrape the seeds out of the bean into the milk mixture
and discard the bean pod. Stir the mixture together thoroughly. Freeze as directed in
the still freezing or food processor method on page 219. If you make this with high fat
dairy products or full-fat coconut milk, still freezing is easy and works very well. Serve
immediately or store the ice cream in your freezer. If it has been frozen for more than
a few hours, remove it from the freezer about 20 minutes before serving. Makes about
1½ pints of ice cream or 6 servings, each of which contains 1¼ carbohydrate units if
made with the liquid sweetener and is free of concentrated carbohydrate if made with
the stevia or Equal.™ (Dr. Cheryle Hart does not count the lactose in milk products).
The fat content varies with the milk used; each serving contains 10 grams of fat each if
made with half-and-half, 20 grams of fat if made with full-fat coconut milk, and 4 grams
of fat if made with whole cow's or goat milk.

*Note on the amount of stevia to use: The amount of stevia used in this recipe varies with the sweetness of the milk. I use ¾ teaspoon Protocol for Life Balance™ stevia
with coconut milk; my husband says ice cream made with half-and-half is best with ⅞
teaspoon of stevia.

Chocolate or Carob Ice Cream

Gluten-Free

2½ cups cream, half-and-half, milk of any kind (cow, goat, soy, etc.), or
    coconut milk (about 1½ 14-ounce cans)
⅜ cup agave, Fruit Sweet™ or honey OR ½ to 1 teaspoon pure white stevia*
    powder such as Protocol for Life™ Balance brand OR 9 to 12 packets of Equal™
3 tablespoons cocoa or 2 tablespoons carob powder
1 teaspoon vanilla extract (optional)

Combine the milk, sweetener, cocoa or carob, and vanilla. Stir the mixture together
thoroughly. Freeze as directed in the still freezing or food processor method on page

219. If you make this with high fat dairy products or full-fat coconut milk, still freezing is easy and works very well. Serve immediately or store the ice cream in your freezer. If it has been frozen for more than a few hours, remove it from the freezer about 20 minutes before serving. Makes about 1½ pints of ice cream or 6 servings, each of which contains 1¼ carbohydrate units if made with the liquid sweetener and is free of concentrated carbohydrate if made with the stevia or Equal.™ (Dr. Cheryle Hart does not count the lactose in milk products). The fat content varies with the milk used; each serving contains 10 grams of fat each if made with half-and-half, 20 grams of fat if made with full-fat coconut milk, and 4 grams of fat if made with whole cow's or goat milk.

*Note on the amount of stevia to use:** The amount of stevia used in this recipe varies with the sweetness of the milk. I use ¾ teaspoon Protocol for Life Balance™ stevia with coconut milk; my husband says ice cream made with half-and-half is best with ⅞ teaspoon of stevia.

STRAWBERRY ICE CREAM

Gluten-Free

A little more than 1 pint of ripe strawberries
1 cup cream, half-and-half, milk of any kind (cow, goat, soy, etc.), or coconut milk
⅜ cup agave, Fruit Sweet™ or honey OR ¾ cup apple juice concentrate
    OR ½ to 1 teaspoon* pure white stevia powder such as Protocol for Life™
    brand OR 9 to 12 packets of Equal™

Wash and stem the strawberries. Puree them with a hand blender, blender, or food processor. Measure out 1 cup of puree. Combine the cream or milk, sweetener and strawberry puree. Freeze the ice cream using one of the methods on page 219. Because of the fiber in the strawberries, the still freezing method works quite well with this ice cream. Serve immediately or store the ice cream in your freezer. If it has been frozen for more than a few hours, remove it from the freezer about 20 minutes before serving. Makes about 1½ pints of ice cream or 6 servings, each of which contains 1¼ carbohydrate units if made with the liquid sweetener and is free of concentrated carbohydrate if made with the stevia or Equal.™ (Dr. Cheryle Hart does not count the lactose in milk products and the fruit sugar in the strawberries adds a negligible amount of carbohydrate per serving). The fat content varies with the milk used; each serving contains 4 grams of fat each if made with half-and-half, 8 grams of fat if made with full-fat coconut milk, and 2 grams of fat if made with whole cow's or goat milk.

*Note on the amount of stevia to use:** The amount of stevia used in this recipe varies with the sweetness of the strawberries and the type of milk used. Coconut milk needs less sweetener than the other types of milk.

Comfort Desserts and Treats

The following desserts and treats are foods that are homey and comforting. The pomegranate tapioca pudding on the next page and "Super-Fruit Gel Dessert" below give us a healthy dose of anti-inflammatory phytonutrients as well. "Healthy Home-made Popcorn," page 225, is one of my husband's favorite treats. Making it with this recipe avoids the unhealthy fats in microwave and movie theater popcorn. The fiber fills him up and makes him feel satisfied. This is such an easy way to make popcorn that, once you've done it, you will wonder why you ever spent the extra money for microwave popcorn.

SUPER-FRUIT GEL DESSERT

Gluten-Free

These desserts are delicious and great for fighting inflammation. If you are allergic to the beef or pork from which gelatin is made, you can use agar to make this recipe.

Blueberry

½ cup Knudsen™ blueberry concentrate (See "Sources," page 279).

1½ cups water

1 tablespoon gelatin powder or ¼ cup agar* flakes

¹⁄₁₆ to ⅛ teaspoon pure white stevia powder such as Protocol for Life™ brand, or to taste (optional)

Cherry

½ cup Knudsen™ cherry concentrate (See "Sources," page 279).

1½ cups water

1 tablespoon gelatin powder or ¼ cup agar* flakes

¹⁄₁₆ to ⅛ teaspoon pure white stevia powder such as Protocol for Life™ brand, or to taste (optional)

Pomegranate

¼ cup Cortas™ pomegranate molasses or ⅜ cup Knudsen™ pomegranate concentrate (See "Sources," page 279).

1¾ cups water

1 tablespoon gelatin powder or ⅜ cup agar* flakes with Cortas™ pomegranate molasses OR 1 tablespoon gelatin powder or ¼ cup agar* flakes with Knudsen™ pomegranate concentrate

⅛ to ³⁄₁₆ teaspoon pure white stevia powder such as Protocol for Life™ brand with Cortas™ pomegranate molasses OR to ¹⁄₁₆ to ⅛ teaspoon stevia powder, with Knudsen™ pomegranate concentrate, or to taste (optional)

Combine the fruit juice concentrate and water in a saucepan. Sprinkle the gelatin or agar over the surface of the liquid and let it stand for a minute or two until it is moistened. Bring the liquid to a boil. If you are using the gelatin, once it is at a full boil, turn it down to a simmer and immediately proceed with the next paragraph. For the agar, after it comes to a boil, lower the heat and simmer for 5 minutes.

Sprinkle the smaller amount of the stevia over the surface of the liquid in the pan and simmer it for about 30 seconds while stirring. Taste it to see if you like the sweetness level. If not, add a tiny pinch more stevia to taste, simmering after each addition. Pour the hot liquid into a container and refrigerate it until it is thoroughly cooled off and has gelled. Makes 4 servings. Each serving of blueberry dessert contains ¾ carbohydrate unit, a serving of cherry dessert contains 1½ carbohydrate units, a serving of pomegranate dessert made with Knudsen™ concentrate contains 1 carbohydrate unit, and a serving of pomegranate dessert made with Cortas™ concentrate contains ¾ carbohydrate unit.

* **Note about agar:** The amount of agar you will need to get this dessert to gel can be unpredictable, probably due to the difference in how loose and flakey the agar flakes are. If the recipe doesn't gel when it is cold, put it back in the saucepan, add 50% more agar, cook it again, and see if it that is enough to make it gel. Record how much agar you use for the next time you make this. If you can get agar powder, which is not easily available, it will work in the recipe but you will need much less. In addition, acidity seems to affect the gelling with agar. I have not been able to get this dessert made with the Cortas™ pomegranate to set firmly, but it is still delicious.

TANGY POMEGRANATE TAPIOCA PUDDING
Gluten-Free

This is my favorite fruit pudding because of its deliciously unique tangy flavor.

¼ cup Cortas™ pomegranate molasses* (See "Sources," page 279).
⅓ cup agave, Fruit Sweet™ or honey OR ¼ teaspoon pure white stevia powder such as Protocol for Life™ brand, to taste
Water – 1⅔ cups with the liquid sweeteners or 2 cups with the stevia
Quick-cooking (Minute™) tapioca – ⅓ cup with the liquid sweeteners or ¼ cup with the stevia

Stir together all the ingredients in a saucepan. Allow them to stand for at least five minutes. Bring them to a full boil over medium-high heat, stirring occasionally. Then cook and stir constantly for one minute. Remove the pan from the heat and allow it to stand for at least 20 minutes before serving. If you want to serve this dessert soon, for optimal taste and texture of the tapioca, allow it to stand long enough to reach lukewarm. Refrigerate the tapioca pudding if you prefer to serve it cold. Makes 4 servings, each of which is 1¾ carbohydrate units if made with the liquid sweetener or 1 carbohydrate unit if made with the stevia.

*Note on alternatives to pomegranate molasses: If you are unable to get Cortas™ pomegranate molasses, you can still have delicious pomegranate tapioca. Use a brand of good-tasting pure pomegranate juice purchased refrigerated (not canned or room-temperature stable) such as Pom Wonderful™ or Earthly Delights™ brand. Combine 2 cups of the juice with ¼ cup minute tapioca, allow it to stand for at least five minutes, and cook and serve as above. Makes 4 servings, each of which contains the amount of carbohydrate in ½ cup of the pomegranate juice you used plus ½ carbohydrate unit.

ROASTED CHESTNUTS

Gluten-Free

Try this for a real treat when fresh chestnuts are in season in the fall and early winter.

    1¼ pounds of raw chestnuts

Preheat your oven to 350°F. Lay each chestnut on its flatter side on a cutting board. With a small sharp knife, cut a slit most of the way around the upper side of each chestnut. Place the prepared chestnuts on a baking sheet and bake them for 30 to 35 minutes. Remove one chestnut from the oven and peel it. Taste it, and if it is soft, they are done; remove the rest of the chestnuts from the oven. If the test chestnut is still quite hard, bake them for an additional 5 minutes and then test another chestnut. After you remove the chestnuts from the oven, wrap them in a kitchen towel for a few minutes and then peel them while they are warm. (If they cool to room temperature it may be difficult to remove the inner membrane). Makes about 10 2-ounce servings of about 5 chestnuts each. Each serving contains 1 carbohydrate unit, ¼ protein unit and 1 gram of fat.

Out-of-season chestnuts: If you are a chestnut fan who misses them when they are not available fresh, order dried chestnuts from Parthenon Foods. (See "Sources," page 277). Place them in a pan with enough water to generously cover them and soak them overnight. In the morning, drain the water and replace it with fresh water twice. Then add enough water to the chestnuts to generously cover them and bring them to a boil. Reduce the heat and simmer for 30 to 45 minutes. Taste a chestnut at 30 minutes and every 5 minutes after that to see if they are no longer hard. (They will not have the same mealy texture as roasted fresh chestnuts). When they are done, drain the water from the pan and put the chestnuts on paper towels to dry. Eat them as they are or, for a more roasted texture, coat them lightly with oil and bake them at 350°F for 15 minutes. Each 2-ounce serving contains 1 carbohydrate unit, ¼ protein unit and 1 gram of fat.

HEALTHY HOMEMADE POPCORN

Gluten-Free

I recently discovered that grocery store brand white popping corn pops to a much larger volume than the yellow popcorn I had been using. I can make my husband a large bowl with ¾ of an ounce of popping corn which satisfies him, makes him feel like he's had a real treat, and is only one carbohydrate unit.

> 2 teaspoons oil, preferably olive oil because it is heat stable
> ¾ ounce or about ³⁄₁₆ cup of unpopped popcorn
> A dash of salt, or to taste
> 1 teaspoon of butter, melted (optional)

Put the oil in a 3 quart or slightly larger saucepan. Add three kernels of popcorn to the pan, put the lid on the pan and heat it over medium heat on your stove. When you hear the three kernels of popcorn pop, add the rest of the popcorn to the pan. Move the pan back and forth on the burner. In a few minutes you will hear the corn beginning to pop. Keep moving the pan and when the popping slows down and nearly stops, remove the pan from the heat. Pour the popcorn into a bowl, sprinkle it with salt, and drizzle it with the optional butter if desired. Makes one large serving of popcorn which contains 1 carbohydrate unit and 9 grams of fat if you do not use the butter or 13 grams of fat if you use the butter.

*Note on popcorn's potential effect on your blood sugar stability: The GI score of popcorn can fall in either in the medium or high range.[1] If you are allergic to corn, skip the popcorn because it will destabilize your blood sugar. One GI control diet totally prohibits popcorn, possibly because their experience involved people with undiagnosed corn allergy. I suspect that the Kroger™ brand popcorn I buy (both white and yellow) has a medium GI score because my husband's experience – the reason I have included this recipe here – is that popcorn as the carbohydrate part of his dinner makes him feel very stable and satisfied. This might occur because the fiber in the popcorn slows down the absorption of his meal. Listen to your body and eat popcorn only if it is right for you.

---

[1] Lieberman, Shari. *Dr. Shari Lieberman's Easy-To-Use Glycemic Food Index Guide,* (New York: Square One Publishers, 2006), 99.

BEVERAGES

Delicious beverages can add much enjoyment to your early morning or to a meal. Wise beverage choices are also a good way to add anti-inflammatory foods to your diet. Some of the beverage recipes below contain carbohydrates and therefore must be balanced with a protein food rather than consumed alone.

GINGER TEA BY THE CUP

Gluten-Free

This is the way to drink ginger tea if you want great flavor and the full benefit of its anti-inflammatory gingerols. Skip the ginger tea bags and make your own potently anti-inflammatory ginger tea using this recipe or the recipe below.

    1 ounce fresh ginger root
    1 cup water

Wash the ginger root and cut off any bad spots. Peel and grate the ginger root. (If you are rushed for time you can skip the peeling). Combine the ginger and water in a saucepan and bring it to a boil. Reduce the heat and simmer it for 10 to 15 minutes. Strain out the ginger and enjoy the tea immediately. This recipe may be doubled, tripled, etc. if you are serving more than one person. If you want to drink ginger tea often without grating and boiling fresh ginger every time, make a large batch of ginger concentrate using the recipe on the next page. Makes one serving which contains a negligible amount of carbohydrate.

PLAN-AHEAD GINGER TEA

Gluten-Free

With this recipe you can enjoy ginger tea often without it taking much preparation time.

    Ginger concentrate, recipe on the next page
    Water

Fill a cup or mug about ¼ full with liquid ginger concentrate or about ⅓ to ½ full with frozen ginger concentrate cubes. Add water to finish filling the cup or mug. Transfer the mixture to a saucepan to bring it to a boil or warm it in a microwave oven. Makes one serving which contains a negligible amount of carbohydrate.

GINGER CONCENTRATE

Gluten-Free

If you have a food processor, use it to easily make enough ginger concentrate for a large supply of ginger tea. Then you can have tea quickly when time is tight. Use the freshest ginger you can find – heavy and smooth skinned – for this recipe.

2 to 2¼ pounds fresh ginger root
10 cups water

Scrub the ginger root and cut off any bad spots. Cut the ginger into chunks that will fit into the feed tube of your food processor. Grate it with the processor, cleaning the fibrous material out of the holes in the blade two or three times as you are processing. Save the ginger you remove from the holes to cook with the grated ginger.

Combine the grated ginger with the water in a large stockpot and bring it to a boil over medium heat. Reduce the heat and simmer it for 30 to 40 minutes. Cool the mixture at room temperature until it is lukewarm or cooler. Working with about two cups of the cooked ginger mixture at a time, strain it through a wire mesh strainer, pressing the grated ginger with the back of a spoon to extract all of the liquid. Freeze the concentrate in small jars containing enough concentrate for you to use in two or three days or put it into ice cube trays to freeze. When the ginger concentrate cubes are frozen, transfer them to a labeled bag or freezer container. Makes 9 to 10 cups of concentrate or enough for about 40 cups of tea, each of which contains a negligible amount of carbohydrate.

GINGER ALE

Gluten-Free

1 cup carbonated water
2 to 4 tablespoons ginger concentrate, above, to taste
½ to 1 stevia spoon* of pure white stevia powder OR 2 to 3 teaspoons of
    agave, to taste
3 or 4 ice cubes

To make the ginger ale, place 2 tablespoons of the ginger concentrate and the smaller amount of the sweetener in a glass and stir them together thoroughly. Add the carbonated water and stir. Taste the ginger ale and add more ginger concentrate or sweetener if desired. Record how much you use for the next time you make this. Add the ice cubes and serve. Makes one serving which contains a negligible amount of carbohydrate if made with stevia or ⅔ carbohydrate unit if made with agave.

*Note on the stevia spoon measurement: Protocol for Life Balance™ and several other brands of pure white stevia powder come with a small plastic spoon that holds an amount of stevia equivalent to about 2 teaspoons of sugar in sweetening power. Use this plastic spoon to measure the stevia in this recipe.

CRANBERRY TEA

Gluten-Free

Although cranberries are not on the anti-inflammatory food lists I've seen, they are closely related to blueberries (which are on the lists) and this tea contains anti-inflammatory spices. It's also delicious!

3 tablespoons Knudsen™ cranberry concentrate (See "Sources," page 279).
1 cup water
$\frac{1}{16}$ to $\frac{1}{8}$ teaspoon each ground cinnamon, ginger, and cloves, to taste
1 tablespoon lemon juice (optional)
$\frac{1}{4}$ cup orange juice or additional water
1 stevia spoon* of pure stevia powder, or to taste (optional)

Bring the cranberry concentrate, 1 cup of water and the spices to a boil. Reduce the heat and simmer 5 to 10 minutes. Stir in the additional $\frac{1}{4}$ cup of water or optional orange and lemon juices and stevia if desired. Return the tea to a boil. Serve as soon as it boils. Makes one serving, or enough tea for a large mug, which contains 1 carbohydrate unit if made with the orange juice or $\frac{1}{2}$ carbohydrate unit if made without the orange juice.

*Note on the stevia spoon measurement: Protocol for Life Balance™ and several other brands of pure white stevia powder come with a small plastic spoon that holds an amount of stevia equivalent to about 2 teaspoons of sugar in sweetening power. Use this plastic spoon to measure the stevia in this recipe.

CAFFEINE-CONTROLLED GREEN TEA

To get the anti-inflammatory effect of green tea with less caffeine, you can either purchase decaffeinated green tea or prepare regular green tea as directed in this recipe.

    1 tea bag or 1 rounded to heaping teaspoon of loose tea
    2 cups boiling water

If you are using loose tea, put it in an infuser or large tea ball. Place the loose tea or tea bag in a glass jar. (A wide mouth jelly canning jar is an ideal size if you are using an infuser). Pour 1 cup of the boiling water over the tea and steep it for 1 minute. You may warm a cup with boiling water before using it at this point if you wish. Remove the tea infuser, ball, or bag and place it in the cup. Pour the rest of the boiling water over the tea in the cup and steep for 3½ to 4 minutes or the time directed on the tea package plus 30 to 60 seconds. Consume the tea in the cup for tea that is lower in caffeine, or you may add some of the tea from the jar to the cup for a small caffeine boost. Although the evidence for removing caffeine with this tea brewing method is anecdotal, I personally feel like I am getting all the flavor with less caffeine when I prepare tea this way. I often enjoy my early morning tea with half of the first brew added back and then re-infuse the leaves later without adding back any of the higher-caffeine first brew. Makes 1 cup of tea which contains no carbohydrate.

*Note on tea: The Tea Spot, Inc. is a wonderful source for loose tea. Their Thin Mint Green™ tea is a long-time favorite of mine. It is very flavorful and also very low in caffeine, containing about 10 milligrams per 8-ounce cup of tea. I feel a great sense of well-being when I drink their Green Twisted Spears tea. See their wide variety of excellent teas at http://theteaspot.com. Their website also contains instructions on how to best brew each variety of tea with the correct water temperature and brewing time.

Dr. Galland's "Slim Chai Tea" variation: Add 3 to 4 whole cloves to the tea when you infuse it. After removing the tea, add a scant ⅛ teaspoon each of cinnamon and cardamom and stir. Green tea alone is anti-inflammatory but will be even more helpful for inflammation with the addition of these spices.

SUPERFOOD SODA

Satisfy your desire for soda pop with these sodas and get a dose of anti-inflammatory anthocyanins at the same time. Since these beverages contain rapidly absorbed carbohydrate, enjoy them with a protein-containing snack or a meal.

Blueberry soda
¼ cup Knudsen™ blueberry concentrate (See "Sources," page 279).

¾ cup carbonated water

3 or 4 ice cubes

1 stevia spoon* of pure stevia powder such as Protocol for Life Balance™ brand, or to taste (optional)

Cherry soda

¼ cup Knudsen™ black cherry concentrate (See "Sources," page 279).

¾ cup carbonated water

3 or 4 ice cubes

A sprinkle of pure stevia powder such as Protocol for Life Balance™ brand, or to taste (less than 1 stevia spoon* – optional)

Pomegranate soda
3 tablespoons Knudsen™ pomegranate concentrate or 2 tablespoons Cortas™ pomegranate molasses (See "Sources," page 279).

¾ cup carbonated water

3 or 4 ice cubes

1 stevia spoon* of pure stevia powder such as Protocol for Life Balance™ brand, or to taste (optional)

Put the juice concentrate into a large drinking glass. If you want to use the stevia,** thoroughly stir it into the juice concentrate. If you are using very thick the Cortas™ pomegranate molasses, stir 1 to 2 tablespoons of warm water into the juice mixture. Add the carbonated water and stir gently. Add the ice cubes and enjoy. Makes one serving which contains 1½ carbohydrate units if you use the blueberry or Cortas™ pomegranate concentrate or 2 carbohydrate units if you use the cherry or Knudsen™ pomegranate concentrate

*Note on the stevia spoon measurement: Protocol for Life Balance™ and several other brands of pure white stevia powder come with a small plastic spoon that holds an amount of stevia equivalent to about 2 teaspoons of sugar in sweetening power. Use this plastic spoon to measure the stevia in this recipe.

**Note on the use of stevia in this soda: If you are not used to drinking sweet soda pop, you may not need stevia in this soda, especially if it is made with the cherry concentrate. Omit the stevia the first time you make the soda. Taste it and if it is not sweet enough, add the stevia, gradually increasing the amount added. Once you have decided to use the stevia routinely and know how much you prefer to use, to keep your soda as fizzy as possible, stir the stevia into the fruit juice concentrate thoroughly before you add the carbonated water. Some brands of stevia tend to clump together and need more stirring to dissolve. Others, such as Protocol for Life Balance™ stevia, dissolve quite easily.

Stevia-Sweetened Lemonade

Gluten-Free

Having acid with your meal can slow down its digestion and absorption, thus decreasing its glycemic impact. You can add acid by having a salad containing several teaspoons of vinegar or have this beverage with your meal. The first time you make this recipe, use the smaller amount of stevia. If it is not sweet enough for you, add more to taste and make a note of how much you added for next time.

> 2 lemons or ⅓ cup lemon juice
> ⅛ to ¼ teaspoon pure stevia powder such as Protocol for Life Balance™ brand,
>   to taste
> 1⅓ to 2 cups cold water
> Ice cubes

Mix the juice and stevia together until the stevia is completely dissolved. Add enough water to make the lemonade the strength you prefer, mix thoroughly, and serve over ice. Makes 2 servings which contain a negligible amount of carbohydrate. For a larger batch, use 6 lemons or 1 cup of lemon juice, ¾ to 1 teaspoon stevia (or more to taste), and 4 to 6 cups of water to make 4 to 6 servings.

SAUCES, SPREADS AND OTHER RECIPES

The recipes in this chapter add a special touch to your meals and snacks. Here you will find no-sugar cranberry sauce for your Thanksgiving turkey or sandwiches, mayonnaise and an egg-free alternative to mayonnaise, pizza sauce, pesto, and more. Also, if are allergic to eggs and are baking with almond flour so need eggs to hold your recipe together, try the flaxseed egg substitute on page 237.

CRANBERRY SAUCE

Gluten-Free

This is great on meat sandwiches and if made with stevia contains just a few grams of carbohydrate. The cranberries are so tangy that you will not realize you are using stevia.

- 1 12-ounce package of fresh cranberries, about 4 cups of berries
- 1 cup agave, Fruit Sweet™ or honey OR 2 cups apple juice concentrate OR 1 cup water plus ¼ to ½ teaspoon pure white stevia powder such as Protocol for Life Balance™ brand

Wash and pick over the berries, discarding any shriveled or soft berries. If you are using the apple juice concentrate, put it into a saucepan and bring it to a boil over medium-high to high heat. Reduce the heat to medium and boil it down until it reaches 1 cup in volume. Add the berries to the boiled-down apple juice concentrate or to the water, agave, Fruit Sweet™ or honey in a saucepan. Bring them to a boil over medium heat; then reduce the heat and simmer, stirring often, for 15 to 20 minutes or until all of the cranberries have popped. If you are using the stevia, stir it into the sauce thoroughly, making sure it has completely dissolved. Pour the cranberry sauce into a jar and refrigerate. Makes about 2 cups of cranberry sauce or 16 2-tablespoon servings each of which contains ⅕ carbohydrate unit if made with the stevia or 1 carbohydrate unit if made with the liquid sweeteners.

Easy Pizza Sauce

Gluten-Free

Make your gluten- or allergen-free pizza especially delicious using this easy homemade sauce.

> 1 6-ounce can tomato paste
> 1 8-ounce can tomato sauce
> ½ cup water
> 1 teaspoon oregano
> ½ teaspoon thyme
> ½ teaspoon sweet basil

Combine all of the ingredients in a saucepan and simmer them for 45 minutes, stirring about every 10 minutes until the sauce thickens. Makes enough sauce for 2 12-inch pizzas. The carbohydrates in this recipe are from vegetables so do not have to be added to the carbohydrate units of the dish in which you use this sauce.

Pesto

Gluten-Free

Try this on your pizza if you are allergic to tomatoes, or serve it on spaghetti squash with a little cooked ground meat to make an especially satisfying main dish.

> 3½ cups sweet basil leaves, washed, stemmed, and dried (about ¼ pound as
>   purchased)
> 1 to 2 cloves of garlic (optional)
> ½ cup pine nuts or other nuts
> ½ cup olive or other oil
> ¼ to ½ teaspoon salt, or to taste
> ⅛ teaspoon pepper (optional)

Chop the garlic in a food processor or blender using a pulsing action. Add the sweet basil and pulse to chop the leaves as finely as possible. Add the nuts and process continually until they are ground. Add the oil gradually while processing. Add the seasonings and process until they are blended in. Serve the sauce over warm cooked pasta or spaghetti squash or use it instead of tomato-based sauce on pizza. This sauce is very rich, so a little goes a long way. Makes about 1 cup of sauce or 8 servings, each of which contain ¼ protein unit and 18 grams of fat.

SUPER-SMOOTH SAUCE

This is a great alternative to mayonnaise for those who are allergic to eggs. If you are allergic to lemon or lime juice, use the vitamin C.

Cashew sauce
¼ cup cashew butter
¼ cup lemon or lime juice OR ¼ cup water plus 1½ teaspoons unbuffered
     vitamin C powder
⅛ teaspoon salt
¼ cup oil

Almond sauce
¼ cup almond butter
¼ cup lemon or lime juice OR ¼ cup water plus 1 teaspoon unbuffered
     vitamin C powder
⅛ teaspoon salt
¼ cup oil

Macadamia sauce
¼ cup macadamia nut butter
¼ cup lemon or lime juice OR ¼ cup water plus 1 teaspoon unbuffered
     vitamin C powder
⅛ teaspoon salt
¼ cup oil

Chose one set of ingredients from the list above. Combine the nut butter, lemon or lime juice or water plus vitamin C, and salt in a 2-cup glass measuring cup, the cup that comes with a hand blender, or the bowl of a food processor or blender. Blend until the ingredients are thoroughly combined. With the blender or processor running, add the oil very gradually in a thin steam until it has all been added and the sauce is thick, smooth, and creamy. Store in the refrigerator. Makes about ¾ cup of sauce or 18 2-teaspoon servings. Each serving of almond or cashew sauce contains 5 grams of fat; the macadamia sauce contains 6 grams of fat per serving.

MAYONNAISE

Here's real mayonnaise for those of you who can eat eggs. It is made without vinegar for those who are allergic to yeast. Although not exactly a "with ease" recipe, it is free of additives and sugar and is so delicious that it's well worth the time it takes to make it.

1 pasteurized egg* or ¼ cup GF egg substitute such as EggBeaters™ (if you tolerate the ingredients*)*
1 teaspoon dry ground mustard
1 teaspoon salt
Dash of pepper
1 teaspoon agave, Fruit Sweet™ or honey (optional)
1 cup oil, divided, preferably walnut or canola because they are high in essential fatty acids
3 tablespoons lemon juice

Combine the egg or egg substitute, mustard, salt, pepper, sweetener, and ¼ cup of the oil in the bowl of a food processor or blender. Turn on the food processor or blender. After the ingredients are thoroughly mixed (this takes just a few seconds), very slowly, pouring in a trickle, add half of the remaining oil while processing continuously. At this point, stop processing. Add the lemon juice and begin processing again. After the lemon juice is mixed in (again, this takes just a few seconds), very slowly, pouring in a trickle, add the rest of the oil while processing continuously. Transfer the mayonnaise to a glass jar with a tight-fitting lid and store it in the refrigerator. Makes about 1½ cups of mayonnaise, or 36 2-teaspoon servings which contain 6 grams of fat each.

*Note on egg or egg substitute: Pasteurized eggs are available in a few areas of the country and hopefully will become more widely available soon. If this mayonnaise will not be eaten by anyone in a high-risk population for serious illness due to *Salmonella* (the very young or the elderly), the USDA now says it is all right to use a regular raw egg in mayonnaise. EggBeaters™ and similar egg products are pasteurized, eliminating the problem of illness from using the egg raw, but they contain the egg white and other allergenic ingredients, some of which may be derived from wheat. At the time of this writing, EggBeaters™ is wheat- and gluten-free but contains maltodextrin which comes from corn.

EFA BUTTER
(ESSENTIAL FATTY ACID BUTTER)

Gluten-Free

This is a great spread for toast, tasty to put on vegetables, and an all around easy-to-spread good substitute for butter or margarine. With EFA-butter you get the taste of butter plus omega-3 fatty acids from the walnut or canola oil for good health.

½ cup walnut or canola oil
½ cup (1 stick) butter or goat butter at room temperature

Allow the butter to come to room temperature. (If you forget to take it out of the refrigerator, carefully microwave it on low power for 5 to 10 seconds without letting it melt). Put the oil and butter in a 2-cup glass measuring cup or small bowl and thoroughly combine them with a hand blender, or use a blender or food processor. Pour the EFA butter into a jar and refrigerate. Makes a little over 1 cup of EFA-butter or about 50 1-teaspoon servings which each contain 4 grams of fat.

AGAVE NUT BUTTER

Gluten-Free IF
made with GF nut butter

The addition of a little agave and cinnamon to natural nut butter makes it a real taste treat. It also keeps the oil from separating from the nut solids making it ready to use at any time. This is great for quick breakfasts and snacks!

1 cup of pure natural nut butter, any kind (almond, cashew, peanut, etc.)
1½ to 2 tablespoons agave, or to taste
⅛ to ¼ teaspoon cinnamon, or to taste (optional)

Thoroughly stir the nut butter and measure it into a bowl. Add the smaller amount of agave and cinnamon. Stir thoroughly and taste the nut butter. Add more agave and cinnamon to your taste preference if needed. Makes 9 2-tablespoon servings, each of which contains ½ protein unit and 17 grams of fat.

Flaxseed Egg Substitute

If you are allergic to eggs, you can use this to hold almond flour crackers together.

½ cup ground flaxseeds or flax meal (such as Bob's Red Mill™ flaxseed meal)
1½ cups water

Stir together the ground flaxseeds or flax meal and water in a saucepan. Cook over medium heat until the mixture begins to simmer. Then reduce the heat to keep it at a simmer and cook for 5 minutes. If you wish to use this shortly after making it, measure out the amount needed and put the measuring cup in the refrigerator until the mixture reaches room temperature. For later use, stir the mixture thoroughly, put it in a glass jar and store it in the refrigerator to be used within the next week or two. Stir it thoroughly again before using it. Makes 1½ cups or the equivalent of 6 eggs. Each serving contains a negligible amount of protein, carbohydrate and fat.

Recipes for Non-Allergic Companions

Being on a special diet can make you feel isolated. While your friends and family members are enjoying celebratory meals and treats, you may be nibbling on gluten- or allergen-free fare that you brought along for yourself. If you are trying to lose weight in addition to being on an allergy or gluten-free diet, the feeling of being alone can be even worse.

Your transition to this healthy eating plan may be easier if you have a friend or family member join you. There are so many people who want to lose weight that if you don't insist on finding a gluten-free or allergy-free companion, you can probably find someone who would like to sign on. The experience, especially sharing stories of weight lost and improved health, can be good for both of you. You can also encourage each other in the harder times. "Two are better than one, because they have a good return of their work; If one falls down, his friend can help him up." (Ecclesiastes 4:9-10)

Groups like Weight Watchers™ provide valuable social support for those trying to lose weight. This is one reason for their popularity. The nature of the Weight Watchers™ diet may be problematic, but the camaraderie of the group enables some people to lose weight (although often temporarily) in spite of the diet. An ideal plan would combine the physiological principles presented in this book with the psychological advantages provided by a weight loss support group.

If your companion(s) on the healthy eating plan do not need to avoid gluten or food allergens, this chapter is for them — and maybe for you as the cook. Use the recipes here plus commercially made 100% stone ground whole wheat bread or crackers, and your companion(s) can join your journey with ease and very little additional cooking required. See "Sources," page 283, for bread and cracker recommendations. (The Ak-Mak crackers are great!) The recipes below for light but high-fiber, low GI breads and treats will help your companion(s) enjoy their meals on the plan.

To make joint meals for you and your companion(s), use the main dish and other recipes in the previous chapters. The few recipes below and commercially made foods will provide them something to eat while you eat your wheat or gluten- or wheat-free baked goods. With the support you provide each other and the understanding you have of your own physiology, you will succeed in improving your health and losing weight.

Bread Machine 100% Stone Ground Whole Wheat Bread

This whole wheat bread is delicious and near-effortless to make with almost any bread machine. However, due to the high level of fiber it contains, the middle of the loaf may fall a little. If you are fussy about how the loaf looks, try the recipe for oven-baked bread on the next page

1⅛ cup warm water
1 tablespoon single source honey, agave or Fruit Sweet™
1½ tablespoons oil or 1 tablespoon oil plus ½ tablespoon lecithin
1 teaspoon salt
3 cups stone ground whole wheat flour such as Bob's Red Mill™ brand
3 tablespoons vital gluten such as Bob's Red Mill™ brand
2¼ teaspoons active dry yeast

Add the ingredients to the pan in the order listed in your bread machine's instruction manual. (For most machines this will be the order given above). Chose a loaf size of 1½ pounds and start the basic cycle or a quick wheat cycle* if your machine has one. (I use the quick wheat cycle on my Zojirushi machine). Start the machine. After 5 to 10 minutes of vigorous mixing, touch the dough. If it is sticky, add 1 tablespoon of flour. After a few more minutes of mixing, re-check the consistency of the dough and if it is still sticky, add another 1 tablespoon of flour. If it is just tacky, you have added enough flour. If you live in a humid climate and your flour absorbs moisture from the air, you may need to add a total of 1 to 3 additional tablespoons of flour to the dough to achieve the right consistency – tacky but not sticky. In a dry climate during a dry season, you may need to add 1 to 3 teaspoons of water (one at a time) to make the dough supple.

Allow the cycle to run to completion. Remove the bread from the machine and allow the loaf to completely cool on a wire rack before slicing it. Store it in a plastic bag. Slice it thinly into 16 slices. Makes one 1½ pound loaf, or about 16 1½-ounce slices each of which contains 1 carbohydrate unit and 2 grams of fat.

*Note on the cycle to use with this bread recipe: Because this bread has a high fiber content, it may fall a little. If this happens with the first cycle you try on your bread machine, switch to another cycle that has a shorter last rise time. If you have a programmable machine, try using a cycle similar to this: Knead – 20 minutes; Rise 1 and 2 – Off; Rise 3 (or the last rise) – 30 minutes; Bake – 60 minutes. Be prepared to tweak this cycle to fit your machine and baking conditions such as climate and elevation. If the loaf over-rises and falls, decrease the time of the last rise. If it comes out dense, increase the last rise progressively – such as 5 minutes each time you make the bread – until it falls in the middle. Then decrease it to the previous setting. Another possible help for the problem of over-rising and then falling is to add an extra ½ tablespoon of gluten. Experiment with the various cycles on your machine, especially any that have a short (30 minute or less) last rise. The whole wheat cycle on most machines includes a lot of rising time, which is not what you want when your bread over-rises and falls. The basic cycle for white bread is more likely to work well.

Oven-Baked 100% Stone Ground Whole Wheat Bread

My husband likes his bread tall and with a perfectly domed top because if the bread isn't tall enough, he ends up with a skimpy sandwich. Since I cannot always get the perfect shape and height in a bread machine, I make his sandwich bread with this recipe.

> 1⅛ cup warm water
> 1 tablespoon single source honey, agave or Fruit Sweet™
> 1½ tablespoons oil or 1 tablespoon oil plus ½ tablespoon lecithin
> 1 teaspoon salt
> 3 cups stone ground whole wheat flour such as Bob's Red Mill™ brand
> 3 tablespoons vital gluten such as Bob's Red Mill™ brand
> 2¼ teaspoons active dry yeast

Prepare this dough by the mixer method as described in the second and third paragraphs of the spelt bread recipe on page 193 or with the dough cycle of a bread machine. When using a bread machine, add the ingredients to the pan in the order listed in your bread machine's instruction manual. (For most machines this will be the order given above). Start the dough cycle. After 5 to 10 minutes of vigorous mixing, touch the dough. If it is sticky, add 1 tablespoon of flour. After a few more minutes of mixing, re-check the consistency of the dough. If it is still sticky, add another 1 tablespoon of flour. If it is just tacky, you have added enough flour. If you live in a humid climate and your flour absorbs moisture from the air, you may need to add a total of 1 to 3 additional tablespoons of flour to the dough to achieve the right consistency – tacky but not sticky. In a dry climate during a dry season, you may need to add 1 to 3 teaspoons of water (one at a time) to make the dough supple. Allow the dough cycle to run to completion.

While the cycle is running or your mixer-made dough is rising, oil a loaf pan that is, if possible, 4 to 4 ½ inches wide and 8 to 10 inches long,* line it with waxed or parchment paper, and oil the paper. Prepare your oven to be a cozy rising place (85 to 90°F) as described on page 188. When the cycle is finished or the mixer-made dough has doubled in size, remove the dough from the machine or rising place, knead it, and form it into a loaf. Place it in the prepared pan. Let rise for 30 to 45 minutes or until it is a little more than doubled;** then remove from the oven. Preheat oven to 350°F. Put the loaf back into the oven and bake it for 45 minutes, covering after the first 30 minutes with foil to prevent excessive browning. Remove the loaf from the pan. It should sound hollow when tapped on the bottom with your knuckles. After it has cooled for a few minutes, peel the wax or parchment paper from the loaf and allow the loaf to completely cool on a wire rack before slicing it. Makes one 1½ pound loaf, or about 16 1½-ounce slices each of which contains 1 carbohydrate unit and 2 grams of fat.

*Note on the pan size: Narrow slices of bread make it possible to slice the loaf more thickly without exceeding about 1½ ounces per slice of bread, or one 15 gram carbohydrate unit serving per slice. You may want to use a Norpro™ bread pan as described on page 133.

**Note on the second rise: When I let this loaf rise in the bread pan, my goal is to product the tallest loaf I can without letting it rise for so long that it will fall. For my pans, I allow it to rise until it is about ¾ inch above the top of the pan; the time that this takes varies. This is probably nearly triple the volume of the original tightly wrapped, totally deflated roll of dough I put in the pan. You may want to experiment to see how much you can let your loaf rise before it falls in the oven.

WHOLE WHEAT BLUEBERRY MUFFINS

2¼ cups stone ground whole wheat flour such as Bob's Red Mill™ brand
3 teaspoons baking powder
¼ teaspoon salt
⅓ cup water
⅔ cup apple juice concentrate, thawed
⅓ cup oil
1 cup fresh or frozen blueberries

Preheat your oven to 350°F. Oil 12 muffin cups or line them with paper liners. If you are using frozen blueberries, put them in a strainer and run cold water over them. In a large bowl mix together the flour, baking powder, and salt. Combine the water, apple juice and oil in a separate bowl or measuring cup. Stir the liquid ingredients into the dry ingredients until just mixed. Gently but quickly fold in the blueberries. Fill the muffin cups ⅞ full to full with the batter. Bake for 20 to 24 minutes. Remove the muffins from the pan and allow them to cool on a wire rack. Makes 12 muffins each of which contains 1½ carbohydrate units and 7 grams of fat.

PIZZA

Pizza is the food that people on restricted diets seem to miss most. See pages 153 to 155 for a wheat and gluten-free pizza recipe, and make this recipe below for your non-allergic eating plan companions. Leftovers of both types of pizza freeze well for when you need a treat later.

Dough for a regular crust

½ cup water
1½ teaspoons single source honey, agave, or Fruit Sweet™
2½ teaspoons oil
½ teaspoon salt
1⅓ cups stone ground whole wheat flour such as Bob's Red Mill™ brand
1 tablespoon plus 1 teaspoon vital gluten such as Bob's Red Mill™ brand
1 teaspoon active dry yeast

Dough for a thin crust

⅓ cup water
1 teaspoon single source honey, agave, or Fruit Sweet™
1¾ teaspoons oil
⅜ teaspoon salt
⅞ to 1 cup stone ground whole wheat flour such as Bob's Red Mill™ brand
1 tablespoon vital gluten such as Bob's Red Mill™ brand
Scant ¾ teaspoon active dry yeast

Toppings

½ batch of pizza sauce, recipe on page 153
4 ounces (about 1 cup) grated mozzarella cheese, preferably part-skim or
   low-fat
2 tablespoons Romano cheese
4 to 5 ounces cooked turkey, lean ground beef or other cooked meat
Vegetables toppings such as sliced bell peppers, olives, etc. (optional)

Prepare the pizza sauce as directed on page 154 if you are using homemade sauce. Use the half-batch of leftover sauce for a wheat- or gluten-free pizza or freeze it for future use.

Choose one set of crust ingredients above. Prepare the dough by the mixer method as described in the second and third paragraphs of the spelt bread recipe on page 193 or with the dough cycle of a bread machine. If you use a bread machine, add the ingredients to the pan in the order listed in your bread machine's instruction manual using the smaller amount of the flour. (For most machines this will be the order given above). Start the dough cycle. After 5 to 10 minutes of vigorous mixing, touch the dough. If it is sticky, add a teaspoon of flour. After a few more minutes of mixing, re-check the consistency of the dough and if it is still sticky, add another teaspoon of flour. If it is just tacky, you have added enough flour. If you live in a humid climate and your flour absorbs moisture from the air, you may need to add a total of 1 to 4 additional teaspoons of flour to the dough to achieve the right consistency – tacky but not sticky. In a dry climate during a dry season, you may need to add ½ to 2 teaspoons of water (½ teaspoon at a time) to make the dough supple. Allow the dough cycle to run its course. As it nears completion, prepare your oven to be a cozy rising place (85 to 90°F) as described on page 188. Very lightly oil a 12-inch pizza pan by rubbing it with paper towel with just a little oil on it.

When the dough cycle has reached completion or the mixer-made dough has doubled in size, transfer it to the pizza pan. Stretch dough thinly in the pan. (See the note* below about stretching the dough for a thin crust pizza). Let it raise in a warm oven 5 minutes, top it with the toppings, and then let it rise again for an additional 5 to 10 minutes. Preheat your oven to 400°F. Bake the pizza for 18 to 20 minutes or until it is nicely browned. Cut the pizza into six slices. If you made regular crust pizza, two slices per serving equals 2 carbohydrate units. If you made thin crust pizza, three slices per serving equals 2 carbohydrate units. (The carbohydrates in the vegetables and sauce do not need to be counted). The protein units per serving are the number of ounces of meat plus cheese used on that serving size. For a regular pizza with 5 ounces of meat used, each 2-slice serving contains 4 protein units and 16 grams of fat. For a thin pizza with 4 ounces of meat used, each 3-slice serving contains 5 protein units and 21 grams of fat.

*Note on thin crust pizza: Do not over-oil the pan or punch down the dough before putting it in the pan. The dough must be stretched very thin – less than ¼ inch – in the pizza pan. This is best done using a pizza dough roller. (See "Sources" page 279 to purchase a roller). If the dough will not stretch enough to fill the pan by using the roller, let it rest for a few minutes and then roll it some more. The next time you make this pizza, allow the dough to rest after removing it from the bread machine; your machine may have kneaded it down too much at the end of the dough cycle.

Hamburger Buns

1⅛ cup warm water

1 tablespoon single source honey, agave or Fruit Sweet™

1½ tablespoons oil or 1 tablespoon oil plus ½ tablespoon lecithin

1 teaspoon salt

3 cups stone ground whole wheat flour such as Bob's Red Mill™ brand

3 tablespoons vital gluten such as Bob's Red Mill™ brand

2¼ teaspoons active dry yeast

Prepare this dough by the mixer method as described in the second and third paragraphs of the spelt bread recipe on page 193 or with the dough cycle of a bread machine. If you use a bread machine, add the ingredients to the pan in the order listed in your bread machine's instruction manual. (For most machines this will be the order given above). Start the dough cycle. After 5 to 10 minutes of vigorous mixing, touch the dough. If it is sticky, add a tablespoon of flour. After a few more minutes of mixing, re-check the consistency of the dough and if it is still sticky, add another tablespoon of flour. If it is just tacky, you have added enough flour. If you live in a humid climate and your flour absorbs moisture from the air, you may need to add a total of 1 to 3 additional tablespoons of flour to the dough to achieve the right consistency – tacky but not sticky. In a dry climate during a dry season, you may need to add 1 to 3 teaspoons of water (one at a time) to make the dough supple. Allow the dough cycle to run its course. As it nears completion, prepare your oven to be a cozy rising place at 85 to 90°F as described on page 188. Oil a large baking sheet.

When the cycle is finished or the mixer-made dough has doubled in size, transfer the dough to a lightly oiled surface. Use a lightly-oiled rolling pin to roll the dough ½ inch thick. Then cut it into circles with an oiled 3½ inch round biscuit cutter (You can use a pineapple can with the end removed in a pinch). Transfer the buns to the oiled baking sheet, leaving room between them so they can expand. Let them rise until doubled, 30 to 35 minutes. Remove them from the oven (if that was your warm rising place) and preheat your oven to 375°F. Bake the buns for 17 to 20 minutes or until brown. Remove the pan from the oven and transfer the buns to a cooling rack. When they are cool, store them in a plastic bag. Any leftover buns freeze well. Makes 8 3-ounce buns, each of which contains 2 carbohydrate units and 4 grams of fat.

Chocolate Cake or Torte

This is a real cake for your non-allergic companions to have on birthdays. Keep in mind, however, that white flour is high on the GI scale, so this should be a rare treat rather than a commonly eaten food.

Fruit or agave sweetened cake

1¼ cups unbleached or all purpose flour

½ cup cocoa

1⅜ teaspoon baking soda

⅝ teaspoon baking powder

⅛ teaspoon salt

2 large eggs

¾ cup + 1 tablespoon agave or Fruit Sweet™

⅔ cup buttermilk

⅓ cup oil

Stevia sweetened cake

1¼ cups unbleached or all purpose flour

½ cup cocoa

1 teaspoon baking soda

⅝ teaspoon baking powder

⅛ teaspoon salt

2⅛ teaspoons pure white stevia powder such as Protocol for Life Balance™ brand, to taste

3 large eggs

⅝ cup milk

⅔ cup buttermilk

⅓ cup oil

Choose one set of ingredients above. Grease and flour two 8-inch round cake pans for a torte-shaped cake or three 7-inch round cake pans for a 3-layer cake. Cut parchment or waxed paper to fit the bottom of the pans and place it in the pans. Preheat your oven to 375°F. Measure the flour, cocoa, baking soda, baking powder, salt, and stevia (if you are using it) into a large bowl and stir them together. Break the eggs into the large bowl of your electric mixer and beat them for about ½ minute until the white and yolk are thoroughly mixed. Add the liquid sweetener (if you are using it), milk (if you are using it), buttermilk and oil and beat again briefly until thoroughly mixed. Add the flour mixture and mix on low speed. Then beat on medium speed for 1½ to 2 minutes. Divide the cake batter between the prepared pans. Bake the cake for 18 to 22 minutes or until a toothpick inserted into the cake comes out dry. Do not over-bake! It is easy to make chocolate cakes dry by over-baking, so test the cake with a toothpick at the minimum time and remove the cake as soon as the toothpick comes out dry. Remove the pans from the oven. The stevia-sweetened cake may fall a little after removing it from the oven, but the flavor will still be good. (When made with stevia, the cake tends to form an upper crust that traps large air bubbles and may result in an uneven top). Let the cake cool on a wire rack for 10 minutes. Then remove the cake layers from the pans and allow them to cool completely. Frost with chocolate or vanilla cream cheese frosting below if desired. Makes 12 servings. If made with the liquid sweetener, each serving contains 2 carbohydrate units and 8 grams of fat. If made with stevia, each serving contains ⅘ carbohydrate unit and 8 grams of fat. Remember also to add the carbohydrate units and fat grams from the frosting if you use it. If this cake is made with the liquid sweetener and you want to use frosting, you will need to use a non-nutritive sweetener in the frosting or decrease the serving size to stay at or under 30 grams of carbohydrate per serving.

CHOCOLATE CREAM CHEESE FROSTING

Gluten-Free

This is the ideal chocolate frosting – beautiful, smooth, fluffy and delicious. It will not add to the carbohydrate content of a cake if you sweeten it with stevia or Equal.™

  1 8-ounce package cream cheese at room temperature
  ½ cup (1 stick) butter at room temperature
  ⅜ cup cocoa
  ⅝ to ⅞ cup agave, Fruit Sweet™ or single source honey, to taste

Use an electric mixer, blender, food processor or hand blender to mix together the cream cheese, butter and cocoa. Beat until fluffy. Mix in ⅝ cup of the agave, Fruit Sweet™ or honey. Taste it and see if it is sweet enough for you. If not, add the remaining agave, Fruit Sweet™ or honey one tablespoon at a time, tasting it as you add the sweetener until you get it to your preferred level of sweetness. If you add enough sweetener to make the frosting too thin to spread easily, refrigerate it for 15 minutes or more until it is of good spreading consistency. Frost the cake. This frosting will be soft but it gets firmer when chilled. Store any cake frosted with this frosting in the refrigerator. Makes about 2 cups of frosting or enough to frost an 8-inch two-layer torte or a 7-inch three-layer cake. If the cake is divided into 12 servings, each serving of frosting contains 2½ carbohydrate units and 12 grams of fat. If used to frost about 30 linzer cookies, each serving of frosting contains ½ carbohydrate unit and 5 grams of fat.

Stevia or Equal™ sweetened chocolate frosting variation: Omit the liquid sweetener. Instead use ¼ cup milk plus 18 to 21 packages Equal™ OR ¾ to 1 teaspoon of pure white stevia powder such as Protocol for Life Balance™ brand, to taste. If used to frost a cake which is divided into 12 servings, each serving of frosting contains negligible carbohydrate and 12 grams of fat. (If you wish to frost the cake generously, you may want to make a extra half-batch of frosting; then each serving of frosting will contain 18 grams of fat). If used to frost about 30 linzer cookies, each serving of frosting contains negligible carbohydrate and 5 grams of fat.

Vanilla Cream Cheese Frosting

This frosting tastes divine – full of rich flavor that shines through because it is not overwhelmingly sweet like bakery frosting.

> 1 8-ounce package cream cheese at room temperature
> ½ cup (1 stick) butter at room temperature
> 4 to 6 tablespoons agave, Fruit Sweet™ or single source honey, to taste
> 1 teaspoon vanilla extract

Use an electric mixer, blender, food processor or hand blender to mix together the cream cheese and butter. Beat until fluffy. Mix in the vanilla extract. Add the agave, Fruit Sweet™ or honey one tablespoon at a time, tasting it as you add the sweetener until you get it to your preferred level of sweetness. If you add enough sweetener to make the frosting too thin to spread easily, refrigerate it for 15 minutes or more until it is a good spreading consistency. Frost the cake. This frosting will be very soft but it gets firmer when chilled. Store any cake frosted with this frosting in the refrigerator. Makes about 1¾ cups of frosting, or enough to frost an 8-inch two-layer torte or a 7-inch three-layer cake. If the cake is divided into 12 servings, each serving of frosting contains 1 carbohydrate unit and 12 grams of fat. If used to frost about 30 linzer cookies, each serving of frosting contains ⅙ carbohydrate unit and 4 grams of fat.

Stevia or Equal™ sweetened vanilla frosting variation: Omit the liquid sweetener. Instead use 3 tablespoons milk plus 6 to 9 packages of Equal™ OR ¼ to ⅜ teaspoon of pure white stevia powder such as Protocol for Life Balance™ brand, to taste. If used to frost a cake which is divided into 12 servings, each serving of frosting contains negligible carbohydrate and 12 grams of fat. (If you wish to frost the cake generously, you may want to make a extra half-batch of frosting; then each serving of frosting will contain 18 grams of fat). If used to frost about 30 linzer cookies, each serving of frosting contains negligible carbohydrate and 4 grams of fat.

CHOCOLATE CUT-OUT COOKIES

Here's the recipe to use when your non-allergic companions must have a cookie. However, as with the cake on pagd 245, remember that white flour is high on the GI scale, so this should be a rare treat rather than a commonly eaten food.

2 squares (2 ounces) unsweetened baking chocolate

¼ cup butter

¼ cup Spectrum Naturals™ non-hydrogenated shortening (See "Sources," page 281)

1 large egg

1 teaspoon vanilla extract (optional)

⅞ cup all purpose or unbleached flour

1½ teaspoons pure white stevia powder such as Protocol for Life Balance™ brand, to taste

½ teaspoon baking powder

¼ teaspoon salt

Melt the chocolate in a double boiler or melt it carefully in the microwave. Set it aside to cool. Cream the butter and shortening with a mixer on medium speed. Add the egg and vanilla to the mixer bowl and beat. Stir together the flour, stevia, baking powder and salt. Gradually add about ⅔ of the flour mixture to the mixer bowl while it is running on low or medium speed. Beat until the flour mixture is thoroughly mixed in. Add the melted and cooled chocolate and beat it in thoroughly, scraping the bowl to make sure it's uniformly mixed into the dough. Beat in the rest of the flour mixture.

Preheat your oven to 400°F. Roll the dough out about ⅛ inch thick on a lightly floured board. Cut the dough into cookies and transfer them to an ungreased baking sheet with a spatula. Bake about 6 to 10 minutes, or until the cookies feel set and dry. (They will bubble as they bake and the baking time will vary with the thickness of the cookies). Remove them from the baking sheet and cool them on paper towel. Makes about 3 dozen 3-inch cookies, each of which contain ⅕ carbohydrate unit and 4 grams of fat.

LINZER COOKIES

Put the chocolate cookies on the previous page together with cream cheese frosting and one or two will satisfy without adding too much carbohydrate to a meal. They look like Oreos™ if you use vanilla frosting.

Make the cookies on the previous page but cut them with linzer cookie cutters, or cut them into circles about 2 inches in diameter. To make linzer cookies, cut half of the cookies as solid bottoms and the other half with a heart, star, etc. shaped hole in the cookie. Make cream cheese frosting or chocolate cream cheese frosting, pages 246 to 247. Put two cookies together with the frosting, using a cookie with a shape cut out of it for the top cookie if you are making linzer cookies. Refrigerate the cookies until serving time. You can frost them 24 hours ahead and they will be good. If you make the frosting ahead and plan to frost them right before serving time, let the frosting stand at room temperature to soften for at least ½ hour before using it to prevent breaking the cookies as you frost them. Makes about 24 2-inch cookie pairs, each of which contains ⅓ carbohydrate units and 6 grams of fat. Remember also to add the carbohydrate and fat units for the frosting you use.

Glycemic Index & Link-and-Balance Data for Foods Commonly Eaten on Food Allergy and Gluten-Free Diets

This table contains GI values and carbohydrate and protein units mostly for unprocessed foods. Unfortunately, GI scores for foods made especially for gluten-free and allergy diets – including grain-based foods such as breads and pasta – are usually unavailable. This is because GI scores can be determined only by testing using human volunteers, and very little of this is done in the United States.[1] Without testing specific brands or foods made with specific recipes, it is not possible to accurately know a food's GI score because, for example, two brands of tapioca bread will be made with different ingredients and different leavening systems or yeast rising times. These differences will then affect the glycemic impact of the bread.

The information in this table was derived from several sources.[2] Some values are missing from the data for some foods because either it is not available (i.e. many vegetables have such a low carbohydrate content that they cannot be tested for a GI score) or it does not apply to that food (i.e. GI scores do not apply to foods which contain no carbohydrate).

Do not allow this table to induce you to weigh your food routinely. If you are uncertain about how large a serving size should be, weigh it out once, and then judge the portion by appearance and size the next time you eat that food. The best practice is to eat foods that are as close to nature as possible and only use these tables as a guideline for choosing low GI carbohydrate foods and for linking and balancing your carbohydrate and protein foods. Practice listening to your body rather than becoming legalistic about your food.

---

[1] GI scores for Australian brands of bread, etc. are found in the *New Glucose Revolution* series of books. In addition, GI scores from many countries around the world are found on www.mendosa.com/gilists.htm.

[2] Hart, Cheryle R., MD and Mary Kay Grossman, RD, *The Insulin Resistance Diet,* (New York: McGraw-Hill, 2001, 2007), 44-61; Brand-Miller, Jennie, PhD, Kate Marsh , and Phillipa Sandall, *The New Glucose Revolution: Low GI and Gluten-Free Eating Made Easy,* (Cambridge, MA: Da Capo Press, 2008), 224-243; Brand-Miller, Jennie, PhD and Kay Foster-Powell. MND, *The New Glucose Revolution Shoppers Guide to GI Values,* (Cambridge, MA: Da Capo Press, 2009 and 2010); www.montignac.com/en/ig_tableau.php; www.mendosa.com/gilists.htm; and *Food Processor for Windows, Version 7.7,* by ESHA Research, Inc., P.O. Box 13028, Salem, OR 97309.

Food	Serving Size	Carb Units	Glycemic Index Score	GI Range

CARBOHYDRATE FOODS

Fruits

Food	Serving Size	Carb Units	Glycemic Index Score	GI Range
Apple, raw	1 medium (5 oz.)	0[3]	36	LOW
Applesauce, unsweetened	½ cup	1	42	LOW
Apples, dried	4 rings (1 oz.)	1	29	X-LOW[4]
Apricots, raw	2 large or 4 small (6 oz.)	1	38[5]	LOW
Apricots, dried	7 halves (1 oz.)	1	30	X-LOW
Banana	½ small (4") or ½ cup slices (2¾ oz.)	1	52	LOW
Blueberries	¾ cup (4 oz.)	1	53	LOW
Cantaloupe	⅓ of a 5" melon (6 oz.)	1	65	MED
Cherries, dark	⅝ cup (3½ oz.)	1	63	MED
Cherries, sour	⅝ cup (3½ oz.)	1	22	X-LOW
Dates, pitted	3 medium (1 oz.)	1	45	LOW
Grapefruit	1 small (3½") or ½ large (6 oz. without peel)	0[3]	25	X-LOW
Grapes	1 cup (3½ oz.)	1	53	LOW
Kiwi fruit	2 small (4 oz.)	1	53	LOW
Mango	½ medium (3½ oz.)	1	51	LOW
Nectarine	1 medium (5 oz.)	1	43	LOW
Orange	1 3-inch diameter (5 oz.)	1	42	LOW
Papaya	½ large (7 oz.)	1	59	MED
Peach, raw	2 small or 1 large (8 oz.)	0[3]	42	LOW
Peach, canned in juice	2 small halves (5 oz.)	1	45	LOW
Peach, dried	2 halves (1 oz.)	1	35	LOW

[3] Raw apple, pear, peach, plum, and grapefruit don't have to be balanced with protein in a meal or a snack because they are very high in fiber and the carbohydrate they contain is mostly fructose. Therefore, the impact these fruits have on blood sugar and insulin levels is low and slow. However, if these fruits are cooked, juiced, canned, or otherwise processed, the carbohydrate they contain is absorbed more quickly, so they must be balanced with protein. In that case, the serving size given in this table will count as one carbohydrate unit.

[4] X-LOW indicates that the glycemic index score of this food is extremely low (less than 35). These foods are usually included in the low range. On this chart, LOW means a score of 35 to 55, MED means 56 to 69, and HIGH means 70 or greater. See page 66 for more about the ranges assigned to GI scores.

[5] The GI score of raw apricots on mendosa.com is 34. *The New Glucose Revolution: Low GI and Gluten-Free Eating Made Easy* gives it a score of 38 and *The New Glucose Revolution Shopper's Guide* gives it a score of 57 (medium range).

Food	Serving Size	Carb Units	Glycemic Index Score	GI Range
Pear, raw	1 small (4¼ oz.)	0[3]	38	LOW
Pear, canned in juice	2 halves (5 oz.)	1	44	LOW
Pear, dried	1½ halves (5 oz.)	1	43	LOW
Pineapple chunks, fresh	¾ cup (4½ oz.)	1	66	MED
Pineapple chunks, canned with juice	⅜ cup (3½ oz.)	1	59	MED
Plum, raw	2 medium (4½ oz.)	0[3]	39	LOW
Plum, dried (prune)	3 medium (1 oz.)	1	29	LOW
Raisins	2 tbsp. (¾ oz.)	1	64	MED
Strawberries, fresh	15 large, 1½ cups (6 oz.)	1	40	LOW
Strawberries, frozen unsweetened	¾ cup thawed (6 oz.)	1	40	LOW
Watermelon, cubed	1½ cups (8 oz.)	1	76	HIGH

Cooked Whole Grains

Food	Serving Size	Carb Units	Glycemic Index Score	GI Range
Barley, pearled	⅓ cup (2½ oz.)	1	25	X-LOW
Buckwheat	½ cup (3 oz.)	1	54	LOW
Millet	⅓ cup (2½ oz.)	1	71	HIGH
Milo (sorghum)	½ cup (3 oz.)	1	39	LOW
Polenta (cornmeal)	⅓ cup (2¾ oz.)	1	68	MED
Quinoa	½ cup (3½ oz.)	1	53	LOW
Rice, brown (most)	⅓ cup (2¾ oz.)	1	50 to 69	MED-HIGH
Rice, brown basmati	⅓ cup (2¾ oz.)	1	58	MED
Rice, white (most)	⅓ cup (2¾ oz.)	1	76 to 98	HIGH
Rice, white, Uncle Bens™ converted	⅓ cup (2¾ oz.)	1	45	LOW
Rice, wild	½ cup (3 oz.)	1	57	MED
Wheat, cracked (bulgur)	½ cup (3½ oz.)	1	46	LOW
Whole wheat kernels	½ cup (4 oz.)	1	41	LOW

Food	Serving Size	Carb Units	Glycemic Index Score	GI Range

Grain-based Baked Goods
(Bread, Tortillas, Crackers, etc.)

This section probably lacks the information you most want – the one-carbohydrate unit serving size and GI score for your favorite gluten-free bread.[6] Lacking that, I suggest you use the GI scores of cooked whole grains above plus the information below to determine trends that you can use in your food choices. Notice that whole wheat and white bread share very similar GI scores (because most flour is very finely milled with metal rollers; thus whole wheat flour is as fine and rapidly digested as white flour) but that the GI score for bread made from stone ground whole wheat flour is lower. Therefore, you might read labels and purchase or bake bread and crackers containing stone ground flour of other kinds, such as Bob's Red Mill™ stone ground quinoa flour. You could also extrapolate which baked goods might be lower on the GI scale from the GI scores of cooked whole grains on the previous page. In addition, note the one-carbohydrate unit serving sizes as you decide which grains you wish to eat most often, either as cooked grains or in bread products. In the absence of GI testing on many grain-based foods, the advice given by Dr. Jennie Brand-Miller for choosing a commercially made low GI gluten-free bread is to use bread that contains a high amount of legume flours (garbanzo or chickpea flour, fava bean flour, soy flour, etc.) and/or that includes additions such a psyllium husks, whole grain kernels, nuts or seeds.[7]

Food	Serving Size	Carb Units	Glycemic Index Score	GI Range
Bagel, white wheat	½ of a 4" or ⅓ of a 5"	1	72	HIGH
Barley bread[8]	1 slice (1-1½ oz.)	1	43 to 67	LOW-MED
Buckwheat bread[8]	1 slice (1-1½ oz.)	1	47 to 67	LOW-MED
Chickpea bread[8]	1 slice (1-1½ oz.)	1	55 to 67	MED
Corn tortilla	1 thin 6-inch tortilla	1	46 to 52	LOW
Rice bread[8]	1 slice (1 oz.)	1	72	HIGH

[6] Since very little GI testing is done in the United States, American brands are not found in the information that was available for compiling this table. This list of GI scores for breads contains only general information, not information from testing American brands, and scores can vary from brand to brand. The rice bread listed here is of unknown composition so its GI score could easily be higher than 58. Read the label on your bread to insure that your serving contains 15 grams of net carbohydrate (total grams of carbohydrate minus grams of fiber) and thus is the amount of bread to equal one carbohydrate unit. The list of GI scores for cooked whole grains is also woefully incomplete because some very useful gluten-free foods such as amaranth have never been tested.

[7] See question 19 on the FAQs page from the glycemicindex.com website.

[8] The GI scores from several alternative grain breads in this section of the table are from these breads made in other countries. The scores came from mendosa.com/gilists.htm and *The New Glucose Revolution: Low GI and Gluten-Free Eating Made Easy.*

Food	Serving Size	Carb Units	Glycemic Index Score	GI Range
Rice cake, puffed	¾ ounce	1	82	HIGH
Rice crackers	¾ ounce	1	91	HIGH
Rye bread, sourdough	1 slice (1-1½ oz.)	1	42	LOW
Rye bread, whole grain[8, 9]	½ to 1 slice (1-1½ oz.)	1	40 to 72	LOW-HIGH
Rye crispbread	½ ounce	1	63	MED
Sourdough wheat bread[8]	1 slice (1-1½ oz.)	1	54	LOW
Spelt bread[8]	1 slice (1-1½ oz.)	1	54 to 74	LOW -HIGH
White bread (average)	1 slice (1-1½ oz.)	1	75	HIGH
Whole wheat bread (average)	1 slice (1-1½ oz.)	1	74	HIGH
Whole wheat bread, stone ground	1 slice (1-1½ oz.)	1	59 to 66	MED
Whole wheat crackers with sesame seeds	½ ounce	1	54	LOW
Whole wheat tortilla[8]	½ 10-inch tortilla	1	30	LOW

Pasta

Pasta may be a low to medium GI food if it is prepared properly; the scores in this table reflect proper preparation. See page 163 for how to cook pasta *al dente*. If it is over-cooked, it will have a higher GI score and more adverse impact on blood sugar levels.

Food	Serving Size	Carb Units	Glycemic Index Score	GI Range
Corn pasta	½ cup (2 oz.)	1	78	HIGH
Mung bean noodles	⅓ cup (2 oz.)	1	59	MED
Rice pasta	⅓ cup (2 oz.)	1	61	MED
Semolina (durum wheat) pasta	½ cup (2 oz.)	1	35 to 59	LOW-MED
Soba (buckwheat) pasta	⅝ cup (2½ oz.)	1	59	MED

Beverages

Food	Serving Size	Carb Units	Glycemic Index Score	GI Range
Apple juice	½ cup (4 oz.)	1	44	LOW
Beer	12 ounces (1 can)	1	66 to 110	MED-HIGH
Carrot juice, fresh	1 cup (8 oz.)	1	43	LOW
Coffee, unsweetened[10]	8 ounces	0[10]	-	-
Cranberry-apple juice, unsweetened	½ cup (4 oz.)	1	52	LOW

[9] The GI scores on mendosa.com/gilists.htm were as low as 40 for several types of rye bread.

[10] Diet soda and coffee or tea prepared without sugar or nutritive sweeteners contain no carbohydrate. However, caffeinated beverages and diet sodas should be consumed with food to prevent an impact on blood sugar stability. See pages 66 to 68 for more about this.

Food	Serving Size	Carb Units	Glycemic Index Score	GI Range
Grape juice, 100% juice	⅜ cup (3 oz.)	1	53	LOW
Grapefruit juice, unsweetened	⅞ cup (7 oz.)	1	45	LOW
Pineapple juice, unsweetened	½ cup (4 oz.)	1	46	LOW
Prune juice	⅓ cup (2⅓ oz.)	1	43	LOW
Rice milk, unsweetened[11]	½ cup (4 oz.)	1	86	HIGH
Soy milk, unsweetened[11]	1 cup (8 ounces)	0[12]	43	LOW
Soda, diet	12 ounces (1 can)	0[10]	-	-
Soda, not diet	4 ounces	1	48 to 58	LOW-MED
Tea. unsweetened[10]	8 ounces	0[10]	-	-
Tomato juice, sugar-free	1½ cups (12 oz.)	1	38	LOW
Wine, dessert type	4 ounces	1	not available	MED-HIGH
Wine, no added sugar	8 ounces	0[13]	-	-

Vegetables

Most vegetables are low in carbohydrate, high in vitamins, phytochemicals and other nutrients, and can be eaten in any quantity you'd like on this healthy eating plan. Therefore, the serving size listed in this section of the table for most vegetables is "to satiety." Many vegetables are so low in carbohydrates that they cannot be tested for a GI score, so the score and GI range data for these vegetables is blank. A few vegetables are sources of concentrated carbohydrates, so the portion size must be kept to an amount supplying 30 grams of carbohydrate or less and must be balanced with protein. Dried legumes are high in protein and count as protein foods when balancing meals or snacks. The carbohydrate they contain is mostly indigestible so you may eat these in a quantity sufficient to satisfy your hunger. For more about legumes, see page 78. If you want a vegetable you do not see here, search for its GI score at mendosa.com/gilists.htm, or – unless it seems starchy – eat as much of it as you want.

---

[11] Check the labels on rice and soy milk for sweeteners. If they are sweetened, use the net carbohydrate content to calculate the correct serving size, which will be smaller than for unsweetened milk. See the dairy product section of this table for more about the protein content of soy milk. Rice milk contains a negligible amount of protein and a large amount of high GI carbohydrate.

[12] The carbohydrate in unsweetened soy milk comes from soybeans and, like all carbohydrates from beans, doesn't need to be counted or balanced with protein.

[13] The carbohydrates in the grapes used to make wine are completely changed to alcohol during fermentation. This alcohol may or may not (depending on the expert) affect blood sugar balance. Although the zero number of carbohydrate units implies that you do not need to balance wine with protein foods, it is advisable to drink wine with a protein-containing snack.

Food	Serving Size	Units	Glycemic Index Score	GI Range
Artichokes	To satiety	-	-	-
Arugula	To satiety	-	-	-
Asparagus	To satiety	-	-	-
Beans, baked	⅓ cup (3 oz.)	1 prot	47 to 55	LOW- MED
Beans, green, wax, etc.	To satiety	-	-	-
Beans, green baby lima	To satiety	-	32	LOW
Beets	To satiety	-	52	LOW
Broccoli	To satiety	-	-	-
Cauliflower	To satiety	-	-	-
Cabbage, any kind	To satiety	-	-	-
Carrots, raw	To satiety	-	16	X- LOW
Carrots, boiled	To satiety	-	41	LOW
Cassava (yucca), boiled	⅓ cup (1½ oz.)	1 carb	94	HIGH
Collards	To satiety	-	-	-
Corn, kernels	½ cup (3 oz.)	1 carb	37 to 46	LOW
Corn on the cob	1 small	1 carb	48	LOW
Cucumber	To satiety	-	-	-
Eggplant	To satiety	-	-	-
Fennel	To satiety	-	-	-
Garlic	To satiety	-	-	-
Green beans, any kind	To satiety	-	-	-
Kale	To satiety	-	-	-
Legumes, dried, cooked	⅓ cup	1 prot	22 to 42	X-LOW- LOW
including black, cannellini, garbanzo, kidney, navy, pinto, soy, and white lima beans, lentils and split peas				
Legumes, chana dal	⅓ cup	1 prot	8 to 11	X-LOW
Lettuce, any kind	To satiety	-	-	-
Mushrooms, any kind	To satiety	-	-	-
Onions, any kind	To satiety	-	-	-
Parsnips	To satiety	-	52	LOW
Plantain, boiled	⅓ cup (1¾ oz.)	1 carb	40	LOW
Peas	To satiety	-	45	LOW
Peppers, all kinds	To satiety	-	-	-
Potato, Russet, baked	1 small (4½ oz.)	1 carb	76	HIGH
Potatoes, mashed with fat	½ cup (4 oz.)	1 carb	71	HIGH
Potato, new red, boiled	4 1-inch (5 oz.)	1 carb	59	MED
Potato, sweet	½ large (3½ oz.)	1 carb	59	MED
Pumpkin, boiled	To satiety	-	64	MED
Spinach	To satiety	-	-	-
Squash, any kind	To satiety	-	-	-
Swiss chard	To satiety	-	-	-
Taro root	¼ cup (2 oz.)	1 carb	56	MED
Tomatoes, raw, cooked, canned, paste, sauce, or puree	To satiety	-	-	-
Turnips	To satiety	-	-	-
Water chestnuts	To satiety	-	-	-
Yam, true (bitter)	½ cup (2½ oz.)	1 carb	74	HIGH

(See "Potato, sweet" for the vegetable called a yam in American stores).

Food	Serving Size	Units	GI Score	GI Range	Grams of Fat/serving

PROTEIN FOODS

Dairy and Egg Products

Dairy products make delicious and convenient protein snacks for your healthy eating plan. Be careful of how much "hidden" fat you are consuming with them, however. This table gives approximate grams of fat per serving, but read the label from your cheese, milk, or yogurt to determine how much fat you are ingesting.

Food	Serving Size	Units	GI Score	GI Range	Grams of Fat/serving
Buttermilk	1 cup	1 prot	-	-	2
Cheese, hard, fat-free	1 ounce	1 prot	-	-	0
Cheese, hard, low-fat	1 ounce	1 prot	-	-	2
Cheese, hard, regular	1 ounce	1 prot	-	-	9
Cheese, mozzarella, part skim	1 ounce	1 prot	-	-	4
Cottage cheese, 1% fat	¼ cup	1 prot	-	-	0.5
Cottage cheese, 2% fat	¼ cup	1 prot	-	-	1
Cottage cheese, creamed	¼ cup	1 prot	-	-	2
Cottage cheese, dry curd	⅓ cup	1 prot	-	-	0
Cottage cheese, nonfat	¼ cup	1 prot	-	-	0
Cream cheese, nonfat	3 tbsp.	1 prot	-	-	0.5
(See page 260 for regular or reduced fat cream cheese).					
Egg substitute	¼ cup	1 prot	-	-	2
Egg, whites	2	1 prot	-	-	0
Egg, whole (large)	1	1 prot	-	-	5
Ice cream, sweetened with corn sweeteners or sugar	½ cup	½ prot/1 carb	51	LOW	4 to 12
Ice cream, no sugar added	1 cup	1 prot	-	-	4 to 12
Milk, cow's, 1% fat	1 cup	1 prot	-	-	3
Milk, cow's, 2 % fat	1 cup	1 prot	-	-	5
Milk, cow's, nonfat	1 cup	1 prot	-	-	0
Milk, cow's, flavored and sweetened	1 cup	1 prot/2 carb	26 to 31	LOW	0 to 10
Milk, cow's, whole	1 cup	1 prot	-	-	8 to 10
Milk, goat's, whole	1 cup	1 prot	-	-	10
Milk shake	⅔ cup	½ prot/2 carb	GI data not available		5
Milk, soy, sweetened	1 cup	1 prot/1 carb	31	LOW	5 to 20
Milk, soy, unsweetened	1 cup	1 prot	-	-	5 to 20
Pudding, sugar free	1 cup	1 prot/1 carb	40	LOW	3 to 8
Pudding, sweetened with corn sweeteners or sugar	½ cup	½ prot/1½ carb	40 to 47	LOW	3 to 8
Ricotta cheese, part skim	¼ cup	1 prot	-	-	5

Food	Serving Size	Units	GI Score	GI Range	Grams of Fat/serving
Ricotta cheese, regular	¼ cup	1 prot	-	-	8
Romano cheese	⅓ cup (1 oz.)	1 prot	-	-	8
Yogurt, flavored, no sugar added	1 cup	1 prot	-	-	0 to 8
Yogurt, plain	1 cup	1 prot	-	-	0 to 8
Yogurt, sweetened with corn sweetener, sugar or honey	1 cup	1 prot/2 carb	14 to 54	LOW	0 to 8

Meat, Poultry and Fish

Since meat, poultry and fish contain no carbohydrate, they may be eaten in a quantity sufficient to satisfy. The amounts given below for "serving size" are usually one ounce or the amount that will yield 1 protein unit (7 grams of protein) for the purpose of balancing these protein foods with the carbohydrate foods on the previous pages. However, for a meal you will probably eat 3 or 4 ounces of meat; the amount must be equal to or greater than the number of carbohydrate units you eat at that meal, which is two units at the most. Processed meats are usually high fat and may contain sugar or corn sweeteners so should not be eaten on a regular basis. To be certain how much processed meat equals one protein unit (7 grams of protein) and how much fat you will also get, read the nutrition label on the meat package.

As long as the meat, poultry or fish you are eating is unprocessed and low fat, do not be overly concerned about the portion size, but rather listen to your body and eat until your hunger is satisfied. As you can see from the listing for chicken or turkey, removing the skin (as recommended by standard weight loss diets) saves you just one gram of fat per ounce of meat, so don't deprive yourself if you enjoy the skin. Fat in meat slows digestion and makes your meal satisfy you longer.

Food	Serving Size	Units	GI Score	GI Range	Grams of Fat/serving
Bacon, raw weight	1 strip (0.8 oz.)	¼ prot	-	-	3 to 13
Beef, broiled, or ground beef, broiled or pan-cooked and thoroughly drained					
10% lean ground beef	1 oz.	1 prot	-	-	2 to 3
20% lean ground beef	1 oz.	1 prot	-	-	4 to 5
Ground, "regular" (27%)	1 oz.	1 prot	-	-	7 to 10
Prime rib roast, ¼" trim	1 oz.	1 prot	-	-	8
Round (rump) roast or steak, ¼" trim	1 oz.	1 prot	-	-	3
Sirloin, ¼" trim	1 oz.	1 prot	-	-	3
Well-marbled steak such as T-bone, ¼" trim	1 oz.	1 prot	-	-	6
Bison (buffalo)	1 oz.	1 prot	-	-	1
Bologna	3 pieces (2 oz.)	1 prot	-	-	16

Food	Serving Size	Units	GI Score	GI Range	Grams of Fat/serving
Chicken or turkey, roasted					
Breast meat, no skin	1 oz.	1 prot	-	-	1
Breast meat, with skin	1 oz.	1 prot	-	-	2
Dark meat, no skin	1 oz.	1 prot	-	-	3
Dark meat, with skin	1 oz.	1 prot	-	-	4
Clams (meat only)	1½ oz.	1 prot	-	-	3
Crab or lobster meat	1 oz.	1 prot	-	-	0.2
Duck	1 oz.	1 prot	-	-	3
Elk or venison	1 oz.	1 prot	-	-	1
Ham, baked	1 oz.	1 prot	-	-	1 to 4
Hot dog, all beef	1½ (2¼ oz.)	1 prot	-	-	13 to 16
Hot dog, all turkey	1 (1½ oz.)	1 prot	-	-	8
Lamb leg, ¼" trim	1 oz.	1 prot	-	-	3
Oysters (meat only)	2½ oz.	1 prot	-	-	2
Pork chop, braised, ¼" trim	1 oz.	1 prot	-	-	5 to 7
Salmon, broiled	1 oz.	1 prot	-	-	2
Shrimp (meat only)	1½ oz.	1 prot	-	-	0.5
Trout, baked	1 oz.	1 prot	-	-	1
Tuna, water packed	1 oz.	1 prot	-	-	0.2
Turkey, ground (8% fat)	1 oz.	1 prot	-	-	2
White fish, poached, baked or broiled (cod, flounder, sole, halibut, etc.)	1 oz.	1 prot	-	-	0.2

Nuts, Seeds, and Nut Butters

Nuts, seeds, and nut and seed butters are great carry-along protein snack foods because they require no refrigeration. However, if you are following this eating plan for weight loss, try to keep the amount of nuts, seeds or nut butter you eat within the amount of fat you should eat per day. If your goal is to control inflammation, nuts and seeds are good sources of omega-3 fatty acids, so be sure to include them in your diet.

Food	Serving Size	Units	GI Score	GI Range	Grams of Fat/serving
Almond butter, natural	3 tbsp.	1 prot	-	-	28
Almonds	1½ oz.	1 prot	-	-	22
Cashew butter, natural	2 tbsp.	1 prot	-	-	16
Cashews	1½ oz.	1 prot	-	-	22
Chestnuts	5 (2 oz.)	1 carb/¼ prot	54	LOW	1
Macadamia nuts	3 oz.	1 prot	-	-	65
Peanut butter, natural	2 tbsp.	1 prot	-	-	16
Peanuts, shelled	1 oz.	1 prot	-	-	14
Pecans	3 oz.	1 prot	-	-	61
Pine nuts	1 oz.	1 prot	-	-	14

Food	Serving Size	Units	GI Score	GI Range	Grams of Fat/serving
Pumpkin seeds	1¼ oz.	1 prot	-	-	7
Sunflower seeds, shelled	¼ cup	1 prot	-	-	16
Tahini (sesame seed butter)	2 tbap.	1 prot	-	-	16
Walnuts, black	2 oz.	1 prot	-	-	32
Walnuts, English	1½ oz.	1 prott	-	-	28

OTHER FOODS

Fats

The foods listed in this section do not contain significant amounts of protein or carbohydrates so they are not listed in the carbohydrate or protein food sections of this table and the "units" column below is blank. The information here is to help you control the amount of fat you eat per day. Don't deprive yourself totally however; avocados and many oils are great sources of heart healthy fats and omega-3 fatty acids. See pages 55 to 59 for more about fats.

Food	Serving Size	Units	GI Score	GI Range	Grams of Fat/serving
Avocado	1 medium (7 oz.)	-	-	-	31
Butter	1 pat (1 tsp.)	-	-	-	4
Cream cheese	2 tbsp.	-	-	-	10
Cream cheese, low fat (Neufchatel)	2 tbsp.	-	-	-	6
Cream – table or light	2 tbsp.	-	-	-	6
Cream – whipping	2 tbsp.	-	-	-	11
Oils, cooking such as olive, canola, safflower, grapeseed, and nut oils	2 tsp.	-	-	-	9
Salad dressing					
Blue cheese	1 tbsp.	-	-	-	5 to 8
French	1 tbsp.	-	-	-	6 to 10
Italian	1 tbsp.	-	-	-	3 to 13

Other types of dressing – Read the nutrition label to determine the fat content

Food	Serving Size	Carb Units	GI Score	GI Range	Grams of Fat/serving

Snack Foods

Highly processed snack foods are best eaten as occasional treats and in moderate quantities. However, Dr. Cheryle Hart recommends dark chocolate for frequent controlled splurges because of its high level of nutrients that stimulate the production of neurotransmitters. See pages 45 to 46 for more about this. With the information in this section of the table you will be able determine what size serving of a snack food is within the two carbohydrate unit (30 gram) limit for a meal or snack and how much protein you need to balance it.

Food	Serving Size	Carb Units	GI Score	GI Range	Grams of Fat/serving
Chocolate, dark, plain	1 oz.	1 carb	41	LOW	9 to 11
Chocolate, milk, plain	1 oz.	1 carb	41	LOW	8 to 10
Corn chips	1 oz.	1 carb	42 to 74	LOW- HIGH	8
Jelly beans	6 (¾ oz.)	1 carb	78	HIGH	0
Mars™ fun-size bar	1 oz.	1¼ carb	51	LOW	19
Popcorn, popped with oil	2¾ cups (1.1 oz.)	1 carb	65	MED	8
Potato chips	1 oz.	1 carb	51 to 59	LOW-MED	8

Sweeteners and Spreads

Food	Serving Size	Carb Units	GI Score	GI Range	Grams of Fat/serving
Agave[14]	4 tsp. (¾ oz.)	1 carb	19	X-LOW	0
Corn syrup[15]	1 tbsp. (⅔ oz.)	1 carb	115	HIGH	0
Grape jelly	1 tbsp. (½ oz.)	1 carb	52	LOW	0
Honey, single source	3 tsp. (¾ oz.)	1 carb	35	LOW	0
Maple syrup, pure	3 tsp. (¾ oz.)	1 carb	54	LOW	0
Orange marmalade	1 tbsp. (½ oz.)	1 carb	48	LOW	0
Strawberry jam	1 tbsp. (½ oz.)	1 carb	46	LOW	0
Sugars, pure					
Fructose	1 tbsp. (½ oz.)	1 carb	19	X-LOW	0
Glucose	1 tbsp. (½ oz.)	1 carb	100	HIGH	0
Sucrose (table sugar)	4 tsp. (⅔ oz.)	1 carb	60 to 68	MED	0

---

[14] The GI score given for agave is an average of agave scores which vary between different sources. All are in the extremely low GI range, however

[15] This GI score came from www.montignac.com/en/ig_tableau.php.

Superfoods for Inflammation

Some foods are super for us because they contain a variety of nutrients that moderate inflammation. Nuts, seeds, and high-fat fish such as salmon contain omega-3 fatty acids. (See pages 33 to 34 for more about how omega-3 fats dampen inflammation). Yogurt promotes the establishment of friendly intestinal flora and helps normalize immunity. However, most of the superfoods listed here quiet inflammation because of the wide variety of phytonutrients (bioflavanoids and carotenoids) they contain. Luteolin (found in green bell peppers and possibly other bell peppers) has an anti-inflammatory effect because it blocks the production of interleukin-6, a powerful promoter of inflammation. Green tea has a very potent anti-inflammatory effect due to its high level of catechin polymers, especially epigallocatechin gallate (EGCG).[1] Citrus flavanoids are found in grapefruit and oranges. Darkly colored fruits are potently anti-inflammatory because they contain high levels of anthocyanidins, so eat plenty of blueberries, cherries, and pomegranates. Reservatrol is found in red grapes and red wine. The vitamin A precursor beta-carotene is found in large amounts in carrots, broccoli, and arugula. Celery and celery seed contain over 20 anti-inflammatory compounds including apigenin.[2] Although this is a secondary effect of foods that dampen inflammation, the catechins in blueberries and green tea stimulate fat-burning in abdominal fat cells which promotes weight loss especially in the mid-section of the body.[3]

See pages 33 to 35 for more about inflammation and include a generous amount of the foods below in your diet every day.

Fruits
(Best eaten fresh and raw)
Apples
Blueberries (Use blueberries frozen without sugar if out of season).
Cherries (Use cherries frozen without sugar if out of season).
Grapefruit
Oranges
Pomegranates
Red grapes*

---

* Most of the foods on this list come from the "Top 40 Superfoods" list in *The Fat Resistance Diet* by Leo Galland, M.D. A * denotes that this food was recommended as an anti-inflammatory food by another expert.

[1] Galland, Leo, MD, *The Fat Resistance Diet,* (New York: Broadway Books, 2005), 98.

[2] http://www.care2.com/greenliving/13-foods-that-fight-pain.html

[3] http://www.care2.com/greenliving/12-surprising-reasons-to-eat-more-blueberries.html

Vegetables
Arugula
Bell peppers
Broccoli
Cabbage
Carrots
Celery*
Leeks
Onions
Romaine lettuce
Scallions
Shitake mushrooms
Spinach
Tomatoes

Nuts and Seeds
(Raw, not roasted)
Almonds
Flaxseeds
Sesame seeds
Walnuts

Animal Protein Foods
Egg whites
Flounder
Salmon
Sole
Tilapia
Yogurt (sugar-free and low-fat or nonfat)

Herbs and Spices
Basil
Black pepper
Cardamom
Chives
Cilantro
Cinnamon
Cloves
Garlic
Ginger
Parsley
Turmeric

Beverages
Blueberry juice
Cherry juice
Ginger tea
Green tea[4]
Pomegranate juice
Vegetable juice (mixed or carrot juice)

---

[4] Although this is strictly my personal experience, some varieties of green tea feel more potently anti-inflammatory to me than others. Green Twisted Spears™ tea gives me a great sense of well-being (plus the more objective sign of open sinuses) which begins within a half hour of drinking it and lasts all day. See page 283 of the "Sources" section for information about getting this tea from The Tea Spot.

EXERCISE: DO IT RIGHT

Conventional weight loss advice says, "Just eat less and exercise more," but it is usually given by someone who never needed to lose weight. What you eat, how foods are combined, and when you eat are just as important as how much you eat. Exercise also is not as simple as conventional advice implies. Just as with carbohydrates and fats, all types of exercise are not created equal. Although exercise routines are not my areas of expertise, having read the experts, it seems to me that how much and what kind of exercise is best for YOU is as much an individual matter as what, when, and how much you eat. There actually are types and amounts of exercise that cause fat deposition rather than fat burning.

There are three types of exercise: aerobic (also called cardio), muscle building (such as weight training), and moderate exercise (also called brisk activity). Aerobic exercise receives the most attention because it strengthens the heart muscles, helps the lungs and is beneficial for most people.[1] However, if done to excess or without sufficient food, aerobic exercise can be physically stressful and induce adrenal hormone production which causes the body to deposit rather than burn fat. If done without eliciting the release of adrenal hormones, it promotes weight loss very effectively because it boosts your metabolic rate for about 36 hours after exercising, thus causing you to use more calories regardless of your activity for the next day and a half.[2] If your insulin levels are low and stable during that time, those burned calories can come from stored body fat.

The definition of aerobic exercise is exercise that is strenuous enough to cause your heart to reach a target rate determined by your age. To calculate your target pulse rate, subtract your age from 220 and then multiply that number by three fourths (0.75 using a calculator).[3] There also are pulse rate monitoring wrist watches that can be worn during exercise to easily monitor your pulse, either to keep it at the target rate for aerobic exercise or to keep it in an optimal range for fat burning, which is lower.

Muscle building exercise is also high intensity exercise and can lead to fat deposition if done to excess. However, increasing one's muscle mass in the correct way – without causing the release of adrenal hormones – will raise your metabolic rate overall because muscle tissue consumes more energy than fat. Indeed, muscle loss as a result of dieting is often a reason that people cannot maintain their goal weight. They require less food after their diet than they did originally because they lost muscle while dieting. You can avoid

---

[1] Some people need to first strengthen their heart with more moderate exercise which promotes weight loss. Then they can add strenuous aerobic training after it will no longer interfere with weight loss. See the story about a patient of Dr. Hart's on page 268.

[2] Hart, Cheryle R., MD and Mary Kay Grossman, RD, *The Insulin Resistance Diet,* (New York: McGraw-Hill, 2001, 2007), 192.

[3] Ibid, 193.

muscle loss while losing weight by having sufficient protein intake (for women - 50 to 75 grams or 7 to 11 units per day; for men - 75 to 100 grams or 11 to 14 units per day)[4] and by doing exercise that builds muscle. For best results, strenuous muscle building exercises such as weight training should be done every other day because the recovery day between exercise days is the time when muscle fibers are built.

In my opinion, moderate exercise (also called brisk activity) does not receive the respect from most exercise experts that it deserves. Perhaps this is because no special equipment or advice is needed. There is nothing to sell when a person takes up walking, but those who walk several times a week are most successful at maintaining weight loss after a diet. Walking is often touted as the best way to lose fat[5] perhaps because it is near-impossible to walk too fast to induce an adrenal hormone response that turns off fat burning. In addition to moderate exercise being the best way to burn body fat, it also builds muscle, although you won't end up with bulging biceps as you might from weight training. Another extremely important effect of moderate exercise is that it decreases leptin resistance.[6] (Leptin is the master hormone for the self-regulation of a healthy level of body fat. See pages 43 to 44 for more about leptin resistance).

Formal metabolic activity tests exist that determine an individual's optimal exercise pulse rate for fat-burning. Rather than having a test, Dr. Cheryle Hart says you can approximate your best fat burning zone by leisurely walking or bicycling, and that if you cannot carry on a conversation without sounding winded, you have exceeded that zone.[7]

Some people err on the side of too little exercise and benefit from adding a sensible exercise regime to their healthy eating plan. Always check with your doctor before starting an exercise program especially if you have been sedentary. Dr. Hart recommends starting with 10 minutes of moderate activity such as walking per day for the first week and increasing your time by two minutes per week. If you need motivation to take up exercise, consider these extra benefits. Moderate exercise is good for us in many ways in addition to burning fat: it relieves stress physically, helps remove your mind from distressing thoughts, releases endorphins in the brain,[8] and gives you a chance to do something nurturing for yourself.

So what is the right amount and type of exercise for you? How can you listen to your body to determine this? It helps to understand the physiology of how your body supplies energy when you do strenuous exercise (aerobic or muscle building exercise). First, you

[4] Hart, Cheryle R., MD and Mary Kay Grossman, RD, *The Feel-Good Diet,* (New York: McGraw-Hill, 2007), 183.

[5] Ibid,179.

[6] Galland, Leo, MD, *The Fat Resistance Diet,* (New York: Broadway Books, 2005), 122.

[7] Ibid, 181.

[8] Hart, Cheryle R., MD and Mary Kay Grossman, RD, *The Insulin Resistance Diet,* (New York: McGraw-Hill, 2001, 2007), 189.

burn whatever glucose is in your blood from a meal or snack eaten during the previous half hour to hour. Then your body converts glucose stored in the muscles and liver in the form of glycogen into glucose. We only have enough stored glycogen to supply us with fuel for about 20 minutes of intense exercise. Because fat cannot be converted to glucose rapidly, after the glycogen is gone, our bodies begin converting muscle protein into glucose.

If you exercise moderately, the fat conversion process is able to keep up with your glucose needs so fat will be burned.[9] Thus, the best way to lose fat is to keep your insulin levels low and stable (so you are in the fat-burning mode) and exercise moderately by walking, gardening, cleaning house, or leisurely bicycling. Dr. Hart says, "If exercising makes you hungry, it means you have used up your glucose and glycogen stores. Most likely you started burning muscle. An important thing to remember is that you don't get hungry when you are burning fat."[10] Thus, hunger after exercise is how your body tells you that you were exercising too hard to burn fat.

In *The Insulin Resistance Diet,* Dr. Hart recommends limiting strenuous exercise to no more than 25 minutes per day to avoid losing muscle mass.[11] She says that a mere 12 minutes of aerobic activity six days a week or 25 minutes three days a week is enough to increase your resting metabolic rate all week long. She advises doing stretching exercises or brisk activity (moderate exercise) if you want to exercise more than 75 minutes a week and recommends house cleaning, gardening, walking, and moderately paced swimming or bicycling as excellent ways to burn fat.

Although it is counter-intuitive to the "calories in with food, fat out with exercise" model you may have been living by, exercise without food can undermine efforts to reduce body fat. When you engage in strenuous exercise before breakfast or after work but before dinner (or at least a linked-and-balanced snack), your body releases adrenal hormones to cause the breakdown of glycogen in the liver so you have sufficient fuel for your exercise.[12] These adrenal hormones cause the release of insulin which can, if excessive, result in fat storage. The hormonal response to exercise without food and prolonged strenuous exercise is the same. After your glycogen stores are used up, fat is not mobilized to be burned for energy, but rather muscle mass is broken down for fuel. Since muscle has a higher metabolic rate than fat, if you lose muscle mass due to over-exercise, your overall resting metabolic rate will decrease, making it more difficult to lose weight.

---

9 Hart, Cheryle R., MD and Mary Kay Grossman, RD, *The Feel-Good Diet,* (New York: McGraw-Hill, 2007), 177-178.

10 Ibid, 156.

11 Hart, Cheryle R., MD and Mary Kay Grossman, RD, *The Insulin Resistance Diet,* (New York: McGraw-Hill, 2001, 2007), 192.

12 This is why I felt less hungry after exercise in the story on page 12 and also was, ironically, part of why I could not lose weight on a standard low-calorie diet weight loss diet.

In *The Feel Good Diet,* Dr. Hart tells about a patient of hers who was a fitness trainer and could not lose weight in spite of following a good linked-and-balanced eating plan. Dr. Hart prescribed a test to determine her best fat-burning zone, and the results showed that she should be exercising at a pulse rate of between 100 and 122 beats per minute for best fat loss, which was 30 to 40 beats per minute less than she usually maintained during exercise. When she began doing all of her exercise at the lower pulse rate, she lost 15 pounds in the next month.[13]

In summary, listen to your body about exercise just as you do about what you eat. Be alert for becoming winded during moderate exercise and slow down if you do. Consider buying a pulse monitoring wrist watch to make sure your pulse is where you want it when you exercise. For moderate exercise your pulse should be well below the target range for aerobic exercise and should remain in a good fat-burning range. If your exercise program makes you hungry, you probably are burning muscle rather than fat; diminish the intensity and time. Before you exercise, have a balanced protein and carbohydrate snack if you get hungry after exercise to avoid setting off a hormonal cascade that will lead to storing fat. Eat properly to keep your insulin level low and stable (which keeps you in the fat burning mode) and make much of your exercise moderate. By applying these principles to your exercise program, you should be able to achieve good fat loss and a healthy weight.

---

[13] Hart, Cheryle R., MD and Mary Kay Grossman, RD, *The Feel-Good Diet,* (New York: McGraw-Hill, 2007), 180-181.

A Tale of Two Dieters

This is a tale of two dieters, my friend Deb and my husband Bill (whose names have been changed). As mentioned previously, I don't need to lose weight although I am a good candidate for using this healthy eating plan to help control inflammation. In spite of my lack of recent personal weight loss experience (although I did lose weight on a similar plan over 30 years ago and have maintained the loss), I have observed and advised Deb and Bill and can share their stories with you. Perhaps their experiences will help you.

When I first met Deb, she had severe multiple food allergies which are now well controlled by EPD. (See *The Ultimate Food Allergy Cookbook and Survival Guide* which is described on the last pages of this book for more information about low dose immunotherapy allergy treatment). She eats normal foods most of the time except for when she needs another EPD shot. She has been battling overweight for several years, and until recently was eating very little, exercising a lot, and feeling hungry much of the time. Yet she not only was unable to lose weight but even gained a few pounds on her Spartan regimen. When I finished the rough draft of the first fourteen informational chapters of this book, I gave it to her along with food tables containing information about the serving sizes and carbohydrate and protein units of commonly eaten foods.

She began to implement the eating plan in the rough draft and lost 8½ pounds in two months while – to her delight – never feeling hungry. Aside from a few "off" times when she was on vacation, she has continued to lose weight at a moderate but steady rate. She even reports that her husband, who is following the eating plan with her, is "losing his tummy" and looking very handsome.

As a veteran dieter, Deb is accustomed to controlling portion sizes and eating low fat dairy products and lean meat. Beef is the only food she has not desensitized to on EPD, and her doctor attributes this to her total lack of exposure to it. Although she and her husband eat plenty of chicken, turkey, etc., they have been watching their fat intake for so many years that they have lost their taste for high fat meats, so she never cooked beef for her husband when her diet was so restricted.

My husband Bill does not have food allergies and actually does not need to lose weight. He does not have an apple shaped body (which is a health risk) and at age 58 weighs less than he did over 30 years ago in our first few years of marriage. However, he does have trouble with blood sugar control. He eliminated sugar about 25 years ago, which helped his blood sugar problems some and resulted in about 25 pounds of weight loss. However, he continued to experience ravenous hunger, irritability, etc. when he went too long between meals.

About six months ago, he decided that he wanted to try this healthy eating plan. He switched from eating white bread to 100% stone ground whole wheat bread (made with the recipe on page 240) and limits his carbohydrate intake to 30 grams (2 units) per meal or snack. He felt more stable blood sugar-wise and was not driven to distraction by hunger in the first few weeks. Yet his weight remained stable for the first two months on his healthy eating plan and he lost only five pounds the next two months. Now that he is experiencing what he describes as "a great hunger control system" his appetite has decreased and rate of loss is picking up.

As we have analyzed both his eating habits and his goals for following the healthy eating plan, some patterns have emerged. First, he is a self-proclaimed epicurean, taking an opposite approach to what he eats from Deb's pattern of eating after years of a diet limited by food allergies. The pleasure of eating is a very important part of life for him. Thus, as he eliminated highly refined carbohydrates, he increased his fat intake to derive eating pleasure. He dislikes lowfat cheese and skim milk, although he will eat lowfat yogurt. On weekends, his afternoon cheese snack is often accompanied by potato chips rather than low GI, low fat crackers for a carbohydrate to balance the protein in the cheese. When the weather was warm he was eating a 16-ounce bowl of no-sugar ice cream (recipe on page 220) sprinkled with no-sugar chocolate chips (recipe on page 198) after dinner nearly every night. When the weather is too cold for ice cream, he often eats no-sugar chocolate (recipe on page 198) for dessert. He likes half-and-half in his coffee, butter on his popcorn (recipe on page 225), and has a one-pound rib eye or T-bone steak for dinner once a week.

However, in spite of losing only five pounds, he has achieved his personal goals[1] for being on the eating plan just as Deb has. He is feeling better and enjoying life without "hunger panic," as we called his former experiences. He is enjoying what he eats, and in spite of a generous intake of fat, he has not gained weight but is losing at a slow rate. His hunger is under good control now. Therefore his desire for high-fat foods is lessening and he's eating less potato chips.

These two stories illustrate some principles which may help you with your eating plan. Think about what your goal really is – improvement of your health and decreased inflammation or weight loss. If your goal is weight loss, you should pay attention to hidden sources of fat and keep your fat intake in the recommended range of 45 to 55 grams of fat per day. If it is inflammation control, be sure to maintain the proper balance in the fat you eat, with anti-inflammatory fats well represented.

Furthermore, to lose weight, most of the time you should eat until your hunger is physically satisfied, not until you've derived the maximum possible pleasure from your food. However, past experience has shown most of us that we can't adhere to a diet forever without some pleasure, so don't be afraid to have the small (1 ounce) chocolate splurge that Dr. Hart recommends if you start feeling deprived. (See page 45 for more

---

[1] Do not take Bill's story as a recommendation to exceed Dr. Galland's recommendation to consume 45 to 55 grams of fat per day as given previously in this book. Although Bill seems to be "getting away with" eating more fat, you should consult your physician and monitor your blood fats as well as your weight. Personal goals such as enjoyment need to be subject to medical goals.

about controlled chocolate splurges and see the recipe for stevia-sweetened chocolate on page 198). If you can't eat chocolate and are feeling deprived, have a link-and-balanced snack containing a favorite pleasurable treat food that you tolerate.

Keep most of the carbohydrates that you eat low or moderate on the GI scale if you want to lose weight. *The Complete Idiot's Guide to GI Weight Loss* contains two diets, one of which gives you great freedom in food choices, but requires the calculation and tabulation of glycemic load units every day. This is not possible on a food allergy or gluten-free diet because there is no glycemic index data available for many of the foods we are able to eat. However, the principle of this diet in *The Complete Idiot's Guide to GI Weight Loss* still applies. The glycemic load units are calculated by multiplying the grams of carbohydrate in a food you eat by its glycemic index and dividing by 100. This makes a slice of white bread, which has GI of near 100, count almost twice as much as a serving of cooked quinoa and 50% more than a serving of 100% stone ground whole wheat bread. All carbohydrates are not created equal!

Losing weight on this healthy eating plan depends on listening to your body (which does not want to be unhealthily thin either). Thus, if you are at or near a normal weight, your weight loss may be minimal. This is fine, and is what was experienced by normal-weight patients whom Dr. Galland put on his similar eating plan for control of inflammation.

If your goal is weight loss and you are not noticing your clothes loosening after a couple of months on this eating plan, see pages 116 to 118 of this book and/or *The Insulin Resistance Diet* where Dr. Cheryle Hart offers more troubleshooting advice.

INGREDIENT SUBSTITUTIONS

When you bake for someone with food allergies or on a gluten free diet, you will need to purchase new ingredients. If you are missing an ingredient, you might wonder if you can substitute something else for that new food. Substitutions are tricky in allergy and gluten-free baking. The recipes in this book should work as written (although an unusual batch of flour from a health food store bulk bin can upset any recipe), but if you substitute, there are no guarantees.

People call me and say, "I've got your recipe made with quinoa flour and I want to make it with rice flour. How can I do this?" I usually can't give them a definite answer although I often try to make suggestions that may or may not work. In my experience, there is no rule or conversion factor for substitutions between any two types of flour that always works predictably. The tables you may have seen on how much of various kinds of flour are equivalent to one cup of wheat flour take into account only how much liquid the flour absorbs. The differences between flours extend far beyond how much liquid they require; gluten content and other factors are equally important. In addition, each kind of flour varies in how it behaves in different types of recipes. For example, barley flour behaves much like wheat in pie crust but nothing like wheat in yeast bread. There is no reliable conversion factor for substitutions between wheat and a non-wheat flour or between any two types of non-wheat flour that works in all recipes. Therefore, when baking with non-wheat flour, the easiest and best thing to do is to use a recipe especially developed for the kind of flour you want to use.

The bottom line on flour substitutions is this: If you substitute, be prepared to tweak the recipe at least several times before it is right. In addition, expect that some substitutions may never work. If you are looking for a recipe to make, for example, crackers with buckwheat or tortillas with garbanzo flour, see *The Ultimate Food Allergy Cookbook and Survival Guide* as described on the last pages of this book. Because that book is designed to be the ultimate resource for people whose diets may be extremely limited, I attempted to make each type of flour (including rarely eaten foods such as tuber flours, chestnut flour, starch flours, and the less common non-gluten grain flours) into as many types of recipes as possible and only omitted a certain recipe if it really was not possible to make. For example, the only reason the book does not contain a recipe for sorghum yeast bread is because I was unable, after many tries, to make a loaf that did not collapse. However, it does have a sorghum non-yeast bread recipe made with eggs to help hold it together. (This is one of the very few egg-containing recipes in the book). There are also recipes for fruited sorghum non-yeast bread (where the fiber in the fruit holds the bread together) and sorghum muffins, crackers, tortillas, pancakes, cake, and cookies[1]. As mentioned

---

[1] These recipes are made with sorghum flour only or sorghum flour plus arrowroot, not a mixture of several kinds of flour as used in most gluten-free baking mixes. This single grain principle applies to all of the recipes in the book because it allows people with extensive food allergies to rotate their foods and increases the likelihood that they will find recipes that they can use as written.

earlier, buckwheat can be bitter in some recipes, so buckwheat recipes can be hard to find. However, those who eat buckwheat often become accustomed to its flavor. Since some severely allergic people can eat only one or two grain alternatives, buckwheat recipes that might be considered marginal on taste by people who can eat more are included in *The Ultimate Food Allergy Cookbook and Survival Guide* for those on extremely limited diets. You can save a lot of time and wasted ingredients by getting the recipe you really need rather than experimenting with flour substitutions.

Home ground flour may also behave differently from commercially ground flour, and it can vary from batch to batch of grain. If you use either very finely milled flour or coarsely milled or blender-ground flour, you will have to change the amount of liquid used in the recipe. Unless you have time to experiment with each new batch of grain when you grind your own flour, you will have the most predictable baking results if you purchase flour from a reliable commercial source.

Unlike wheat flour, milk is an ingredient where substitutions in baking recipes usually work. In most recipes, you can replace the milk called for with an equal amount of water. Sometimes you can replace milk with fruit juice, but the acidity of the juice can affect the leavening process and result in a collapse of your baked product. Gluten-free yeast breads, in which the protein content contributed by the milk helps strengthen the structure of the bread, may sometimes be an exception to the rule that water can be substituted for milk.

In allergy baking eggs can usually be replaced with an equal volume of water if the recipe is not depending on the egg for structure. However, in a recipe made with a gluten-free or low gluten flour, the egg sometimes serves to replace part of the structure normally provided by gluten. Therefore, replacing the egg with water may lead to a collapse of your bread or cake.

Refined starches usually can be substituted for each other in the same amounts in baking recipes. You can use arrowroot and tapioca flour interchangeably for baked goods. Water chestnut starch and cornstarch also will usually substitute for the other starches in baking although in a few recipes the amount may need to be adjusted. However, starches behave differently when used to thicken liquids, so you might need more or less than you expect to get the desired result. Don't hesitate to try this substitution, however, because making a sauce is not like baking where there is nothing you can do by the time you see your bread collapsing in the oven! If the sauce you are making is too thick, just add more water; if it seems too thin, add more starch.

Fruit juices and purees may substitute well in some recipes. You can usually substitute an equal volume of a fruit juice, fruit juice concentrate, or fruit puree (such as applesauce) for another fruit juice, concentrate or puree of about the same consistency. For instance, you can substitute apple juice for grape juice or pureed peaches for applesauce. Pureed bananas, however, are much thicker than applesauce, so this substitution will not work as expected. Pineapple is more acidic than the other fruits so substituting pineapple juice concentrate for another juice concentrate often requires adjustments in the leavening, such as leaving out or decreasing the amount of the vitamin C indicated in the recipe. However, pureed pineapple sometimes substitutes without leavening changes because it is less concentrated and therefore less acidic. Again, it depends on the recipe, and the only way to know if it will work is to try it.

Some liquid sweeteners can be substituted for each other in most recipes. For instance, agave, Fruit Sweet™ and honey have about the same sweetening power; therefore, many of the recipes in this book give you a choice between these sweeteners. Because honey is more viscous than Fruit Sweet™ and agave, occasionally it may need to be diluted slightly with water before substituting it in a recipe. Fruit juice concentrates are less sweet and more acidic, and some, such as pineapple juice concentrate, contain a fair amount of fiber, so they can only occasionally be used in place of agave, Fruit Sweet™ or honey. Obviously, dry sweeteners cannot be substituted for liquid sweeteners without making major (and often unpredictable) adjustments in the amount of liquid ingredients and leavening ingredients in the recipe.

The most unpredictable sweetener to substitute is stevia. It lacks many attributes that other sweeteners add to a recipe in addition to sweetness, such as a browning effect and effects on the texture and the leavening process. I have made recipes literally dozens of times in my attempts to use stevia. If I do finally settle on a recipe that seems to be good, the texture is never the same as it was in the original recipe sweetened with a nutritive sweetener. However, if you are substituting stevia in a non-baking recipe and are only interested in the level of sweetness, a starting point for substitution is that one teaspoon of Protocol for Life Balance™ pure stevia powder[2] has about the same sweetening power as one cup of sugar, agave, honey, or Fruit Sweet™. Unfortunately, this "rule" is affected by the other ingredients in the recipe. For example, if chocolate or cocoa is used in the recipe, I have been amazed to discover that the amount of stevia required can be two or three times what I expect. If the recipe does not contain strongly-flavored ingredients, you may need to use less stevia to prevent the licorice-like aftertaste that may be detectable even with the purest stevia. When substituting stevia for a liquid sweetener, you will also have to add more liquid to the recipe (which may be unpredictably less than the full amount of liquid that you used for the other sweetener). If the sweetener was acidic, you may or may not need to add a little more vitamin C to the leavening.

The best advice for success with baking recipes is this: Don't substitute unless you're willing to make a recipe multiple times before it succeeds and are prepared to encounter an occasional recipe that is impossible to convert. With non-wheat flours, the leavening process is easily upset. If you feel you must have the experience of substituting, make ice cream or a non-baked recipe. For best success in baking, use a proven recipe, measure accurately (see pages 97 to 98 for more about this), mix correctly (see pages 98 to 99), and then enjoy what you make on the first try.

---

[2] If you are not using Protocol for Life Balance™ brand of pure white stevia, this rule will be "off." If the stevia is not pure and has been cut with anything else, it will be less potent and you will need to use more – sometimes much more – stevia. Some brands have a more pronounced licorice-like taste and will need to be used in smaller amounts.

TABLE OF MEASUREMENTS

For some of these recipes you will need to measure less-common amounts of ingredients such as ⅜ cup or ⅛ teaspoon. The easiest and most accurate way to do this is to have a liquid measuring cup with ⅛ cup markings, a set of dry measuring cups that contains a ⅛ cup measure, and a set of measuring spoons that has a ⅛ teaspoon. Such kitchen equipment is available from the King Arthur Flour Baker's Catalogue (See "Sources," page 279). While you are waiting for your measuring cups and spoons to arrive or if you need to halve, double, or triple recipes, use this table.

⅛ teaspoon[1]	= ½ of your ¼ teaspoon measure	
⅜ teaspoon	= ¼ teaspoon + ⅛ teaspoon	
⅝ teaspoon	= ½ teaspoon + ⅛ teaspoon	
¾ teaspoon	= ½ teaspoon + ¼ teaspoon	
⅞ teaspoon	= ½ teaspoon + ¼ teaspoon + ⅛ teaspoon	
1 teaspoon	= ⅓ tablespoon	= ⅙ fluid ounce
1½ teaspoons	= ½ tablespoon	= ¼ fluid ounce
3 teaspoons	= 1 tablespoon	= ½ fluid ounce
½ tablespoon	= 1½ teaspoons	= ¼ fluid ounce
1 tablespoon	= 3 teaspoons	= ½ fluid ounce
2 tablespoons[2]	= ⅛ cup	= 1 fluid ounce
4 tablespoons	= ¼ cup	= 2 fluid ounces
5⅓ tablespoons	= ⅓ cup	= 2⅔ fluid ounces
8 tablespoons	= ½ cup	= 4 fluid ounces
16 tablespoons	= 1 cup	= 8 fluid ounces
⅛ cup	= 2 tablespoons[2]	= 1 fluid ounce
¼ cup	= 4 tablespoons	= 2 fluid ounces
⅜ cup	= ¼ cup + 2 tablespoons[2]	= 3 fluid ounces
⅝ cup	= ½ cup + 2 tablespoons[2]	= 5 fluid ounces
¾ cup	= ½ cup + ¼ cup	= 6 fluid ounces
⅞ cup	= ¾ cup + 2 tablespoons[2]	= 7 fluid ounces
	OR ½ cup + ¼ cup + 2 tablespoons[2]	
1 cup	= ½ pint	= 8 fluid ounces
1 pint	= 2 cups	= 16 fluid ounces
1 quart	= 4 cups OR 2 pints	= 32 fluid ounces
1 gallon	= 4 quarts	= 128 fluid ounces

[1]To measure less than ⅛ teaspoon see the next page.

[2]In my experience, measuring tablespoons are all a little scanty of 1/16 cup so 2 tablespoons is a little short of ⅛ cup. Therefore, if you need to measure, for example, ⅜ cup of liquid and do not have a measuring cup with ⅛ cup markings, it will probably be more accurate to eyeball an amount halfway between ¼ cup and ½ cup than to use ¼ cup plus two tablespoons.

Measuring Stevia

Pure white stevia powder often is used in very small amounts in recipes, so when I saw a set of measuring spoons called "Dash, Pinch, Smidgen" at my local What's Cooking store a few years ago, I bought them. They were promoted as measuring $\frac{1}{8}$, $\frac{1}{16}$ and $\frac{1}{32}$ of a teaspoon. I found them very handy for measuring stevia and used them to develop the stevia-containing recipes in this book.

Since some readers do not have access to a well-stocked cookware store, when I began work on the "Sources" section of this book I looked for an online source for these spoons. I found several different varieties of mini-measuring spoons, including one set which claimed to measure $\frac{1}{6}$, $\frac{1}{12}$ and $\frac{1}{24}$ teaspoon. Like various carbohydrate foods and different types of fat, all mini-measuring spoons are not created equal! They obviously do not come in sizes conforming to a universal standard.

I wondered if my mini-measuring spoon set actually measured $\frac{1}{8}$, $\frac{1}{16}$ and $\frac{1}{32}$ of a teaspoon so tried an experiment. I used the $\frac{1}{8}$ teaspoon from a regular measuring spoon set purchased from King Arthur Flour (which kitchen tests all their products thoroughly before selling them) as the standard. When I filled that spoon with salt, leveled it off, and placed the salt in the dash spoon, the dash was just very slightly over-full. I was very relieved that this was not a $\frac{1}{6}$ teaspoon measure! I measured salt in the smidgen spoon four times and poured it into my $\frac{1}{8}$ teaspoon standard and it was a perfect fit. Two pinches also fit perfectly into the $\frac{1}{8}$ teaspoon standard. This set was definitely designed to measure $\frac{1}{8}$, $\frac{1}{16}$ and $\frac{1}{32}$ of a teaspoon.

I was delighted to find an online source for mini-measuring spoons identical to the set I own at www.spoonsisters.com. They sell the mini-measuring spoon set for $4.95 or less when purchased in quantity. The Spoon Sisters also offer a delightful assortment of gifts of all kinds. I wish I had children to shop for when I visit their website. See "Sources," page 280, for more contact information for them.

Sources of Special Foods and Products

This section lists sources of special ingredients and products needed for the recipes in this book which may not always be easy to find locally. Most of these companies sell products in addition to those listed below. Visit their websites for up-to-date information about all of their products.

AGAR FLAKES

Eden Foods, Inc.
701 Tecumseh Road
Clinton, Michigan 49236
888 424-EDEN (3336)
www.edenfoods.com

BEANS FOR SOUP

13-Bean Soup Mix and Chana dal
Bob's Red Mill
5209 S.E. International Way
Milwaukie, OR 97222
(800) 349-2173 or (503) 654-3215
www.bobsredmill.com

BROTH, GLUTEN-FREE

Health Valley Natural Chicken, Beef, and Vegetable Broths
Health Valley Foods
The Hain Celestial Group, Inc.
4600 Sleepytime Drive
Boulder, CO 80301
(800) 434-4246
www.healthvalley.com

Imagine Organic Free Range Chicken Broth
Imagine Foods
The Hain Celestial Group, Inc.
4600 Sleepytime Drive
Boulder, CO 80301
(800) 434-4246
www.hain-celestial.com

CAROB POWDER

Bob's Red Mill
5209 S.E. International Way
Milwaukie, OR 97222
(800) 349-2173 or (503) 654-3215
www.bobsredmill.com

CHESTNUTS, FRESH AND DRIED

Parthenon Foods
9131 W. Cleveland Avenue
West Allis, WI 53227
(877) 301-5522
http://parthenonfoods.com

FLAVORINGS, NATURAL
(gluten-, corn- and alcohol-free)

Frontier™ Alcohol-Free Vanilla Flavor
Frontier Natural Products Co-op
P.O. Box 299
3021 78th Street
Norway, IA 52318
(800) 669-3275
www.frontierherb.com

Some Frontier flavorings such as this vanilla are corn-, alcohol-, and gluten-; free, others are not.

FLOURS, GRAINS, and GRAIN ALTERNATIVES

Amaranth flour and grain

Nu-World Amaranth, Inc.
P. O. Box 2202
Naperville, IL 60540
(630) 369-6819
www.nuworldfoods.com

Bob's Red Mill
5209 S.E. International Way
Milwaukie, OR 97222
(800) 349-2173 or (503) 654-3215
www.bobsredmill.com

Arrowroot

Bob's Red Mill
5209 S.E. International Way
Milwaukie, OR 97222
(800) 349-2173 or (503) 654-3215
www.bobsredmill.com

Barley flour

Arrowhead Mills
The Hain Celestial Group, Inc.
4600 Sleepytime Drive
Boulder, CO 80301
(800) 434-4246
www.hain-celestial.com

Sustagrain™ barley flour
King Arthur Flour Baker's Catalogue
P.O. Box 876
Norwich, VT 05055
(800) 827-6836
www.kingarthurflour.com

Buckwheat flour

Arrowhead Mills
The Hain Celestial Group, Inc.
4600 Sleepytime Drive
Boulder, CO 80301
(800) 434-4246
www.hain-celestial.com

Quinoa flour, grain and pasta

The Quinoa Corporation
P.O. Box 279
Gardena, CA. 90248
(310) 217-8125
www.quinoa.net

Bob's Red Mill
5209 S.E. International Way
Milwaukie, OR 97222
(800) 349-2173 or (503) 654-3215
www.bobsredmill.com

Bob's Red Mill sells whole grain quinoa and quinoa flour, but not pasta.

Rice flour, brown

Arrowhead Mills
The Hain Celestial Group, Inc.
4600 Sleepytime Drive
Boulder, CO 80301
(800) 434-4246
www.hain-celestial.com

Rye flour

Arrowhead Mills
The Hain Celestial Group, Inc.
4600 Sleepytime Drive
Boulder, CO 80301
(800) 434-4246
www.hain-celestial.com

Spelt flour, grain and pasta

Purity Foods, Inc.
2871 W. Jolly Road
Okemos, MI 48864
(517) 351-9231
www.purityfoods.com

Tapioca starch/flour

Bob's Red Mill
5209 S.E. International Way
Milwaukie, OR 97222
(800) 349-2173 or (503) 654-3215
www.bobsredmill.com

Teff flour and grain

Bob's Red Mill
5209 S.E. International Way
Milwaukie, OR 97222
(800) 349-2173 or (503) 654-3215
www.bobsredmill.com

JUICE CONCENTRATES

Blueberry, cherry, and pomegranate, bottled

R. W. Knudsen and Sons, Inc.
1 Strawberry Lane
Orrville, OH 44667-0280
(888) 569 6993
www.knudsenjuices.com

Pomegranate molasses, bottled

Cortas™ Pomegranate Molasses
Parthenon Foods
9131 W. Cleveland Avenue
West Allis, WI 53227
(877) 301-5522
http://parthenonfoods.com

KITCHEN EQUIPMENT

Bread machines, measuring cups and spoons, pizza roller, silicone egg poachers, etc.

King Arthur Flour Baker's Catalogue
P.O. Box 876
Norwich, VT 05055
(800) 827-6836
www.kingarthurflour.com

Long bread pans, pizza roller, etc.

Norpro Cookware
2215 Merrill Creek Parkway
Everett, WA 98203
(425) 261-1000
www.norpro.com

Mini-measuring spoons, etc.

The Spoon Sisters, Inc.
153 West 27th Street, Suite 802
New York, NY 10001
(800) 716-4199
www.spoonsisters.com

LEAVENING INGREDIENTS

Baking powder, corn-free

Featherweight Baking Powder
The Hain Celestial Group, Inc.
4600 Sleepytime Drive
Boulder, CO 80301
(800) 434-4246
www.hain-celestial.com

Freeze-dried French sourdough starter

King Arthur Flour Baker's Catalogue
P.O. Box 876
Norwich, VT 05055
(800) 827-6836
www.kingarthurflour.com

Order item #1040, not the fresh sourdough starter. The freeze-dried starter is wheat- and gluten-free but may contain traces of beef.

Unbuffered vitamin C powder, cassava source

(Made by Allergy Research Group)

Professional Supplement Center
2427 Porter Lake Drive
Sarasota, FL 34230
(888) 245-5000
www.professionalsupplementcenter.com

Yeast, active dry and quick-rise

(gluten-, corn- and preservative-free, in 1 or 2 pound bags)

Red Star Yeast and SAF Yeast
King Arthur Flour Baker's Catalogue
P.O. Box 876
Norwich, Vermont 05055
(800) 827-6836
www.kingarthurflour.com

MEAT, GAME

Game Sales International
P.O. Box 7719
Loveland, CO 80537
800-729-2090
www.gamesalesintl.com

MISCELLANEOUS INGREDIENTS

Gum, guar and xanthan

Bob's Red Mill
5209 S.E. International Way
Milwaukie, OR 97222
(800) 349-2173 or (503) 654-3215
www.bobsredmill.com

No-cook thickener

Signature Secrets™ Thickener
King Arthur Flour Baker's Catalogue
P.O. Box 876
Norwich, VT 05055
(800) 827-6836
www.kingarthurflour.com

This thickener contains corn.

Non-hydrogenated, trans-fat free shortening

Spectrum Naturals™ Organic All Vegetable Shortening
Spectrum Organic Products, Inc.
The Hain Celestial Group, Inc.
4600 Sleepytime Drive
Boulder, CO 80301
(800) 434-4246
www.spectrumorganics.com

This shortening is soy-free and contains palm oil only.

Rye flavor, gluten-free

Authentic Foods
1850 W. 168th Street, Suite B
Gardena, CA 90247
(800) 806-4737 or (310) 366-7612
www.authenticfoods.com

NUT PRODUCTS

Almond flour, blanched and finely ground

Honeyville Food Products
11600 Dayton Drive
Rancho Cucamonga, CA 91730
(909) 980-9500
http://honeyvillegrain.com

Almond, hazelnut and pecan meal

King Arthur Flour Baker's Catalogue
P.O. Box 876
Norwich, VT 05055
(800) 827-6836
www.kingarthurflour.com

Almond meal

Bob's Red Mill
5209 S.E. International Way
Milwaukie, OR 97222
(800) 349-2173 or (503) 654-3215
www.bobsredmill.com

Coconut, unsweetened, finely shredded

Jerry's Nut House, Inc.
2101 Humboldt Street
Denver, CO 80205
(303) 861-2262

Coconut milk, free of guar gum

Natural Value™ Coconut Milk
www.naturalvalue.com

Purchase Natural Value™ coconut milk through your health food store or order it in case quantities on Amazon.com. To find out which stores near you have it or can order it, email Gary@NaturalValue.com. Natural Value "regular" coconut milk is free of guar gum. Their organic coconut milk contains guar.

NUTRITIONAL SUPPLEMENTS

For general nutritional support to help control blood sugar and insulin levels
Metabolic CoFactor™ (made by Allergy Research Group)
Carlson Lab's Nutra-Support Diabetes Formula™

For moderation of cortisol levels
Relora™ (made by Pure Encapsulations)
Relora-Plex™ (made by Douglas Labs)

All four supplements listed here may be purchased from

Professional Supplement Center
2427 Porter Lake Drive
Sarasota, FL 34230
(888) 245-5000
www.professionalsupplementcenter.com

SPICES AND SEASONINGS

Known-source cinnamon, Italian herb blend, chile pequin, etc.

Penzey's Spices
12001 West Capitol Drive
Wauwatosa, WI 53222
(800) 741-7787
www.penzeys.com

SWEETENERS

Agave

Madhava agave nectar, light, dark, amber, and raw
Madhava Honey
4689 Ute Highway
Lyons, CO 80540
(303) 823-5166
www.madhavasagave.com

Coconut sugar

Essential Living Foods
922 Colorado Ave
Santa Monica, CA 90401
(310) 319-1555
http://essentiallivingfoods.com

Date sugar

NOW Natural Foods
395 S. Glen Ellyn Road
Bloomingdale, IL 60108
(800) 283-3500
www.nowfoods.com

Order from NOW Foods through your health food store.

Fruit Sweet™

Wax Orchards, Inc.
P.O. Box 25448
Seattle, WA 98665
(800) 634-6132
www.waxorchards.com

Stevia, pure white powder

NOW Natural Foods
395 S. Glen Ellyn Road
Bloomingdale, IL 60108
(800) 283-3500
www.nowfoods.com

Order from NOW Foods through your health food store. This is not a "next generation" stevia and has a licorice after taste.

Protocol for Life Balance™
(877) 776-8610
Email: sales@protocolforlife.com
www.protocolforlife.com

This stevia has been treated with an enzyme to remove the licorice-like after taste and is allergen- and gluten-free. Use the powder rather than the packets for baking. Their bottled powder contains only stevia, but the packets contain maltodextrin from corn. Protocol for Life Balance™ products are available from health care practitioners. If your health care practitioner does not carry this stevia, email the company for information on where to get it. Also, check the foodallergyandglutenfreeweightloss.com website for more information about its availability or email using the contact form on the website.

TEA

Loose green tea and other teas, all extremely flavorful, steepware

The Tea Spot, Inc.
4699 Nautilus Court South, Suite 403
Boulder, CO 80301
(866) TEA-SPOT or (303) 444-8324
http://theteaspot.com

WHEAT CONTAINING BAKED GOODS
(for your non-allergic diet companions)

Bread

Alvarado Street Bakery Diabetic Lifestyle Bread™
Alvarado Street Bakery
2225 S. McDowell Blvd.
Petaluma, CA 94954
(707) 283-0300
http://www.alvaradostreetbakery.com

One slice of Diabetic Lifestyle Bread™ contains 15 grams of carbohydrate (1 carbohydrate unit) and 5 grams of protein (about ¾ protein unit).

Carb Helper Bread™
Available at Kroger, King Soopers, or City Market Stores

One slice of Carb Helper Bread™ contains 7 grams of carbohydrate (about ½ carbohydrate unit) and 5 grams of protein (about ¾ protein unit).

French Meadow Bakery Men's Bread™
French Meadow Bakery
1000 Apollo Road
Eagan, MN 55121
(651)286-7891
www.frenchmeadow.com

Two slices of Men's Bread™ contain 17 grams of carbohydrate (slightly over 1 carbohydrate unit) and 15 grams of protein (2 protein units).

Crackers

Ak-Mak™ Crackers
The Low-Carb Connoisseur
1208 North Main Street
Anderson, SC 29621
(888) 339-2477
www.low-carb.com

Tortillas

Tumaro's™ Low in Carbs Tortillas
Tumaro's Gourmet Tortillas
313 Iron Horse Way
Providence, RI 02908
(951) 697-5950
www.tumaros.com

REFERENCES
HELPFUL BOOKS, ARTICLES AND WEBSITES

Books and Articles

Beale, Lucy and Joan Clark, MS, RD, CDE. *The Complete Idiot's Guide Glycemic Index Cookbook.* New York: Alpha, 2009.

Beale, Lucy and Joan Clark, RD, CDE. *The Complete Idiot's Guide to Glycemic Index Weight Loss.* New York: Alpha, 2005.

Black, Jessica K., ND. *The Anti-Inflammation Diet and Recipe Book.* Alameda, CA: Hunter House Publishers, 2006.

Brand-Miller, Jennie, PhD, Thomas Wolever, MD, Kay Foster-Powell. MND, and Stephen Colaguiri, MD. *The New Glucose Revolution.* New York: Marlowe and Company, 2003.

Cannon, Christopher P., MD and Elizabeth Vierck. *The Complete Idiot's Guide to The Anti-Inflammation Diet.* New York: Alpha, 2006.

Challem, Jack. "The Omega Factor: Figuring Out Fats." *Better Nutrition,* October 2009, 44.

Dumesnil, Jean G. "Effect of a low-glycemic index – low fat – high protein diet on the atherogenic metabolic risk profile of abdominally obese men," *British Journal of Nutrition*, November, 2001, 86:557-568. A summary of this study is found at www.montignac.com/en/etude_scient_sur_meth_mont.php

Galland, Leo, MD. *The Fat Resistance Diet.* New York: Broadway Books, 2005.

Gallop, Rick. *The GI [Glycemic Index] Diet.* New York: Workman Publishing, 2002.

Hansen, Barbara Caleen, PhD and George A. Bray, MD. *The Metabolic Syndrome: Epidemiology, Treatment, and Underlying Mechanisms.* Totowna, NJ: Humana Press, 2008.

Hart, Cheryle R., MD and Mary Kay Grossman, RD. *The Feel-Good Diet.* New York: McGraw-Hill, 2007.

Hart, Cheryle R., MD and Mary Kay Grossman, RD. *The Insulin Resistance Diet.* New York: McGraw-Hill, 2001, 2007.

Kessler, David, MD. *The End of Overeating.* New York: Rodale, 2009.

Michael Pollan. *In Defense of Food: An Eater's Manifesto.* New York: The Penguin Press, 2008.

Rivera, Rudy, MD and Roger Deutsch. *Your Hidden Food Allergies Are Making You Fat.* Rocklin, CA: Prima Publishing, 1998.

Sears, Barry, PhD. *Enter the Zone.* New York: Regan Books, 1995.

Sears, Barry, PhD. *Mastering the Zone.* New York: Regan Books, 1997.

Sears, Barry, PhD. *The Anti-Inflammation Zone.* New York: Regan Books, 2005.

Stevenson, E.J., N. Astbury, E. Simpson, M. Taylor, I. Macdonald. "Fat Oxidation During Exercise and Satiety During Recovery Are Increased Following a Low-Glycemic Index Breakfast in Sedentary Women." *Journal of Nutrition*, May 2009, 139(5):890-897. Abstract at http://www.ncbi.nlm.nih.gov/pubme d/19321590?itool=EntrezSystem2.PEntrez.Pubmed.Pubmed_ResultsPanel. Pubmed_RVDocSum&ordinalpos=5

Woodruff, Sandra, MS, RD. *The Good Carb Cookbook: Secrets of Eating Low on the Glycemic Index.* New York: Penguin Group, 2001.

Websites

Food allergies, causes, diagnosis, treatments, etc. – www.food-allergy.org

Eating low on the glycemic index – www.glycemicindex.com
  How to buy or make lower GI bread – www.glycemicindex.com, FAQs page, question 19
  See a sample newsletter in PDF form – www.glycemicindex.com/blog/2007 /june2007june.2007.pdf

Glycemic index scores
  www.mendosa.com/gilists.htm
  www.montignac.com/en/ig_tableau.php

The Montignac Method (weight loss based low glycemic index principles) –
www.montignac.com/en/la_methode.php

Weight loss for those with food allergies or gluten intolerance –
www.foodallergyandglutenfreeweightloss.com

INDEX TO RECIPES BY GRAIN USE

To help those on rotation diets find recipes made with the grain they need for each diet day, this index lists the recipes for baked goods according to the major grain or grain alternative that they contain. The recipes that do not contain a grain or grain alternative, such as those for main dishes, vegetables, etc., are not listed in this index but can be found by name in the "General Index" on page 289. Arrowroot and tapioca are used as binders in baking recipes in this book but are not included in the listing below because they may be used interchangeably. Headings which contain **GF** indicate that the grain or grain alternative is gluten-free.

RICE (GF)

RYE

SPELT

TEFF (GF)

GENERAL INDEX

Recipes appear in *italics*. Informational sections appear in standard type.

BOOKS TO HELP WITH YOUR SPECIAL DIET

Food Allergy and Gluten-Free Weight Loss gives definitive answers to the question, "Why is it so hard to lose weight?" It is because we have missed or ignored the most important pieces in the puzzle of how our bodies determine whether to store or burn fat. Those puzzle pieces are hormones such as insulin, cortisol, leptin, and others. Individuals with food allergies or gluten intolerance face additional weight-loss challenges such as inflammation due to allergies or a diet too high in rice. This book explains how to put your body chemistry to work for you rather than against you, reduce inflammation which inhibits the action of your master weight control hormone, leptin, and flip your fat switch from "store" to "burn." It includes 175 recipes and a flexible healthy eating plan that eliminates hunger, promotes the burning of fat, and reduces inflammation.

ISBN 978-1-887624-19-0 . . . .$23.95

Allergy and Celiac Diets With Ease: Money and Time Saving Solutions for Food Allergy and Gluten-Free Diets provides solutions to both the economic and time challenges you face with your diet. It shows how to shop economically, cook without spending all day in the kitchen, stock your kitchen for efficiency and good health, make the best use of your appliances, have good times with friends and family without breaking the bank, get organized, and be able to do this in limited time. This book contains over 160 money-saving, quick and easy recipes for allergy and celiac diets. Over 140 of them are gluten-free. It includes extensive reference sections including "Sources" and "Special Diet Resources" sections to help you find the foods you need. A list of helpful books and websites (even an online celiac/special diet restaurant search database) is also included.

ISBN 978-1-887624-17-6 . . . .$19.95

The Ultimate Food Allergy Cookbook and Survival Guide: How to Cook with Ease for Food Allergies and Recover Good Health gives you everything you need to survive and recover from food allergies. It contains medical information about the diagnosis of food allergies, health problems that can be caused by food allergies, and your options for treatment. The book includes a rotation diet that is free from common food allergens such as wheat, milk, eggs, corn, soy, yeast, beef, legumes, citrus fruits, potatoes, tomatoes, and more. Instructions are given on how to personalize the standard rotation diet to meet your individual needs and fit your food preferences. It contains 500 recipes that can be used with (or independently of) the diet. Extensive reference sections include a listing of commercially prepared foods for allergy diets and sources for special foods, services, and products.

ISBN 978-1-887624-08-4 . . . .$24.95

Gluten-Free Without Rice introduces you to gluten-free grains and grain alternatives other than rice such as teff, millet, sorghum, amaranth, quinoa, buckwheat, tapioca, arrowroot, potato starch, and more. It gives you over 75 delicious recipes for muffins, crackers, bread, pancakes, waffles, granola, main and side dishes, cookies, and desserts. (Even ice cream cones!) With this book you can cook easily for a gluten-free diet without relying on rice. Whether you have celiac disease or food allergies, this book will make it easier and more enjoyable to stay on your diet and improve your health.

ISBN 978-1-887624-15-2 . . . .$9.95

Allergy Cooking With Ease **(Revised Edition)**. This classic all-purpose allergy cookbook was out of print and now is making a comeback in a revised edition. It includes all the old favorite recipes of the first edition plus many new recipes and new foods. It contains over 300 recipes for baked goods, main dishes, soups, salads, vegetables, ethnic dishes, desserts, and more. Informational sections of the book are also totally updated, including the extensive "Sources" section.

ISBN 978-1-887624-10-7 . . . .$19.95

Easy Breadmaking for Special Diets contains over 200 recipes for allergy, heart healthy, low fat, low sodium, yeast-free, controlled carbohydrate, diabetic, celiac, and low calorie diets. It includes recipes for breads of all kinds, tortillas, bread and tortilla based main dishes, and desserts. Use your bread machine, food processor, mixer, or electric tortilla maker to make the bread YOU need quickly and easily.

Revised Edition – ISBN 978-1-887624-11-4 . . . . $19.95

Original Edition Bargain Book – ISBN 1-887624-02-3 . . . .**SALE!** - $9.95

> With the bargain book we will include an insert of updated pages about current bread machines and the tortilla recipes from the new edition.

Do you need more fun in your life? *I Love Dessert but NOT Sugar, Wheat, Milk, Gluten, Corn, Soy, Unhealthy Fat...* can help you rediscover the enjoyment of simple pleasures. If you are on a restricted diet due to food allergies or gluten intolerance, you don't have to miss out on your favorite desserts any more. The book contains more than 300 easily-made recipes for almost any dessert you might want, all free of sugar, wheat, corn, soy, and unhealthy fats. Many of them are gluten-free. A very few of the desserts contain dairy products or eggs, but there are egg and milk-free alternatives for the same desserts. Many recipes are made with healthy new sweeteners such as agave. When your friends or family are having a treat, now you can join in. Don't deprive yourself any more!

ISBN 978-1-887624-18-3 . . . .$22.95

The Low Dose Immunotherapy Handbook: Recipes and Lifestyle Tips for Patients on LDA and EPD Treatment gives 80 recipes for patients on low dose immunotherapy treatment for their food allergies. It also includes organizational information to help you get ready for your shots.

ISBN: 978-1-887624-07-7 . . . .$9.95

How to Cope With Food Allergies When You're Short on Time is a booklet of time saving tips and recipes to help you stick to your allergy or gluten-free diet with the least amount of time and effort.

. . . .$4.95 or FREE with the order of two other books on these pages

Order these books on-line by going to
www.foodallergyandglutenfreeweightloss.com
or **food-allergy.org**,
by mail using the order form on the next page
or from Amazon.com at **www.amazon.com**.

Mail your order form and check to:
Allergy Adapt, Inc.
1877 Polk Avenue
Louisville, CO 80027

Questions? Call 303-666-8253
or email foodalle@food-allergy.org.

Shipping for mail-in orders:

IF YOU ARE ORDERING JUST ONE BOOK, FOR SHIPPING ADD:
$5.00 for any one of the starred (*) books
$3.00 for any one of the non-starred books

TO ORDER MORE THAN ONE BOOK, FOR SHIPPING ADD:
$7.00 for up to three starred* and up to two non-starred books
$9.00 for up to four starred* and up to two non-starred books
$12.00 for up to eight starred* and up to three non-starred books

Call 303-666-8253 for international shipping rates or if you have questions about shipping calculations or large quantity orders.

Thank you for your order!

ORDER FORM

Send to:

Name: _____

Street address: _____

City, State, ZIP code: _____

Phone number (for questions about order): _____

Item	Quantity	Price	Total
*Food Allergy and Gluten-Free Weight Loss**		$23.95	
*Allergy and Celiac Diets With Ease**		$19.95	
*The Ultimate Food Allergy Cookbook and Survival Guide**		$24.95	
Gluten-Free Without Rice		$9.95	
*Allergy Cooking With Ease**		$19.95	
*Easy Breadmaking for Special Diets** – Original Edition Bargain Book / Revised Edition		$9.95 / $19.95	
*I Love Dessert**		$22.95	
The Low Dose How Immunotherapy Handbook		$9.95	
How to Cope with Food Allergies When You're Short on Time		$4.95 or **FREE**	

Order any TWO of the first eight books above and get ***How to Cope* FREE!**	Subtotal	
	Shipping – See chart on the previous page	
	Colorado residents add 4.1% sales tax	
	Total	

CPSIA information can be obtained at www.ICGtesting.com
Printed in the USA
LVOW132009090212

267710LV00002B/43/P

9 781887 624190